M000113720

# SECRET YOGA CLUB

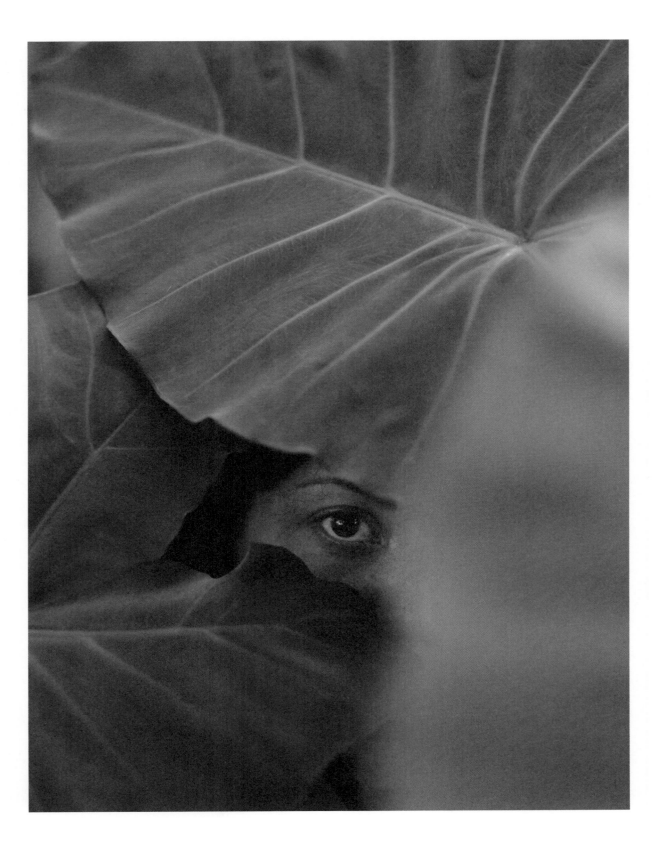

# SECRET YOGA CLUB

## SELF-EMPOWERMENT THROUGH THE MAGIC OF YOGA

GABRIELLE HALES

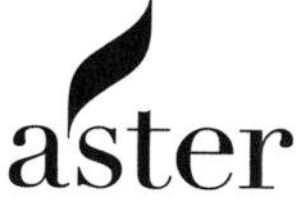

FOR MARLYN, MY MOTHER

**For the decade of longing
and a life spent loving.
Birthing me, bearing me,
breathing me and
believing in me.
Again and again.**

An Hachette UK Company
www.hachette.co.uk

First published in Great Britain in 2020 by Aster,
an imprint of
Octopus Publishing Group Ltd
Carmelite House
50 Victoria Embankment
London EC4Y 0DZ

www.octopusbooks.co.uk
www.octopusbooksusa.com



Distributed in the US by
Hachette Book Group
1290 Avenue of the Americas
4th and 5th Floors
New York, NY 10104

Distributed in Canada by
Canadian Manda Group
664 Annette St.
Toronto, Ontario, Canada M6S 2C8



ISBN 978-1-91202-365-3

A CIP catalogue record for this book is available from the British Library.

Printed and bound in China

10 9 8 7 6 5 4 3 2 1

Consultant Publisher Kate Adams
Art Director Yasia Williams
Senior Editor Alex Stetter
Designer Miranda Harvey
Photography Natasha Marshall
Production Manager Caroline Alberti

# CONTENTS


Secret Yoga Club Mission *6*

INTRODUCTION 11

**1:** BACK TO THE SOURCE 21

**2:** ELECTRIC BODY – THE LIFE FORCE 41

**3:** PRACTICAL MAGIC 59

**4:** SIGHING INTO STILLNESS 153

**5:** IN THE COMPANY OF WOMEN 171

**6:** EXPANDING WITH PURE SENSATION 193

The Divine Feminine 219

Bibliography 220

Index 221

Author's Acknowledgements 224


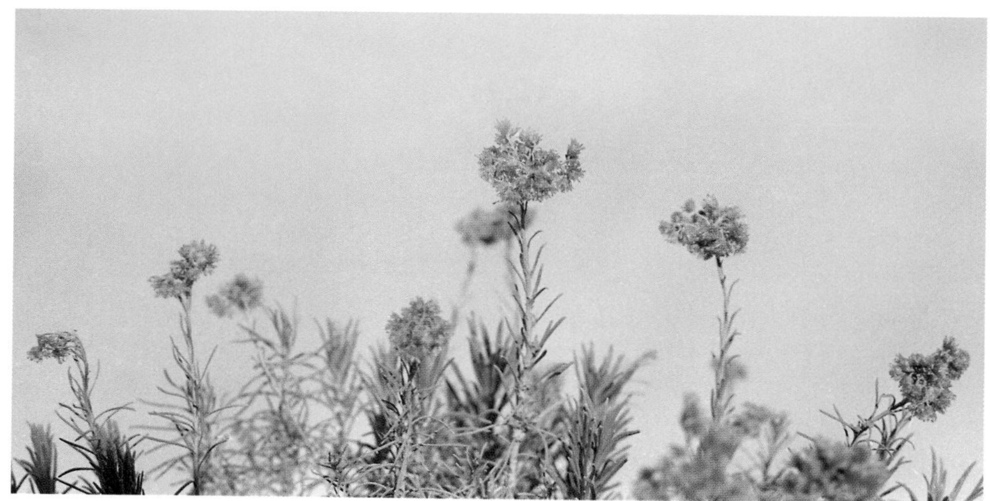

# SECRET YOGA CLUB MISSION

We are a small business run by women.

We work on healing and exploring ourselves, so we can blossom, unfold and endlessly evolve.

We share with each other what and whom we find inspiring and loving.

Most of all, we love to sit with other women and hear the universal from each unique being.

Through the journey of healing ourselves, we've been awed and reassured by our own capacity for regeneration.

We've noticed how, through self-change, we've become proud to take responsibility for our own lives, and how we interact with our fellow beings and Mother Nature.

We know that it's a privilege to have the space, time and resources to receive.

That's why we must empower ourselves to be agents of change.

We begin at home.

In learning to speak our truth, we invite others to voice theirs.

First of all, we celebrate our bodies.

We value them as instruments that conduct our spirit.

We treasure the way they feel, how they move us, breathe us and communicate us.

They are the interface between the core of our being and the world surrounding us.

Through yoga, we have become more confident, fluid and compassionate.

We feel you, you are near to us, you are one of us.

We're happiest when we look round the room and see you light up.

When you step through the door you become our family, whether you feel joyful and sociable, or tender and contracted.

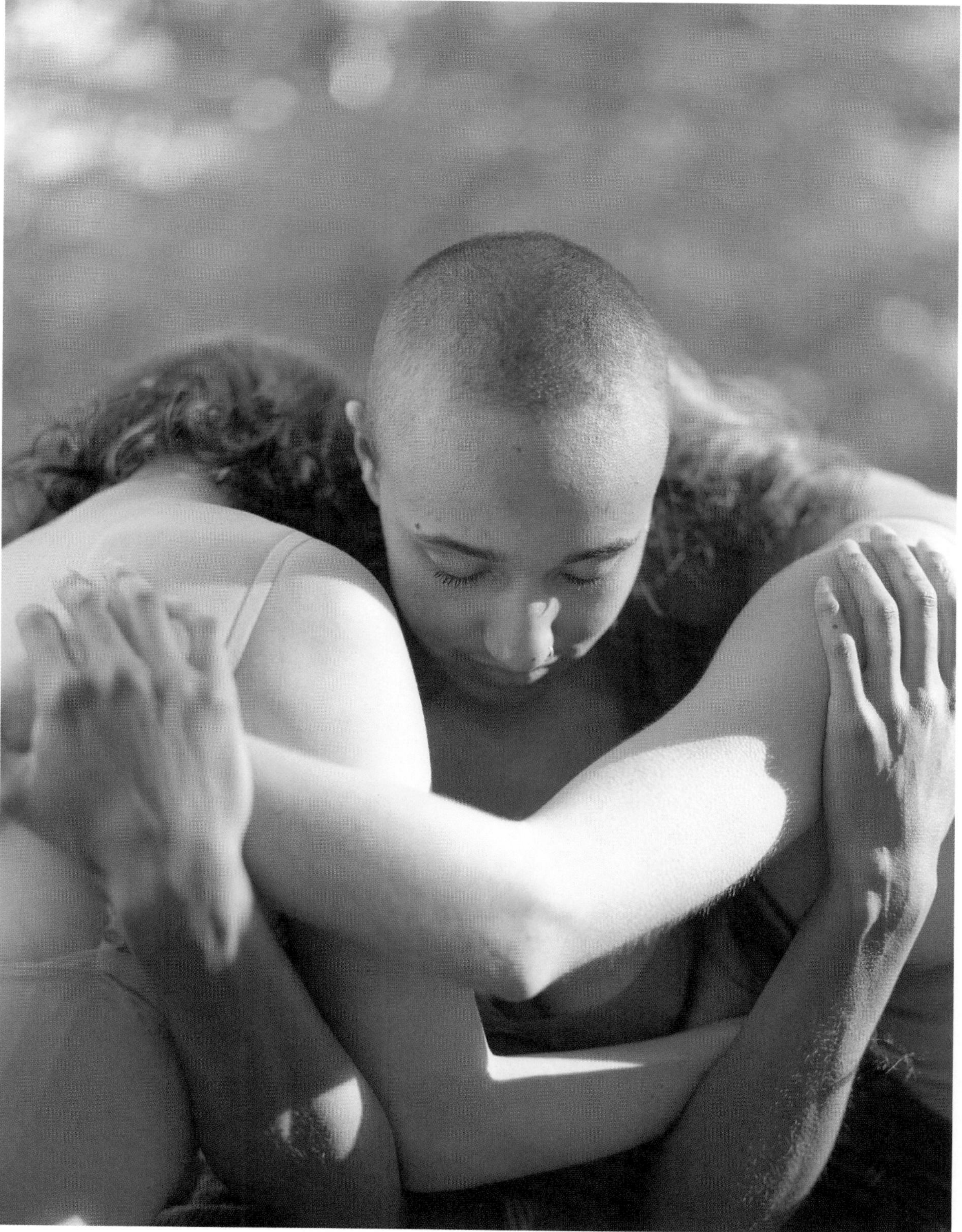

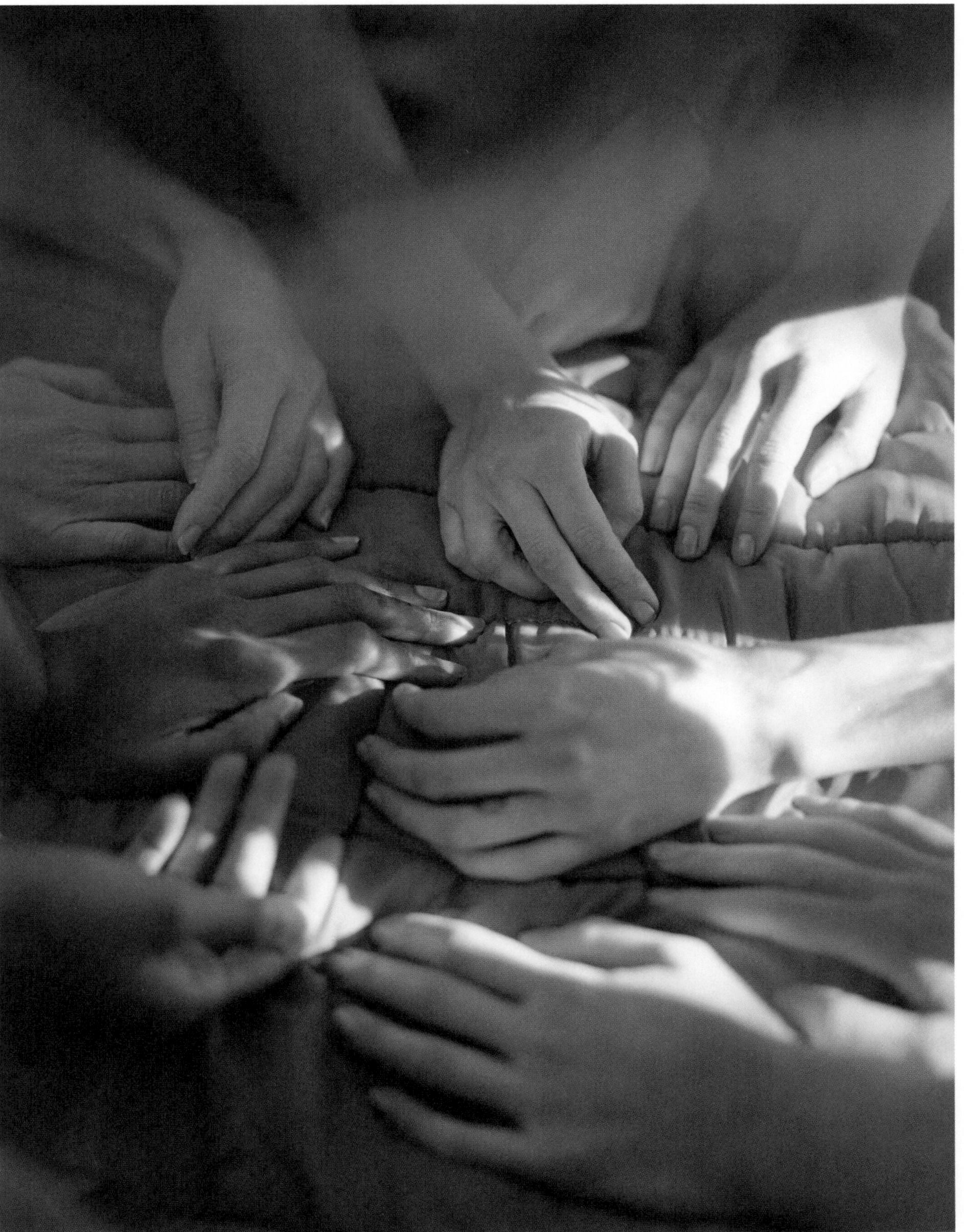

We extend to you the love that we have received.

We believe in you, the way our teachers, family or friends believed in us,
before we believed in ourselves.

We know that you can heal, because we are becoming whole.

We are healing ourselves for our families, lovers, friends, communities, children.

For a future.

To be better, stronger and kinder.

We know that yoga can improve health and wellbeing.

We dream of a world in which everyone has a personal practice,
a toolkit to know and love themselves,
and a community of loving humans where they can be held.

We believe that the future is feminine.

The world needs compassion, intuition, tenderness and peace.

We are empowering ourselves, and each other.

You too can feel it through your body, your voice and the ancient wisdom
of your intuition.

This book contains some wisdom I have learned from elders.

Most of what you will find here is for everyone.

Anyone who identifies as a woman, or loves a woman.

Some of these rituals are for those who identify as women
and were assigned that gender from birth,
for this is an ongoing journey that started with my own body.

I hope you will enjoy what I've found inspiring.

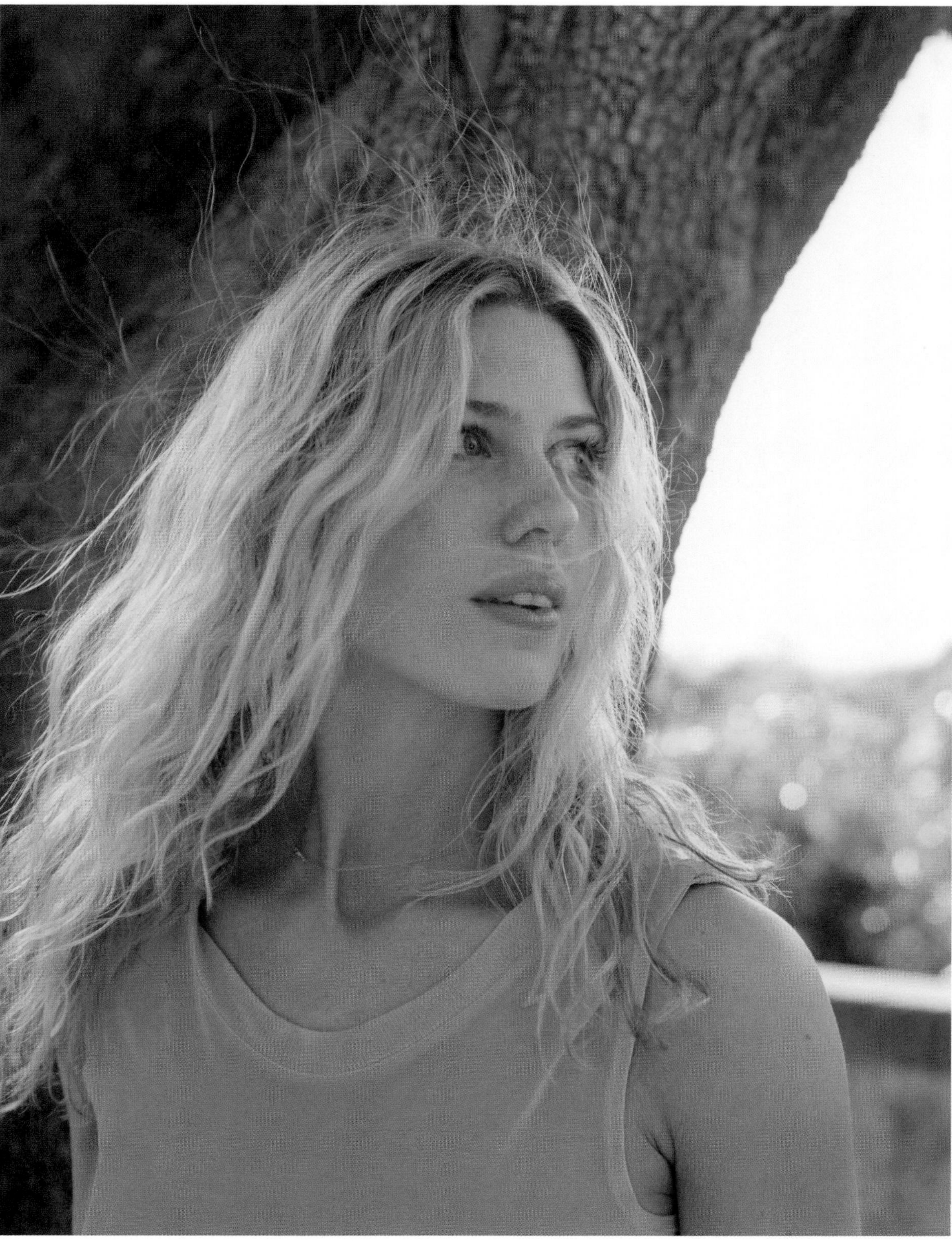

# INTRODUCTION

*"Curving back within myself I create again and again."*

BHAGAVAD GITA

# THE JOURNEY & THE DESTINATION

Everything is yoga, but let's begin where I started – with the body.

Yoga is an intimate, alchemical process in which you discover your own landscape and allow yourself to be explored. Yoga is how you sing yourself back to life. It's in the moments that you witness the sublime wisdom of the body, how it knows before you do, sending out signals, like Morse code. Quick breath. Blush. Contractions. Or how it turns itself into one...long...sigh.

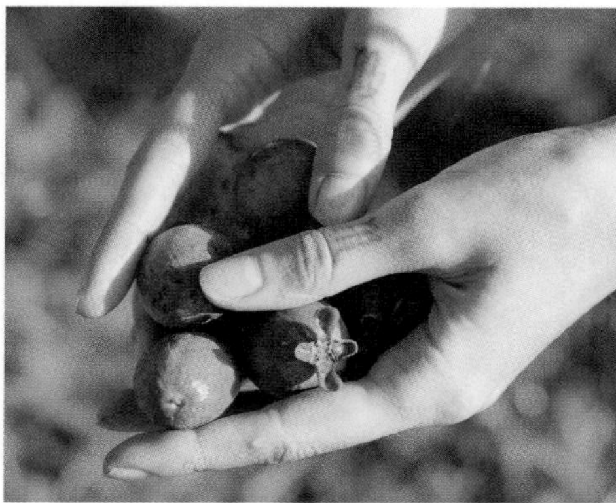

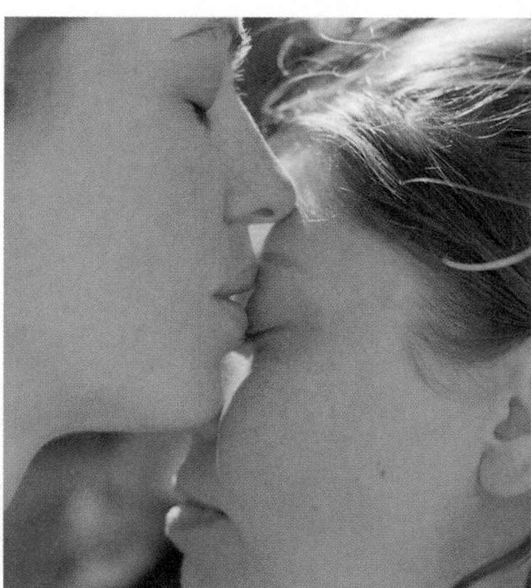

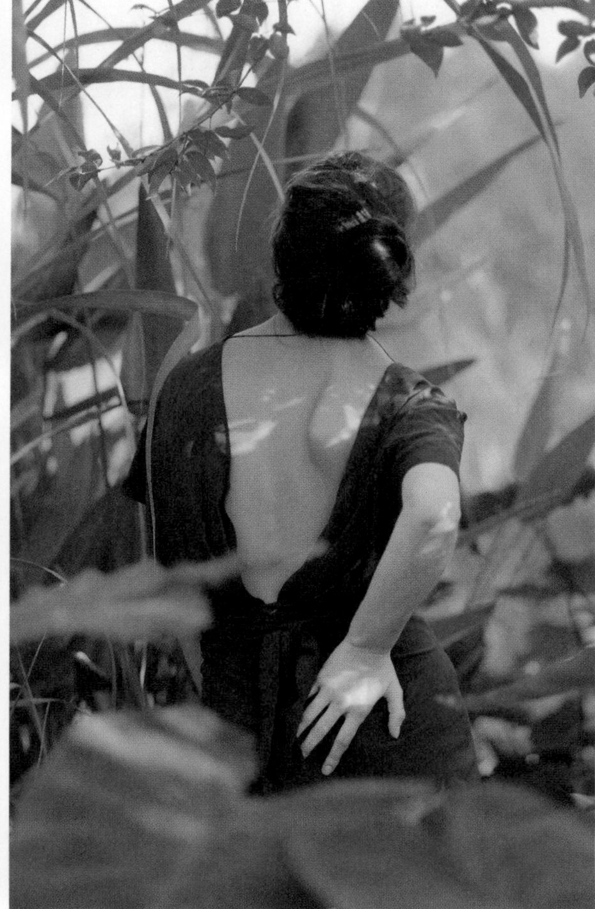

Yoga is when you awaken the mind so that it is able to witness memories, patterns and sensations. You trace your own body, primitively exploring the cartography of your flesh. You reclaim barren continents of your own, naming them with colours, feelings and sounds. Moving back into them gently, honouring what grew there when they were neglected. Calling them in quietly, looking at them tenderly. Letting them go.

Yoga is also when you hold yourself precious, when you keep yourself close. It's when you find the ocean in your breath and see the cosmos in your skull. When you dissolve into space and you experience yourself as energy and vibrations.

It's how you expel the emotions rotting in your body. It's where you find your confessions, when you realize that you have documented every single moment of your life in your flesh and that your ancestors sleep in your bones.

I would not be who I am today if it were not for yoga. Yoga is how I was finally able to mourn my father. How I learned that all the different kinds of grief hide themselves in secret coves of your body and wait for the right tide to flood and spill them out. It's how I realized that the trauma in my parents lived on through me, how I learned to liberate myself from their pain.

It's how I gathered myself back from the vortex of depression and how I coax myself home, when darkness threatens. How I learned to be seen, not to seek to hide. It's when I realized that I had a voice. It's where I stopped being lonely, found a sense of belonging and met a whole community of beautiful souls whom I feel honoured to call my friends. It's how I let go into surrender, and set myself free again and again.

Yoga practice is an intimate thing. It's there to expand your mind, to remind you of the mystery of life. It teaches you how to enjoy your body, to enhance your pleasure and locate your longing. It's there for you when you're heartbroken, when grief has sunk your joy or when work steals your sleep. When you rage at the news, when politics pelts pebbles at your heart, or you feel helpless and disempowered. But not when you just want to hide and insulate yourself from the world. It will empower and energize you to do something, to feel how important you are in the ecosystem. Yoga is your medicine. It's something that you can self-administer with almost no equipment, anywhere and anytime. It is an act of remembering that is often poetic and always cathartic.

With a good teacher, your yoga practice dissolves boundaries, deconstructs prejudices, builds a community and emboldens you to honour yourself and your brothers and sisters. It is through exploration of your inner world that you are able to move with bold compassion in the external one.

# QUESTING

I have been practising yoga for more than a third of my life. Various practices are deeply embedded in me and mapped into my future. Yoga has been so precious to me that I believe everyone should have these tools to help them heal and empower themselves.

My trip began when I fell in love with *āsana*, or postural yoga. I just loved the way it made me feel. The best way I can find to describe this feeling is to ask you to imagine that you never iron anything: you are very happy with your clothes, you don't actually notice they are creased. But then you decide to take your shirt and wash it, putting it through a cycle of twists and turns before laying it out to dry and ironing it carefully, lovingly. You put it on and marvel at how fresh and bright it looks and how light it is. It feels so great that you wonder how you could possibly have made do with such a crumpled old thing before.

It is more than a decade since I had those first experiences. A lot of yogic practices and other more extraordinary rituals have now passed through my body. I still love a sweaty flow, but my attitude to yoga has softened and expanded and is no longer limited to the mat. I've reached a place where I can practise intuitively, by honouring my seasons and prescribing something for myself.

To be able to hear and trust your intuition, you need to touch the space that stands behind all sounds, all thoughts and all words. It speaks to us most fully in silence. Everything comes out of silence and emptiness. Sound, the universe, a painting out of a blank canvas. So in order to know what we want, we need to turn away from distractions, into the internal world. And listen.

Over time, I realized that I wanted my practice to be one of joy and to incorporate different teachings, from all cultures. Instead of punishing or testing my body and living in a constant state of denial or guilt, I wanted to listen to what it needs, when it should be challenged and when it asks to be celebrated or nourished.

Part of a dedicated yoga practice is *svādhyāya*, a Sanskrit term which translates as "self-study". It's found in the ancient Hindu scriptures known as the Vedas, and in Patanjali's *Yoga-sutras*, the collection of writings in which the theory and practice of yoga were first written down in the 2nd century BCE. I realized that if I was to understand myself, I needed to explore many other elements beyond my breath and skin. I thought about feminism and language. How language, culture and conditioning have shaped me and my perspective of the world. I was drawn to more female empowerment events, and found that I wanted to create my own *satsang* with women. *Satsang* is a beautiful Sanskrit word that means association with the wise, or sitting together in truth. This is what we do, when we gather together as women.

The more I tasted my intuition, the more I felt drawn to align with my natural rhythms. I began to learn about my menstrual cycle, so I could discern my emotional landscape more truthfully and begin to synchronize my diary with the ebb and flow of my natural waves of energy. As I tuned in more profoundly, I noticed what felt good and committed myself to bringing more of that into my life. It was only a matter of time before I began to consider the healing powers of what my friend Jayne Goldheart calls "pleasure medicine" and to recognize the female orgasm as a delicious and empowering self-care tool.

I relaxed and diversified my daily rituals. I was already practising meditation, but I realized that there are endless ways to meditate: sometimes it's savouring a cup of cacao in the morning or watching a leaf slowly becoming unstuck and turning its way through the air to the ground.

When I can, when it's necessary, natural or easy, I savour my *āsana* practice and am endlessly discovering myself. I meditate most days and prioritize this and *prāṇāyāma* (breathing exercises – see page 120) over moving my body. It's a fast track to cosmic stillness. I also run a couple of times a week – I get all scratchy if I can't breathe in some nature. I'm almost happiest using my voice with my sisters.

The list really could go on, but the thing all these practices have in common is that they have enabled me to trust and connect, to honour my boundaries, and this supports my expansion. I have found my voice, my direction and my joy in work and life.

Of course, we all have times when we need to retreat into ourselves. We can only give if we are energetically strong, and have something to offer. But my yoga doesn't insulate me from the world and surrounding community. It enhances my experience, connection and desire to contribute to it.

# THE SEED OF SECRET YOGA CLUB

I've been teaching yoga since 2008, and my offering has slowly evolved with my practice. My priority is to create a compassionate space for people to explore their physical landscape and breath as portals into the energy body and the subtler realms within and without. I'm interested in finding different ways to explore the body, seeking different words with which to communicate and new experiences to awaken us all.

I teach a slow, mindful flow, prefaced with some kind of *prāṇāyāma*, to draw people to the inner world. I teach some flows on a breath count; at other times I encourage students to find their own rhythm. Sometimes there is music; in other classes people need to listen to their heart, their breath and the pad of their feet on the floor as they move through space. I close classes with singing with crystal bowls, to create a nourishing space for people to soften more deeply into themselves.

I started Secret Yoga Club as a hobby in 2012, with the intention of gathering together a group of like-minded people. It happened after I had gone out for lunch one day with a friend who is a chef. I distinctly remember feeling the warmth and generosity of the restaurant industry – it seemed as if I was part of a huge family. They had created a space where there was a sense of everyone really looking after each other, as if you were coming into their home and eating at their table.

Not long after, I began cooking for people after class. It seemed natural. Once everyone has relaxed and stretched out of the city, they want to sit, let the practice percolate and have the pleasure of sharing food together. There were no yoga supper clubs going on at the time. Word spread, the classes grew, and I started hosting events in a friend's gallery, with another friend cooking the food.

At the beginning, I really felt that this was all I could ever want out of an evening: a relaxing yoga class with live music, a sound bath and then a delicious meal. A year or so later, we were asked to host three big yoga dinners for one hundred people in the Royal Academy of Arts, as part of their *Sensing Spaces* architecture exhibition, and everything else is history.

Now we host ever more creative events at lots of magical places and continue to be delighted by the glorious people who walk through the doors. Over the years, Secret Yoga Club has become a real community. I work with beautiful and kind practitioners and teachers. It's a very personal business and I often forget that it is my work. I think people really respond to this, or I hope they do. I feel as if I welcome everyone in as if they are an old friend.

It has been incredibly rewarding to see people invest more time in transformational experiences. With so many of us leading such busy lives, it has become all the more important for these experiences to be sociable. At Secret Yoga Club, our ultimate goal is to have a special space to call home, so that we can create a timeless sanctuary for our community, teachers and guests alike.

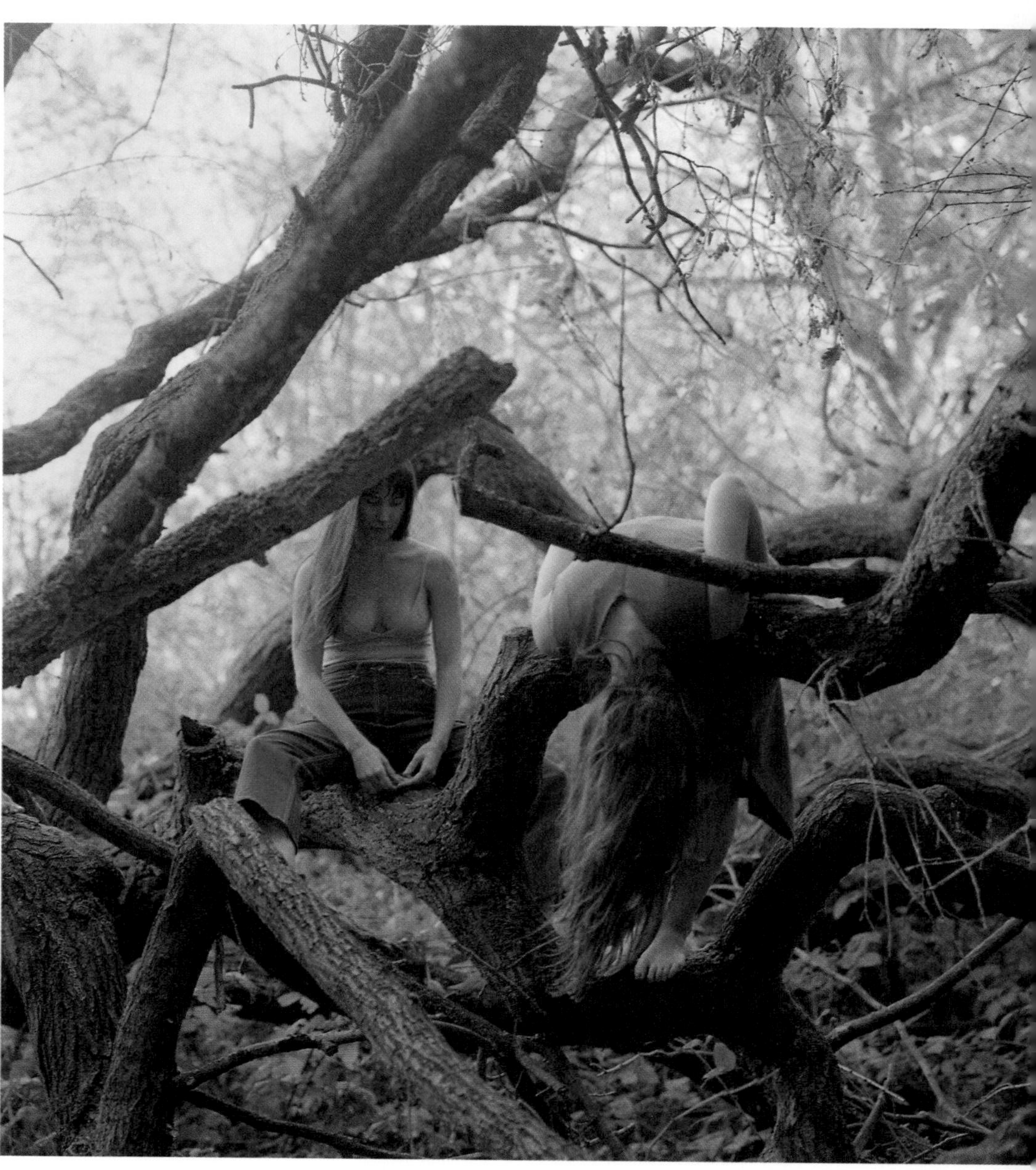

# YOUR JOURNEY & THIS BOOK

Until a few years ago, most of my knowledge of yoga traditions was limited to mystical experiences in meditation, *Śavāsana* (the "corpse pose" often used to end a practice), sound baths and chanting. They are one element, but I needed to ground myself and my practice by clarifying underlying confusion regarding the genealogy and philosophy of the yogas I had been practising, and seeking other teachings that would help me carry the power, joy or peace found on the mat into my life, as I moved though the world or negotiated challenging experiences of growth.

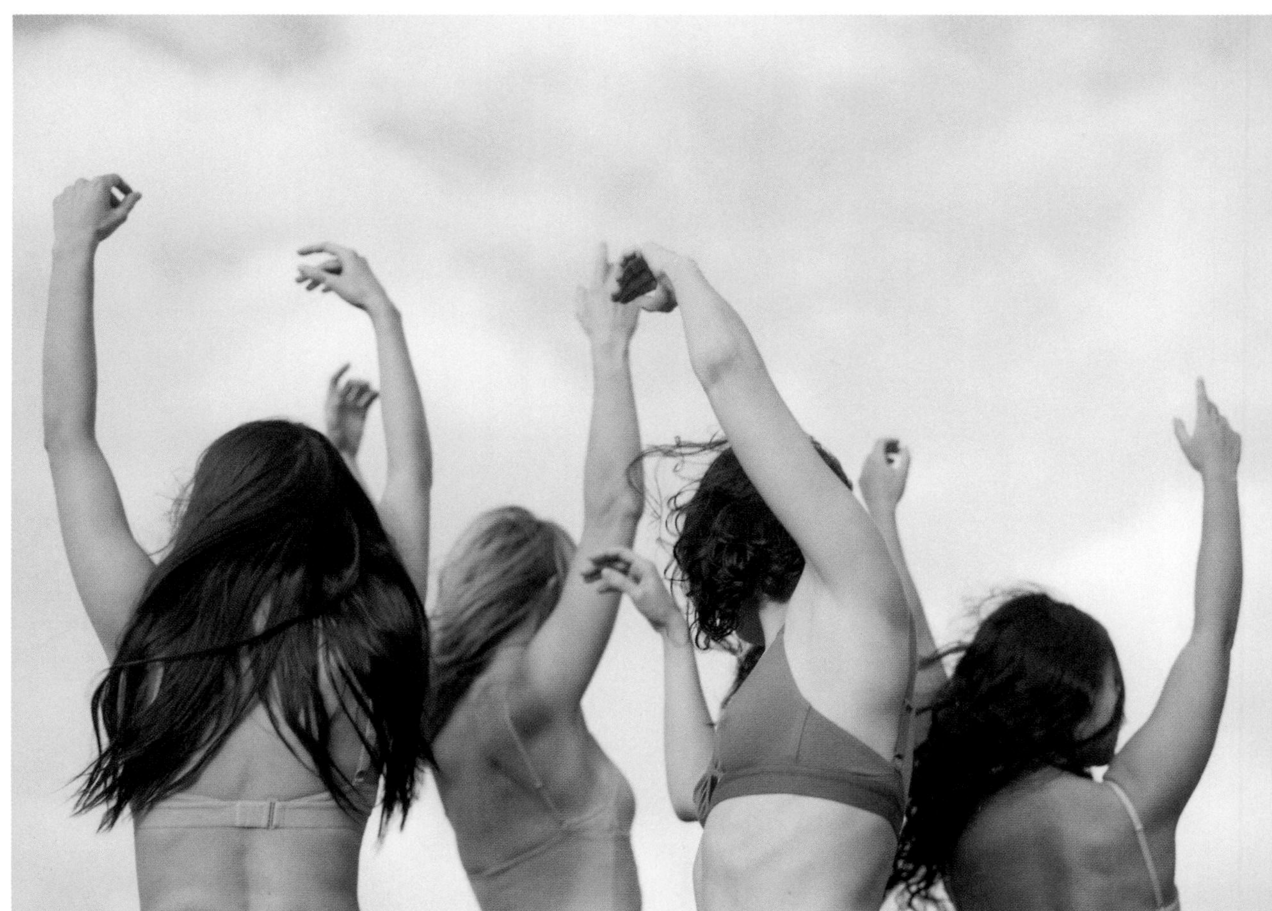

This book is therefore a practical and informative introduction for those who are open to learning more about the lesser known side of yoga from a non-dogmatic perspective. As there is so much to learn, this can be only a starting point for my studies and yours. I have tried to identify the most pertinent of the many things I do not know, and seek out a few answers. I hope it will encourage you to reach for the same books as I did, and start your own treasure hunt.

My research revealed a wonderfully rich and varied philosophy exploring meaningful and elusive questions about existence and consciousness. I discovered that there isn't one yoga, but a broad spectrum that embodies a variety of different philosophies and practices. Some of the traditions are rooted in ritual and dark magic, but their history also reveals an impressive roster of acrobatic showmen and tricksters, so today's Instagram circus is really only a continuation of yogi predecessors manipulating their bodies for the crowds.

Learning about the tradition made me realize that yoga is a living organism, that there has always been a conversation. There's a vast web of interconnecting ideas, a cross-pollination of cultures and doctrines that can embolden us to integrate new physiological, spiritual and practical findings into our own tradition, as long as we honour the date and place of their conception.

This book includes a variety of rituals, *prāṇāyāma* and practices that I have found especially useful and inspirational over the years. I've included quick fixes for rushed mornings, a survival kit for stressful times, as well as more lengthy and indulgent rituals and explorations.

The practices here go beyond *āsana*, not because the postures aren't important, but because yoga is so much more. If you don't have an *āsana* practice yet, I'd definitely recommend that you get your ass to a studio and practise with a human, as opposed to learning from a book. But here you will find some of my favourite shapes and movement sequences.

I will also address questions such as how old is yoga, and where did it come from? What is "authentic" yoga? What aspects of it can help you at different times in your life? What might fire you up or help you sleep? Can yoga improve your sex life? How can you get high on breathing?

My intention is to introduce you to a whole world, so that you know how to look within and identify what you need, what to ask for and where to look for it.

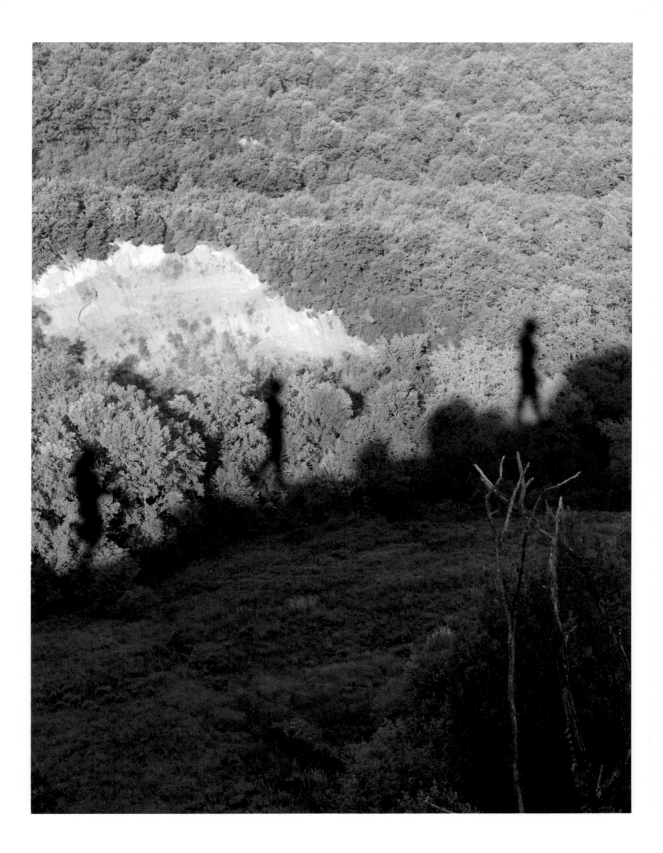

1

# BACK TO THE SOURCE

*"I have been a seeker and I still am, but I stopped asking the books and the stars. I started listening to the teaching of my Soul."*

RUMI

# ANCIENT PRACTICE

Yoga is the worship of mystery, an enquiry into the nature of consciousness, love, death, our very existence and what it means to integrate fully into this world and feel vibrant and alive. It's a path to liberation from the negative thought patterns, habits and conditioning that dim our happiness. It's a vast tradition that weaves together practical techniques, metaphysics, myths and poetry, as a means for us to cleanse our bodies and minds, to understand ourselves, to learn how to value our emotional life, trust our intuition, take pleasure in our physicality and seek to move through the world with compassion and self-respect.

The goal of a sustained yoga practice is to reach a point where you cleanse yourself of any filters of perception that colour your reality, and all the imprints of previous experiences that are etched on your heart. You dwell in the sweetness of the present and merge into the divine. This experience is beyond words: the moment when your knowledge of the absolute lands in your bones, and your true essence reveals itself to you. This moment is the removal of *avidyā*, the idea of not knowing, or ignorance of your true nature. It is the ultimate goal of a yoga practice and is either experienced directly, like a blast of ascension, or slowly, in hovering stages, that increase in length and poignancy. This is what is known as enlightenment, or the sense of liberation that comes after the state of meditative consciousness we call *samādhi*.

This ancient intelligence is an invitation to open into the very human experience of wonder, and explore all the facets of longing, love, fear – the deepest questions about the human condition. But if you've just found yourself on a mat for the first time, moving attentively with a more profound sense of your own breath, then that is enough. That, already, is poetry. Let the rest unfold as it comes – like falling in love. Just savour the beginning, the precious time when you experience your body anew and awaken to your own latent potential, with the joy of knowing that there is much more to come.

*...like falling in love. Just savour the beginning, the precious time when you experience your body anew and awaken to your own latent potential...*

Yoga practices are incredibly powerful. Mastering them will mean that you are able to harness your own personal power, dam up your energy leakages and deploy yourself in full force as you head toward your goals. Practices that weave together the body, mind and breath break through limiting thought patterns and fears. You hone your perceptive skills, have a more profound sense of the energetic realm and experience a deep sense of flow that can lead to feelings of clairvoyance or simply an inner knowing – the body *knows*.

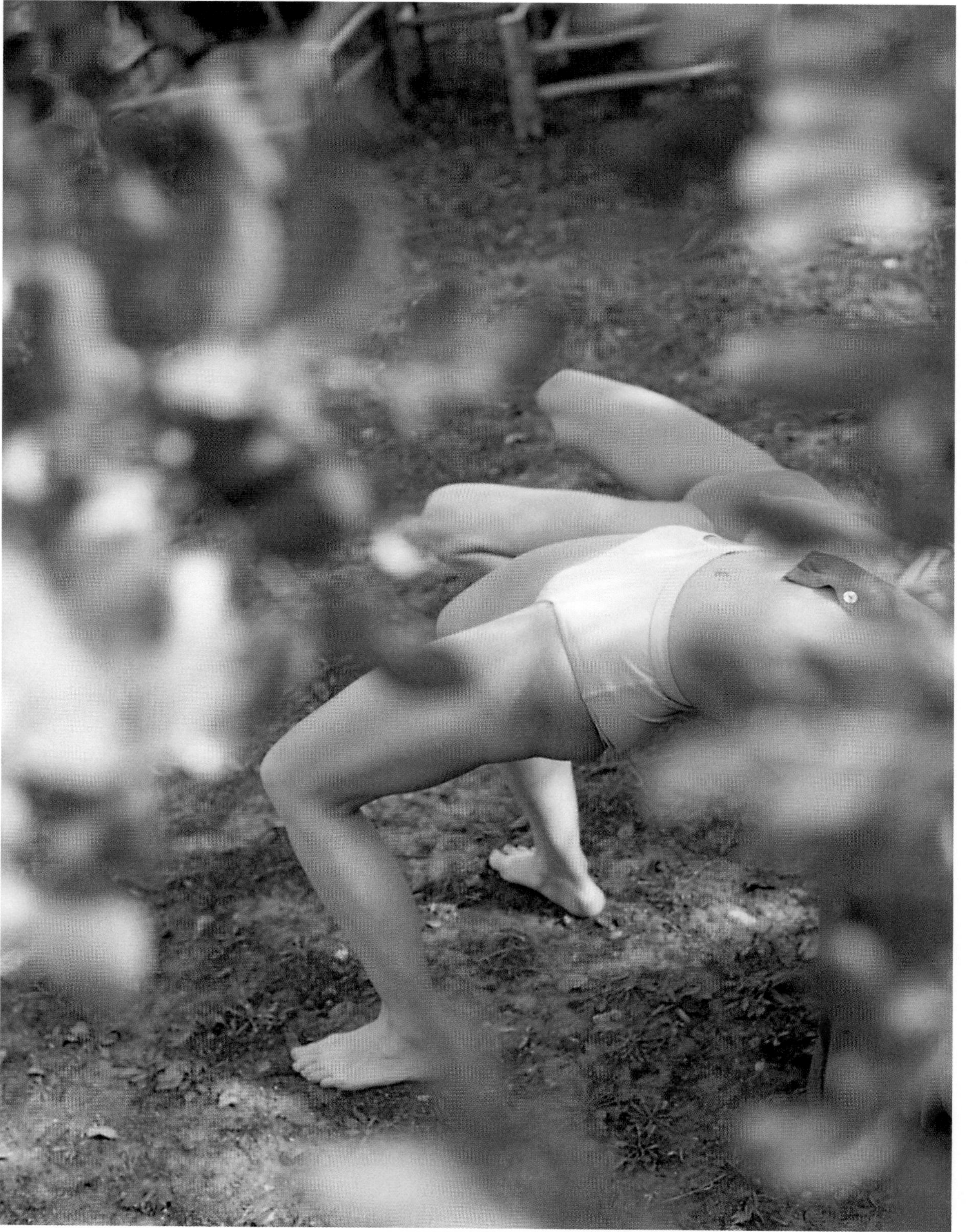

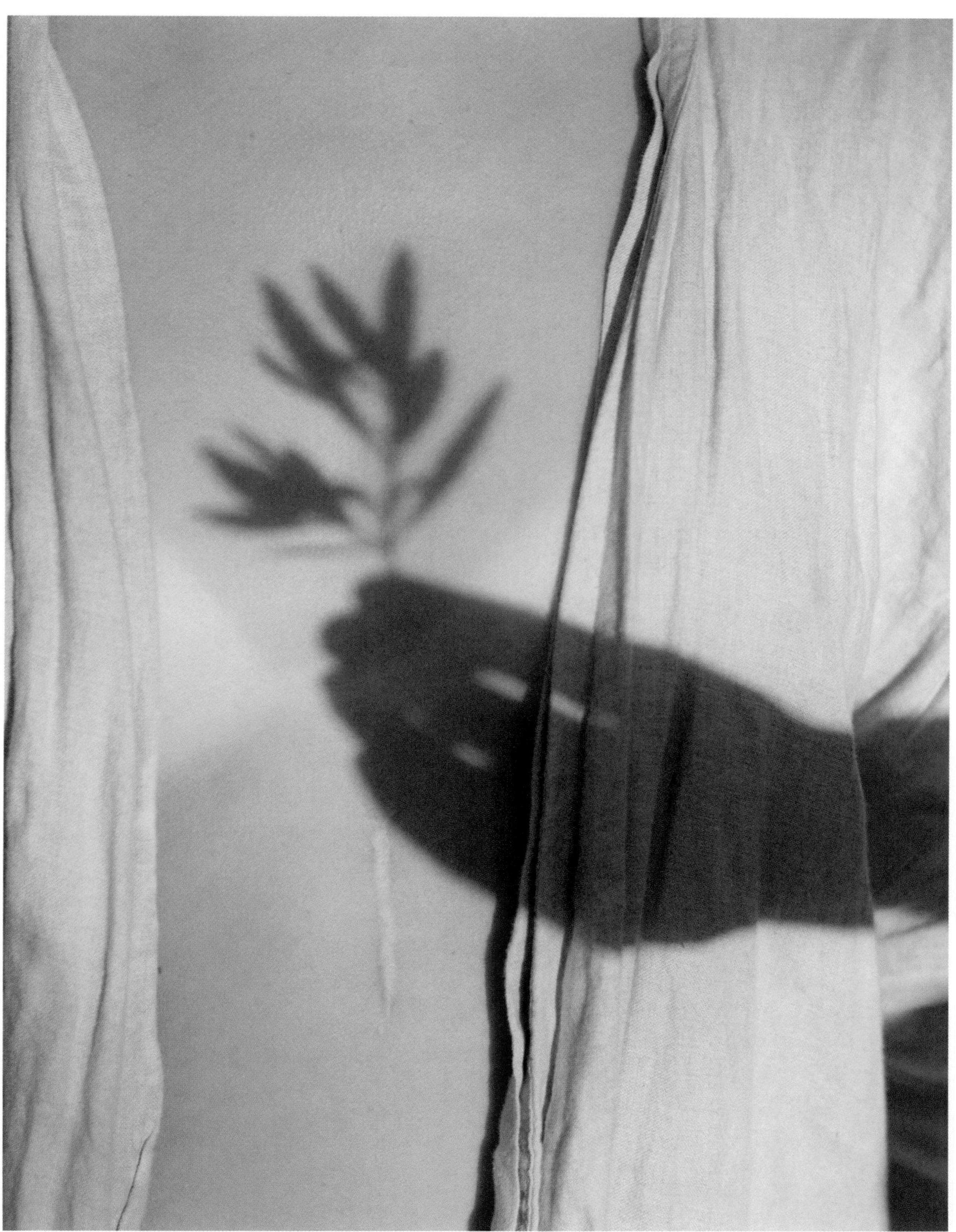

This knowledge of the unseen worlds, and the powers they lend you, are called *siddhis* in the *Yoga-sutras*. They also include time travel, the ability to appear in two places at once, and invisibility. (I'll keep you posted…) But I do agree that they are powerful, and your experiences of flow, clarity of intuition and synchronicity certainly multiply once you dive into a trusting practice.

Everything can be a yoga practice of sorts: eating a delicious meal, walking at a slow, hypnotic pace, drawing lines on a piece of paper, a deliciously slow kiss, breathing in a sea breeze. Definitely making love. Any action that is soaked in awareness. Because it is through developing our awareness that we notice the ripples of energy and emotion that travel through us – maps that are tried-and-tested ways to ascend gradually to a higher consciousness, and which also show the way back home to ourselves.

*Everything can be a yoga practice of sorts: eating a delicious meal, walking at a slow, hypnotic pace, drawing lines on a piece of paper, a deliciously slow kiss, breathing in a sea breeze…*

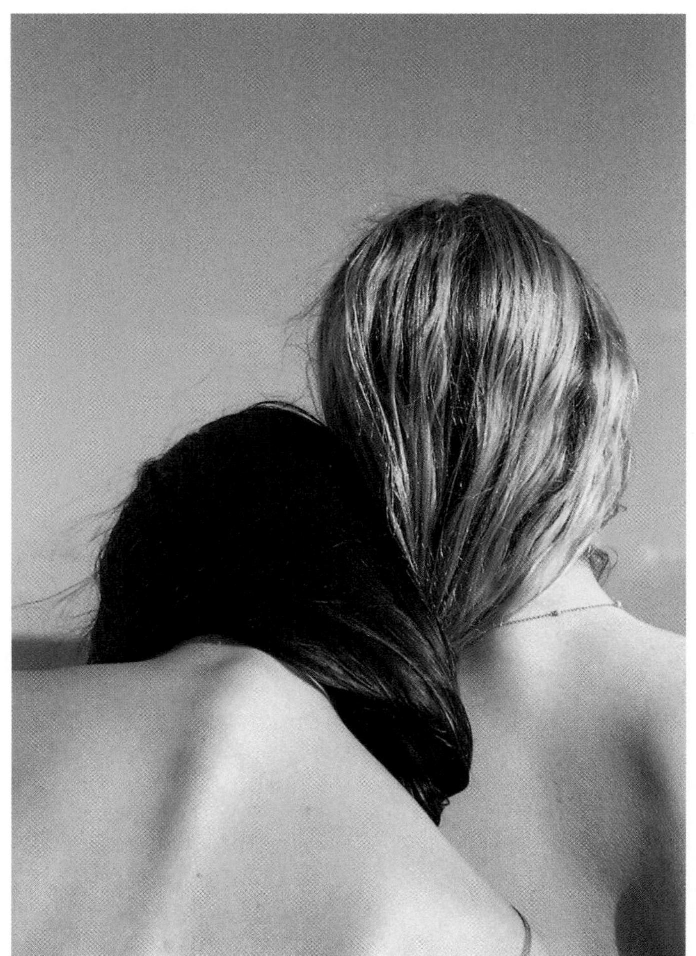

# AUTHENTICITY

*I firmly believe that yoga practices are there to enhance your life and make it as joyful as possible.*

In the last few years yoga has been completely absorbed into mainstream culture. There are multiple "brands" of yoga, and endless claims of authenticity and ownership. There are thousands of training courses; studios are opening up everywhere and yoga is being used to advertise all kinds of things.

With this explosion of interest, how do true yoga lovers continue to honour the tradition? For me, the answer is patiently to educate ourselves and seek out information. So here is a very, very brief summary of the origins of yoga, as a starting point for your own exploration.

As someone who discovered yoga through *āsana*, my research began with questions about the physical practices: how new postures, breathing practices and rituals had been accumulated and whether these could genuinely be considered yoga. What my treasure hunt ultimately revealed to me was that yoga is, and always will be, a living tradition. Although it's important not to disassociate yoga from the rich tradition of wisdom underpinning it, it's also OK to include other rituals of awareness and embodiment. Each human body and mind is unique, and each of us needs to seek out a spectrum of practices that works for our own design.

Yoga has always been a hybrid of philosophies and different religious practices. I don't think that it is disrespectful for each individual to seek a selection of self-care tools and rituals that are best suited to their own, unique journey of self-enquiry and empowerment, as long as they are sensitive and respectful towards the yoga tradition and acknowledge its roots from India.

If you find additional practices and wisdom that heighten your awareness and create awakenings, then that is your yoga and your truth. If it is a new practice that works for you, it's precious. It doesn't matter if it is one thousand years or one year old. You are your own teacher and guru.

As I said earlier, traditional elements such as meditation and *āsana* are very much part of my practice, but so are other, personal additions, such as an exploration of my menstrual cycle as a blueprint for the waxing and waning of my energy (see pages 174—83). This has enabled me to understand my emotional landscape, structure my life and select the most useful rituals to practise within it.

This awareness also acts as a means of personal enquiry, which I interpret as an aspect of *svādhyāya* or self-reflection. This is a key element of a yoga practice, sometimes through the study of literature and following the example of sages and other wise souls. You can use the practice of *svādhyāya* to move through life in an ethical and compassionate way. In my own practice, I have treated it as an invitation to incorporate elements that lead me to a better understanding of myself, in order to seek a more truthful way of living and being.

Another ritual that is very much not an authentic yoga practice (to my knowledge!) is an exploration of the intrinsic value of sexual pleasure and orgasms to heal (see pages 201–17). It is deeply important to me that women reclaim their birthright and vanquish any shame surrounding their sexuality. Not claiming this is denying our truth. The possession of our pleasure demands that we explore, listen to, honour and celebrate our bodies.

Sex and self-pleasure are profound ways to be present, to meditate and release all the juicy hormones that are exciting and nutritious. It's also a test of our confidence, our honesty and our ability to be direct and ask for what we want.

For some, the journey to explore our own body can take time, trust and patience. Using this self-found knowledge, we can liberate ourselves from performing and pleasing. I would also argue that learning how to enjoy our own bodies, and communicating how we like to receive pleasure, is an intimately political act. Equality in the bedroom informs equality in the boardroom.

I firmly believe that yoga practices are there to enhance your life and make it as joyful as possible. I hope this book will serve as a starting point for your journey, and persuade you to gather your own set of survival and pleasure tools.

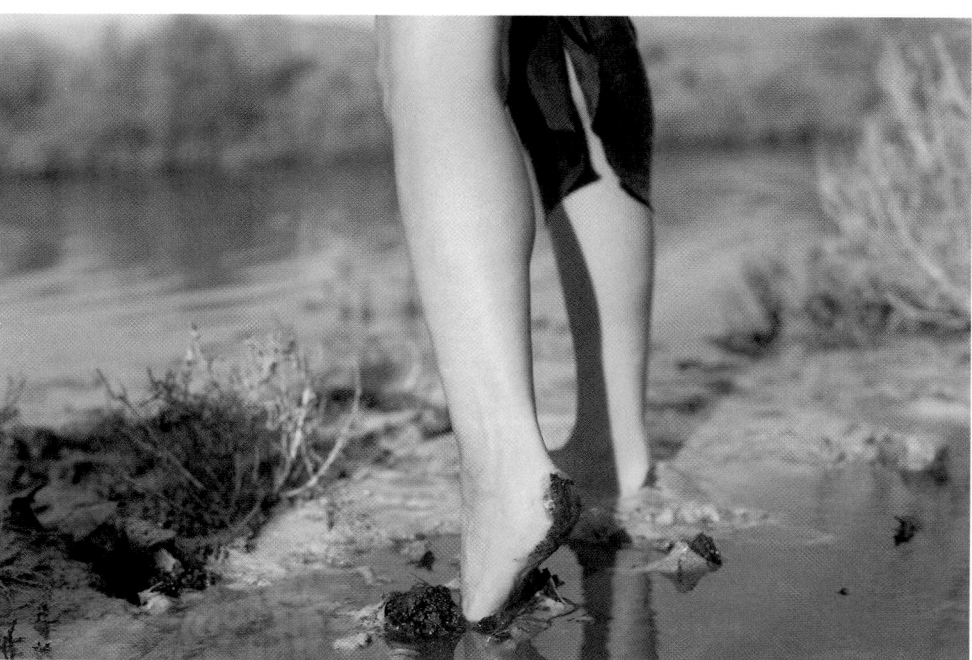

# DEFINITIONS OF YOGA

Most people will tell you that the word yoga means "union" or "yoke", and you may be familiar with B K S Iyengar's description:

> *The union of the individual soul with the universal Spirit is Yoga.*

When people use the word "union" in relation to yoga, they often mean union of the individual to the universal consciousness. But this could imply separation, because two things can only be united if they have been separated. So to me, this can be interpreted as duality and difference and it's not the philosophy to which I subscribe. An *āsana* practice is a never-ending quest to transcend the flesh and, finally, hope to merge with bliss. This turns the body into an obstacle between the union of our soul with the divine.

*Yoga is... a homecoming, an awakening into the pure love that you truly are.*

I prefer the Tantric definition of yoga, which is an awakening and a remembrance. There has been no initial separation from the divine. You yourself are an incarnation of love and godlike consciousness, but you have forgotten your true nature. According to this definition, yoga is therefore a homecoming, an awakening into the pure love that you truly are. Yoga is both the methods used to achieve an awakened state, and the actual state of freedom or *samādhi*.

There are many different lineages and ways of practising yoga, and the huge body of teachings has a deep history of evolution and cross-pollination. Yoga, as a system of practical philosophy and psychology, has always been open to influence. Though it's not a religion, it did co-develop with Hinduism and philosophical schools, including Vedānta, Sāṃkhya, Jainism and Buddhism.

## THE ROOTS OF YOGA

Some schools of yoga work with meditation, sound, prayer, visualization, cleansing and cleaning practices and breath work or movement. All of these can serve as a means to awaken to the divine, which is the Supreme Consciousness within us, sitting behind the thinking and the ego mind, infusing our being with a deeper knowledge and wisdom.

Nobody knows exactly how old yoga is, though the first mention of the word occurs approximately 2,500 years ago in the sacred text known as the Kaṭha Upanishad. There was also the infamous discovery of the Proto-Śiva seal of Mohenjo-daro in the

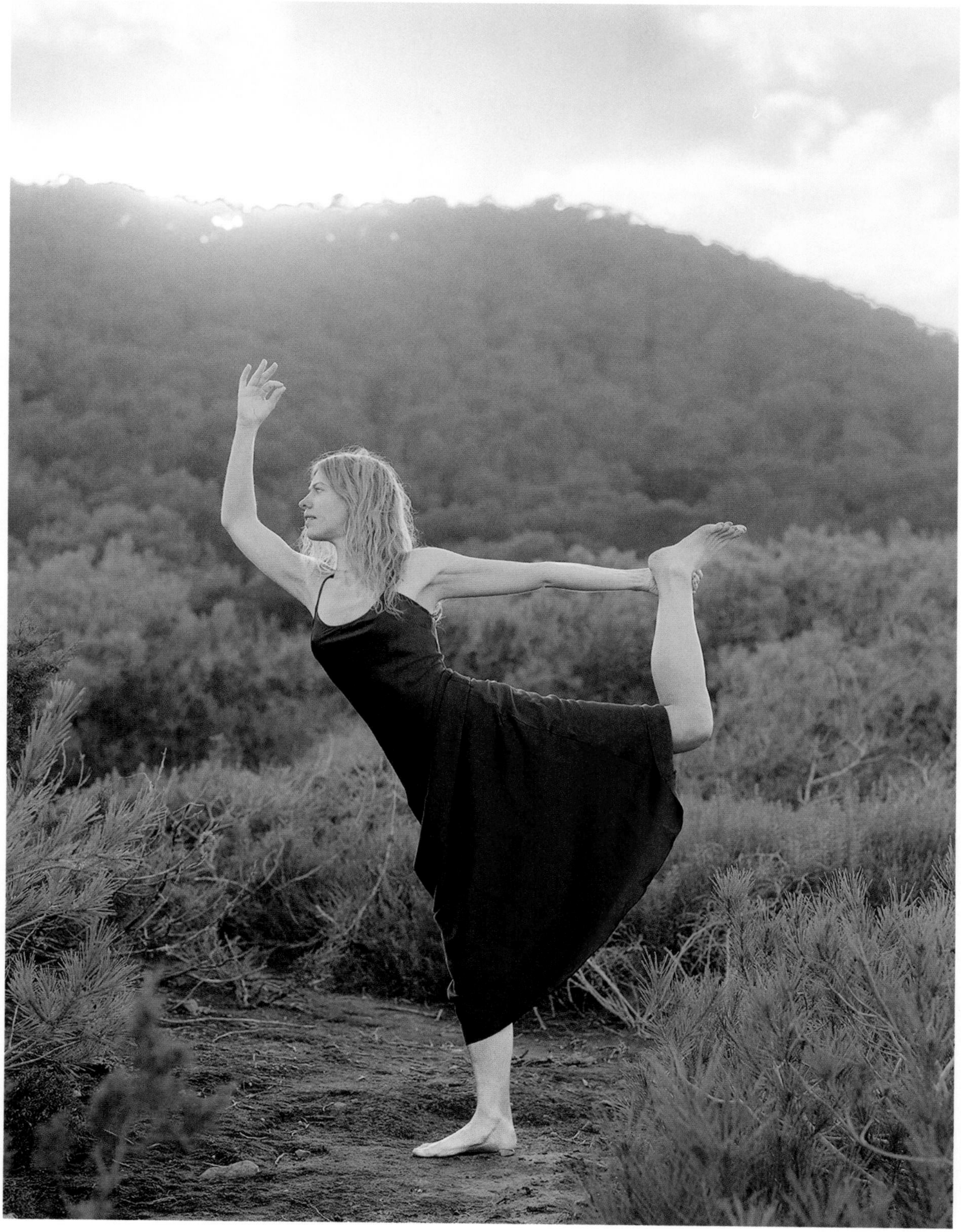

1920s. Mohenjo-daro, in present-day Pakistan, was a large settlement of the Indus valley or Harappan civilization, a culture that flourished in the Indian subcontinent from about 2500 BCE to 1700 BCE. The seal depicts a figure that appears to be sitting in an *āsana* known as *Baddha Koṇāsana*, or Bound Angle pose, with the heels pulled towards the groin, the soles of the feet pressing together and the bent knees opened out to the sides. The arms are stretched, with the hands are resting on the knees.

It is this discovery that prompted the widespread (and generous) claim that yoga is 5,000 years old. However, scholars now generally agree that the figure's posture probably isn't a yoga pose. It is in fact a very common day-to-day resting position in India, and in their book *Roots of Yoga*, James Mallinson and Mark Singleton argue that the seals "offer no conclusive evidence of an ancient yogic culture".

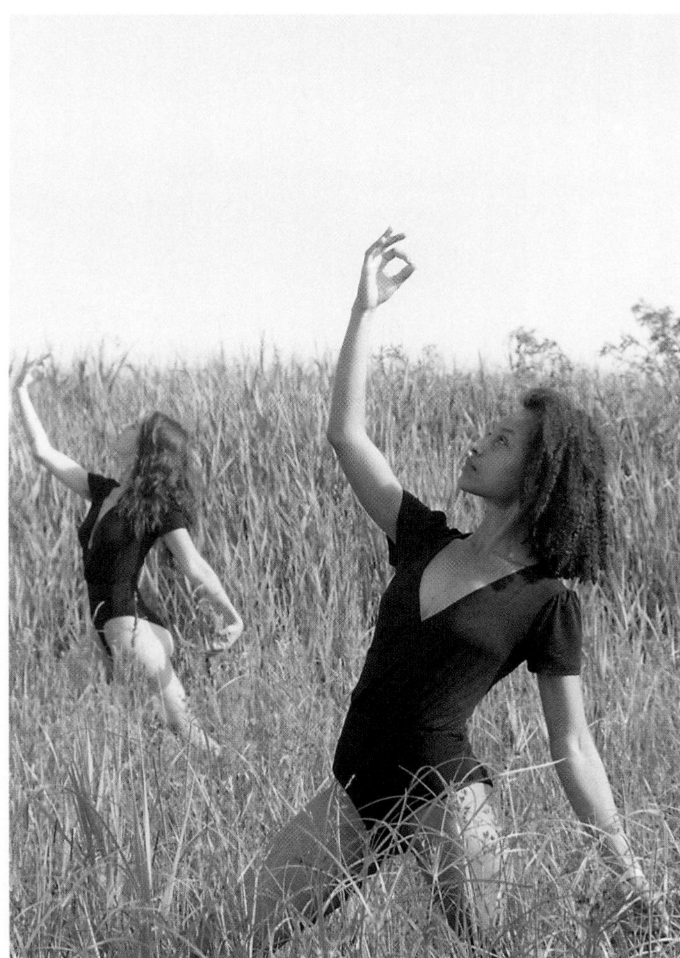

*This beautiful ritual soon sinks into our lives, creating a little oasis at the beginning of our day.*

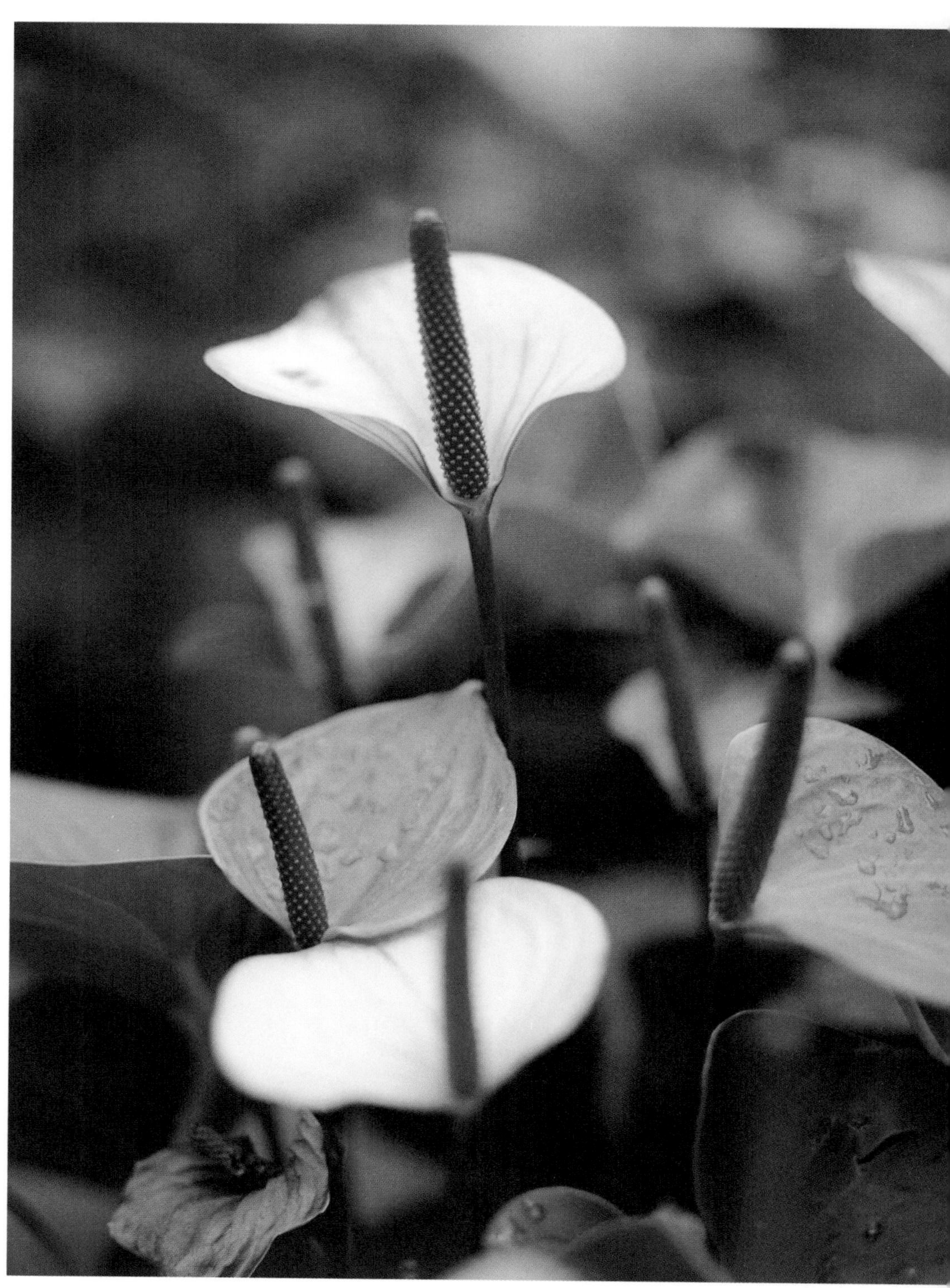

# PĀTAŃJALA YOGA

The *Yoga-sutras* are only one set of a collection of literature, believed to date from the 4th or 5th century CE. But until recently, they've dominated the yoga tradition, mainly because they caught the interest of European scholars in the 19th century, and were widely disseminated by the Hindu monk Vivekananda and the Russian philosopher Helena Blavatsky. It's only recently that it's been understood that the *Sutras* were originally separate from the *Haṭha* tradition (see page 35).

The *Yoga-sutras* are built on the idea of duality, of the body as an obstacle to transcend, which I think can be divisive and counter-productive to living a fulfilled and joyful life. However, they have been fundamental to the development of a number of different yoga practices. Here, we can find the seeds of rituals and philosophies that remain relevant today.

*Sutra* means "string" or "thread" and comes from the word *siv*, which means "that which sews and holds things together". The individual *sutras* have been likened to pearls of wisdom on a thread. Here are a few of elements explored in the *Yoga-sutras*.

## KRIYĀ YOGA

*Kriyā* is rooted in the Sanskrit word *kṛ*, which means action. As outlined in the *Yoga-sutras*, *Kriyā* yoga is the path that leads to *samādhi*. But it later took on a new meaning, and *kriyas* are now generally understood to be cleansing practices that are undertaken to purify the body and, therefore, life. If we are disciplined in the practices that we choose, dedicating ourselves to them daily, meeting the heat of resistance that burns through the clutter of our mind in an act of transmutation; if we dwell in a practice of self-enquiry, one that leads to self-knowledge, a sense of clarity and luminous peace, and if we devote these practices, and surrender ourselves to the Divine, then we will taste bliss.

## GUṆAS

Another Sanskrit word, this translates as "strand" or "thread". In relation to yoga, it means a quality, attribute or property: an attribute of the five elements, each of which has its own peculiar quality or qualities as well as organ of sense.

The three *gunas* evolved from the Yoga-Samkhya tradition, which had a great influence on Hindu philosophy. They describe three forces whose interplay produces all essential aspects of all nature, or *prakṛti*. This includes energy, matter and consciousness. At the highest plane of reality, all three types of *gunas* are perfectly balanced.

### THE THREE FORCES OF *GUNAS*

Each of these forces has its own attributes:

***Sattva***

light, peaceful, truthful, whole, creative, joyous

***Rajas***

stimulating, passionate, mobile

***Tamas***

inert, dull, inactive, concealing

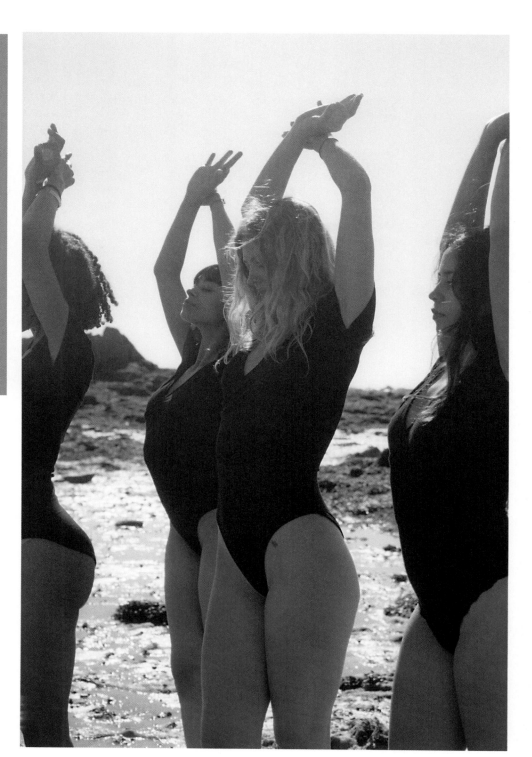

## AṢṬĀṄGA: THE EIGHT LIMBS OF YOGA

The core chapter of Patanjali's *Yoga-sutras* describes the eight paths by which a yogi can attain liberation, only one of which involves the physical postures most commonly associated with modern yoga practice. This eightfold path is called *Aṣṭāṇga* – *aṣṭā* means "eight" and *āṇga* means "limb". Each of the limbs in *Aṣṭāṇga* builds on the previous one and is often depicted as a rung on a ladder leading to *samādhi*. The eight limbs are:

1

***Yama*: restraint**

Moral attitudes that help rein in our instinctual life and instill a sense of moral integrity.

2

***Niyama*: observance**

Purity of the mind through restraint and training with practices such as meditation; contentment with what is within reach; austerity; study of the higher self; devotion to the transcendental, eternal and omnipresent.

3

***Āsana*: posture**

*Āsana* literally translates as "seat", but has come to be understood as therapeutic postures or poses that awaken the body and bring relief and release.

4

***Prāṇāyāma*: breath control**

*Prāṇā* means both "breath' and "life force" in Sanskrit, and *yama* is "control'. In manipulating the flow of the breath, we are able to shape, contain or release the flow of the energy, or life force, within the body.

5

***Pratyāhāra*: sense-withdrawal**

The turning inward of the senses, away from external stimuli, in order to quieten the noise of the outside world, to amplify the experience of the inner realm.

6

***Dhāraṇā*: concentration**

The space to know yourself through witnessing and contemplating the mind in meditation.

7

***Dhyāna*: a state of deep meditation**

A lake-like stillness that comes with practice and dedication.

8

***Samādhi*: ecstasy**

In the Sutras, *samādhi* is meditative absorption, but I translate it as the point at which the individual recognizes the presence of the divine collective consciousness and expands into a space of ecstasy, which leads to ultimate liberation. The goal of the journey of yoga is enlightenment, which leads to aloneness or separation, or *kaivalya*. The state of *samādhi* is intrinsically impossible to put into words. It's a divine, profound and sustained awakening into the bliss of knowing that we are timeless and infinite. It's a sustained blossoming of innate and endless awareness.

# HAṬHA YOGA

If you ask yogis what *Haṭha* means, they will often say that it is the union of the inner sun (*ha*) and moon (*ṭha*). However, the word's literal meaning is "violence" or "force". There has been controversy among scholars as to what this means, but they agree that *Haṭha* bloomed between the 11th and 14th centuries CE. Its goals included a healthy and long life, conserving life-essence, which was believed to reside in physical substances in the body, forcing energy up the body in order to achieve *samādhi*, cultivating supernatural powers, and *jivanmukti*, or liberation while living.

There are exercises and beliefs within this practice that are still relevant today. However, much of it is obscure and not necessarily applicable for contemporary audiences. *Trāṭaka*, a meditation that involves staring at a candle, is one that I've borrowed from the *Haṭha* tradition, as is *kapālabhāti* (see page 128).

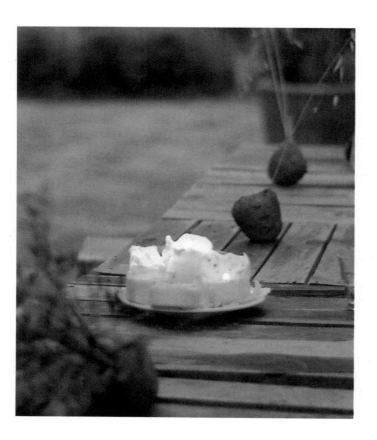

# MODERN POSTURAL YOGA

In the West, postural practice has become the most widespread. In its present form it is only about a hundred years old, and is the result of an unlikely coming together of different yoga lineages, overlaid with a variety of postures and sequences from the Western world. Mark Singleton has described it as "a hybridized product of colonial India's dialogical encounter with the worldwide physical culture movement", emerging from a blossoming of excitement for athletic and gymnastic disciplines in Britain and Europe in the 19th century. Perfection of the physical body and the exhibition of strength were interpreted as an expression of moral purity and superiority that evolved into the cultivation of a national identity.

*I think that any kind of movement can be yoga, if practised mindfully with total presence and grace.*

This culture percolated through to the official training programme of the Indian army under the British, and inspired the "harmonial gymnastic" programme found in the YMCA. It was also disseminated throughout India via the Anglican education system.

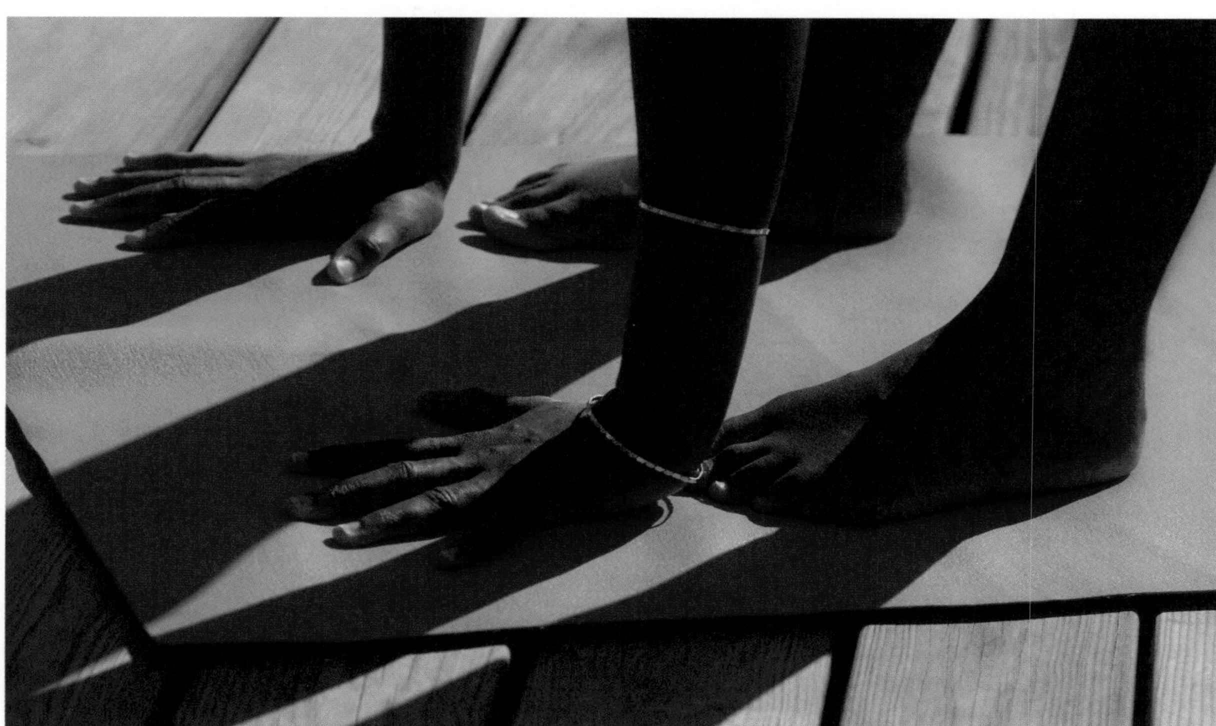

The physical education drillmasters in Indian schools were often ex-military, and perpetuated a military attitude alongside a Westernized system of gymnastics. This system was firmly established well into the 20th century and shaped the structure of modern postural yoga.

Bodybuilding was also a surprising influence. At the end of the 19th and beginning of the 20th centuries, Eugen Sandow was a famous bodybuilder who established a cult following in India. He elevated his physical discipline by suffusing the development of the physical body with religious discourse. The movement was wildly popular, and this merging of the spiritual or religious with the athletic planted the seed for a new physical programme that could claim authority by attaching itself to ancient yogic and Hindu philosophy.

What this demonstrates to me is that there isn't really any "authentic" modern postural yoga. Instead, this is an invitation to us to continue to develop the tradition, with a view to making it as inspiring, nourishing and therapeutic as we possibly can. It's our responsibility to engage with a kinder practice, one that will preserve and celebrate our bodies. I think that any kind of movement can be yoga, if practised mindfully with total presence and grace. Please see the Practical Magic section (see page 59) for more ideas on nutritious movement.

## TANTRA

All of this is a background to the type of Tantric philosophy that I prefer. The Tantric lineage was conceived around 400–800 CE, much later than many yoga traditions. This means that Tantric luminaries were able to cherry-pick what they felt was useful and relevant from a wealth of existing practical, psychological and metaphysical intelligence.

According to Tantra, our bodies are a microcosm of the universe. We contain the five elements, the *pañca mahābhūta*: earth, water, fire, air and ether. We are in constant communication with the world around us. Though we have our own, unique vibration, we long to attune to the orchestra of the earth and its creatures – all the cells in our body naturally want to align in harmony and unity. The fact of our existence is an act of pure love, and we move toward a life as an expression of that love.

*Tantra* means "loom" or "weave" in Sanskrit, which perfectly communicates the interconnective nature of life. Tantric cosmology explains existence as being born of, and sustained by, two fundamental principles: consciousness and energy. The two are inextricably linked, one cannot exist without the other. They are symbolized (apologies for the gender roles!) as the timeless, unchanging masculine element of consciousness, and the feminine element, the creative force that acts in the world energy. These two principles are often depicted as the Hindu deities Śiva and Śakti.

According to Tantra, the whole sublime universe is an act of love, and is steeped in pure love. Tantric yoga practice is an act of remembrance and a process of awakening. Permeating this philosophy of love is the concept of non-duality, the union of each individual soul, *atman*, with the universal soul of Brahman, the Supreme Cosmic Spirit of Hinduism. It's a denial of separation and otherness, while supporting the precious and unique nature of each being.

*Anything that emphasizes our experience of this connection, and the invisible threads connecting our hearts and our futures, is very precious.*

Tantra is essentially saying yes to life. It is human, it is loving, it is pleasure, it is connection, it is similarities, it is individuation, it is embracing, it is nature, it is celebration, it is expansion, it is artistic, it is erotic, it is love.

It is also very practical, and that is essential.

I'm drawn to these teachings because they are life-affirming. The Tantric tradition recognizes a connection between the spirtual experience and the physical experience of the body and the breath. The material world is a perfect incarnation of the divine, infused with a universal Supreme Consciousness that permeates all beings. The path to awakening is not union with the Supreme Consciousness through transcending the physical plane, as there is no separation to be bridged.

This key detail is the difference between Tantra and an ascetic practice, as outlined in the *Yoga-sutras* and projected onto postural practices that seek to conquer the body in order to reach *samādhi*. In Tantra, we are not separate; we are godly beings ourselves. The path is a remembrance, a homecoming.

Tantra believes that we are all inherently godly and luminous. We have the same longing to be loved, to belong, to have families, to find a purpose in life and a way of earning a living that is aligned to our personal values. We all want to be healthy and safe, to have freedom and the opportunity to learn and evolve. There is more that binds than divides. We need to remember that as often as we possibly can – anything that emphasizes our experience of this connection, and the invisible threads connecting our hearts and our futures, is precious.

One of the reasons I love Tantra is that it gives an opening to the bliss of the body and the importance of pleasure. Our bodies are incredibly beautiful and mysterious, something that we forget too readily. Think about the glorious beginning of a romance: there is the potent thrill of hormones that excite your whole body, of course, but there is also the experience of seeing yourself and your body through the dewy awe of a lover. It's the joy of being unwrapped, every dot of you precious, each breath of you intoxicating. The landscape of your body being explored with care and fascination. The thrill of being brand-new again.

It is not just about the lover, but about how they refresh your perception and experience of your own body. But we can do this ourselves: we can treasure and worship our human vessels every day. Practices and rituals are a way to return to our sacred truth, the sublime nature of embodied life. This is truly magical and empowering.

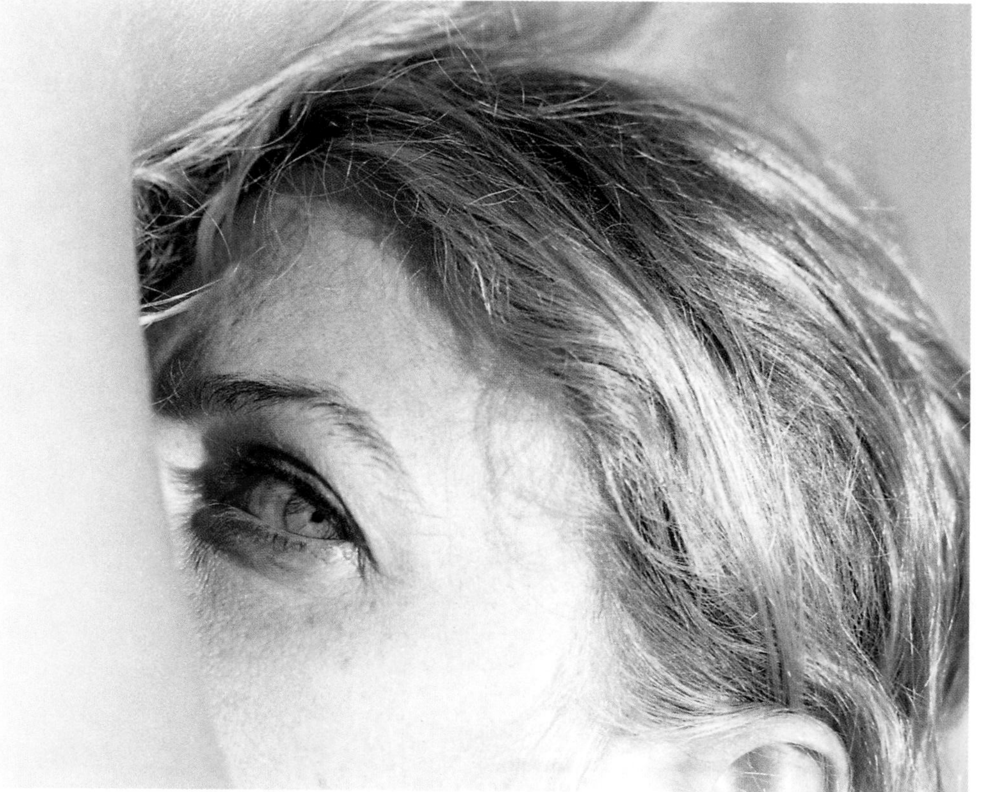

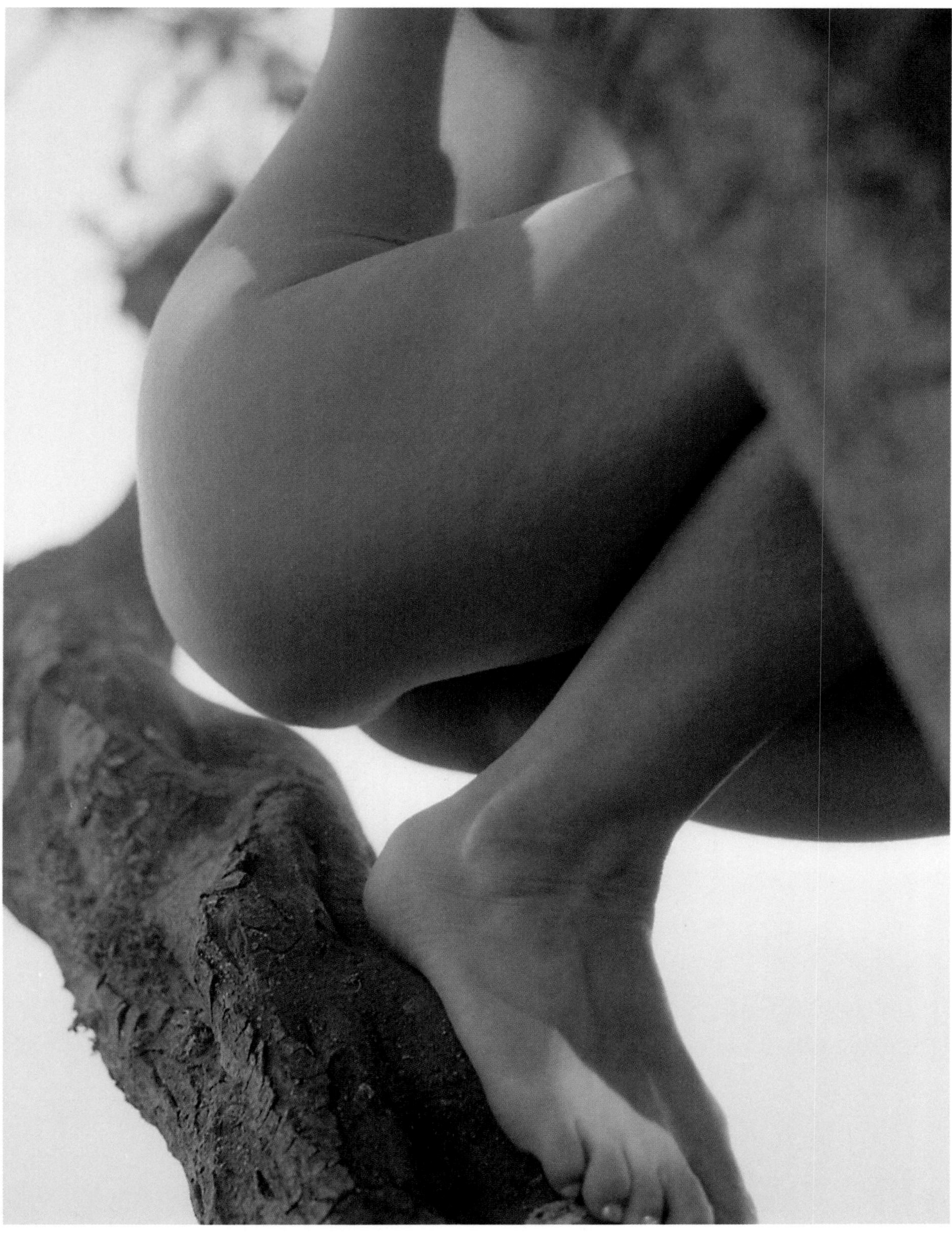

2

# ELECTRIC BODY – THE LIFE FORCE

*"Spirit and energy should be clear as the night air;*
*In the soundless is the ultimate pleasure all along."*

SUN-BUER

# TANTRA, PRĀṆĀ & THE CHAKRAS

Most of us find ourselves drawn to yoga in an effort to move our bodies and create space, release tension and find some kind of physical relief. That's how I started, approaching the practice like gymnastics. I had no idea the teachings would take me from the tangible experience of bones, musculature and lungs into the exciting realm of energetic, mystical and metaphysical explorations. You might have found, too, that your curiosity will carry you from the physical into the unseen. At some point when you meditate, or practise postures or *prāṇāyāma* (see page 120), the cognitive veils of perception drop and you find yourself deep in elastic and expansive moments of cosmic space. This is when the subtler realms also reveal themselves, and you become fascinated with the energy body.

The more I practised and observed my subtle body, the more I realized that what seemed to be abstract and mystical was actually common sense to me. That the physical is an incarnation of the cosmic, the energetic world extroverting itself. The two are inextricably interconnected. It's impossible to create a holistic approach to wellbeing without taking care of the material body, the subtle energy body and the spirit – particularly when we explore the potential of the yogic energy system known as the chakras as an ancient representation of the nervous system.

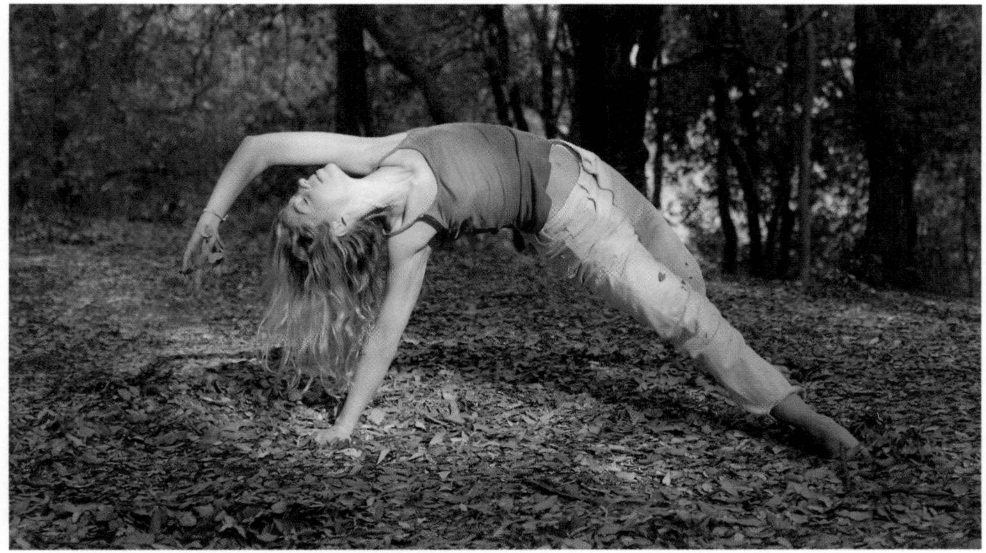

We are so much more than blood and clay. According to Hindu philosophy, all the material world is infused with a dynamic energy called *prāṇā*. This is our "vital life force", like nature's electricity – the invisible energy matrix that animates matter, endlessly shape-shifting in communication with its surroundings. Without this potent energy, there would be no life at all. No sea, no trees, no vegetables, animals or humans. The world of the living is essentially *prāṇā* manifesting itself in a spectrum of forms and qualities.

*When our energy body is healthy and our prāṇā is flowing freely, we feel bright and integrated.*

This mystical force can be difficult to understand, both within and outside the Tantric framework touched on here. It's like catching cognitive butterflies. Experientially, though, it's very simple. Our *prāṇā* body is primal. We feel it most poignantly in flutters, beats, blushes, ripples, flames and flushes. It's also our intuition, our inner wisdom and fire. With this in mind, we can consider our bodies as human-shaped conductors of *prāṇā*, the life force.

When our energy body is healthy and our *prāṇā* is flowing freely, we feel bright and integrated. We are grounded in the physical world, and receptive to the colourful, unseen realm. When *prāṇā* is stagnant or blocked, we become dull or heavy, and lose access to subtlety in areas of the body. A Tantric yoga practice is a wonderful method for us to connect the tangible, ephemeral world of the seen with the timeless world of the unseen. It provides a very useful system that outlines the various colours of *prāṇā* and layers of consciousness and reality, with different practices and rituals for the different stages of awakening.

The energy body is constantly shaping and percolating through our experiences. It informs our thoughts, perception and intuition. It influences our kindness, our capacity to love and our creativity. It guides our way through life, pulling us toward what we need and where we can flourish, dissolving differences and revealing connections. It illuminates and ignites.

Our *prāṇā* is eternally engaging with our friends, lovers, neighbours. It shape-shifts in relation to *prāṇā* everywhere: in the food we eat, the sounds we hear, the natural world or the things we ferociously consume with our eyes. It draws us magnetically to people. It prickles in warning, rushes in arousal or tells us wordless truths.

This energy body is just as vital as the physical body, and they both influence each other constantly. For example, overwork makes us stressed and anxious. We don't take enough free time to allow our brains to slow down and rest, which leads us to sleep too little, or too lightly. Our energetic vibration drops, and we experience ourselves, and are experienced by others, as being less magnetic and empowered. Instead of focusing and harnessing our personal power to achieve our goals and be anchored within the present moment, we leak our precious energy through worrying and thinking negatively about the future.

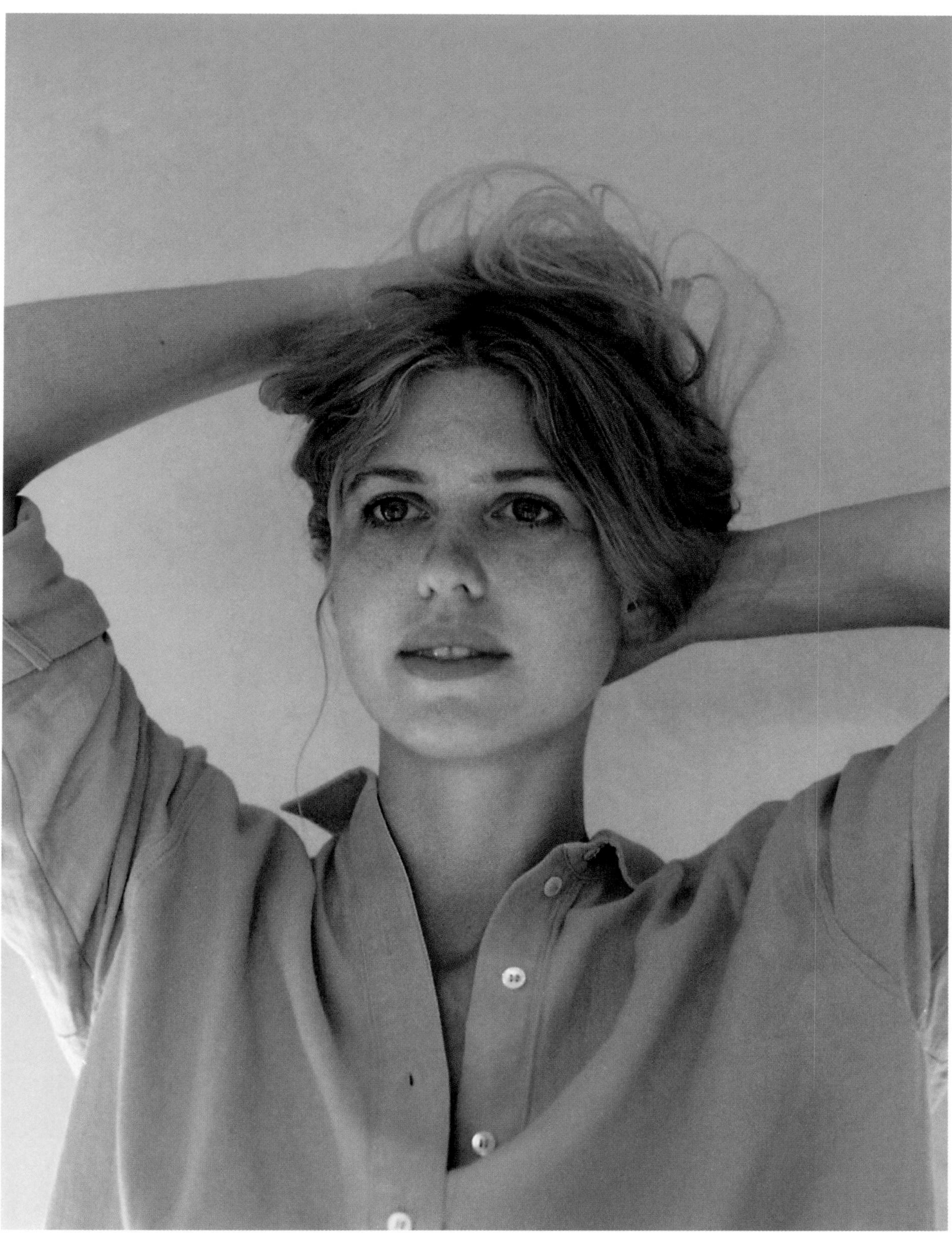

This energetic dimming is exacerbated when our body responds to stress with its most primal response: by activating the sympathetic nervous system. This puts us into the famous "fight or flight" mode. Our glands secrete the hormones cortisol and adrenaline, which prepare our bodies to burst into action – but our bodies are not expending this energy, it has nowhere to go. So it fizzes around, making our hearts beat faster and our breath a little shallower. Our muscles become tense and uncomfortable. Stress tampers with other hormones in the body, affecting our metabolism, digestion and cognitive functioning. And so the cycle continues: external perceived pressures influencing our energetic, chemical and psychological make-up, which will then shape the external world and our performance within it.

## A PATH TO FREEDOM

It's important to realize that it is impossible to isolate any of these elements. The energy body and the physical body are in endless conversation, always renegotiating power and health. One can't exist without the other. The material needs to be permeated with vibrational energy to bring it to life. Energy needs a physical body to animate, mist and vibrate through. Our energy body is affected by our mental and physical health, while our spirit is affected by our energy body.

We can change the vibration of our cells by working with sound and with energetic healing modalities such as acupuncture. This will conduct a visceral realigning. Think about how you experience profound atmospheric shifts without verbal or physical interactions. There are people, places and rituals in our life that intensify our presence.

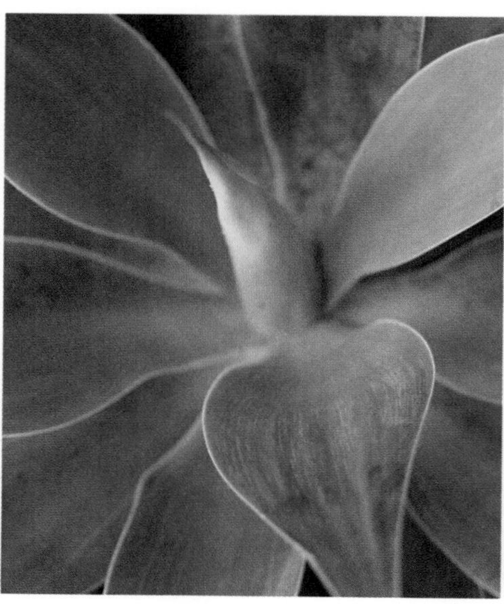

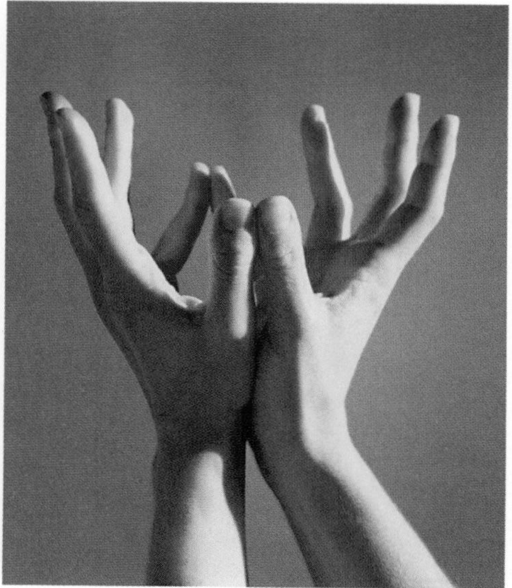

Until I began to practise yoga, I was mostly unconscious of my vital energy. When I began practising, I wasn't able to focus on kindling and exploring *prāṇā* through breath work, meditation and traditional Tantric visualization. So the access point for me was moving my body. It took years for me to awaken in trust, and to understand exactly how to play with, contain and sustain *prāṇā*.

*Until I began to practise yoga, I was mostly unconscious of my vital energy ....the access point for me was moving my body.*

When this work moved into me, I found it equally as powerful as a *yogāsana* practice, and arguably a better tool for self-enquiry and empowerment. I explored a Westernized interpretation of the chakras famously espoused by teachers like Anodea Judith and Carolyn Myss. I find their work a really practical and useful addition to more ancient yoga teachings.

So how does *prāṇā* work?

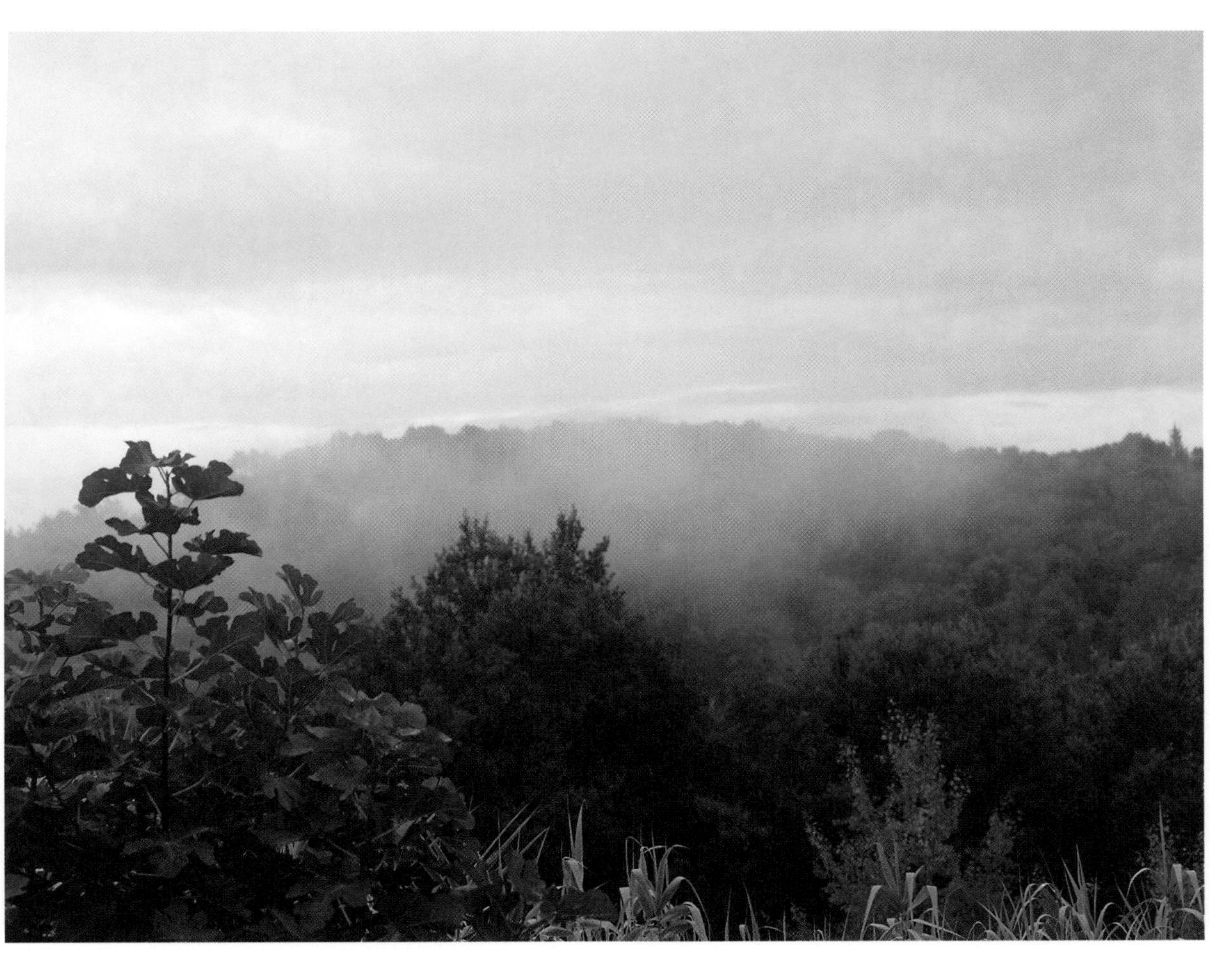

## PRĀṆĀ, NĀḌĪS AND KUNDALINI

According to tradition, *prāṇā* is diffused through the body via a "wireless" system of circuits called *nāḍīs*, "streams", originating from the Sanskrit for movement. This sublime pulsation of energy is understood to have a purely psychophysical force, though some texts suggest that it also includes what are called the "gross channels" – physical systems such as the cardiovascular, lymphatic and nervous systems. There's a lot of conflicting information out there, so really you have to go on your own adventure and make up your own mind.

Though *prāṇā* is said to pervade the whole being, its main highway is the *sushumna nāḍī*, which runs along the spine from the sacrum right up through the crown of the head. Within it is the very delicate *brahma nāḍī*, which is allegedly the carrier of spirit. A spool of dormant spiritual or sexual energy rests at the base of the spine and is called *kundalini*; it's represented as a coiled snake, just waiting to be woken up.

*Kundalini* is the energy that we play with during *prāṇāyāma* (see pages 126–35 for practices), *prāṇā* meaning life force in Sanskrit, and *yama* reining in or control. So *prāṇāyāma* is the restraint and control of the breath. As we practise this, we stir the *kundalini* awake and hope to draw it up the spine through the *sushumna nāḍī*.

Wound around the *brahma nadi* divining rod are two other dominant *nāḍīs* that terminate in the nostrils. The *ida nāḍī* terminates in the left nostril and is activated by breath there; the *pingala nāḍī* is the equivalent on the right. According to the author Harish Johari, the *sushumna nāḍī* is activated only when both nostrils are balanced and working harmoniously. Humans breathe on average fifteen times a minute, so 900 times an hour, and he says that out of those 900 times, only a tiny ten breaths are taken with both nostrils. So 890 out of 900 times, we are activating only one of these threads.

## CHAKRAS

You've probably heard of the chakras, meaning "wheels" or "vortex" in Sanskrit. These are dynamic subtle energy centres. Individual chakras can be isolated and fired by different techniques. When *kundalini* awakens and rises, it is said to activate each chakra, causing it to spin, and finally bursting through the seventh chakra in the crown of the head. When this happens, we experience a sense of blissful euphoria and transcendence.

The chakras are said to act as an energy map to guide us through stages of awakening. There are many different systems, depending on which lineage you study; the most popular one identifies seven main chakras, starting at the base of the spine and working up to the crown. Each chakra is identified with a colour, but again these vary according to the system you follow. Nothing is finite. Your experience is your truth – each of us has our own, unique energy body that changes in temperature, colour and form, depending on our lifestyles and practices.

Although there is a discrepancy regarding the number of chakras, there is a general consensus that everyone holds and experiences their emotions in their lower belly, heart and head. I can run with that. Think of the honeyed heart when there's love, or heaviness in pain, butterflies of excitement in the tummy and the crystallization of anxiety in tenseness of the brow. These points are highly charged, and working on them as such can have a deeply alchemical quality.

If you've seen images of the chakra system, you'll know they're heavily laden with colourful symbolism and poetically illustrated with a glorious array of lotuses, geometric shapes or *yantras*, and archetypal deities. They're intended to be part of yoga practices, mystical visualizations or meditation techniques that create a particular experience. The mythology is meant to convey the indescribable – it's too dampening to gird ether with words; much more accurate to use it to evoke a feeling.

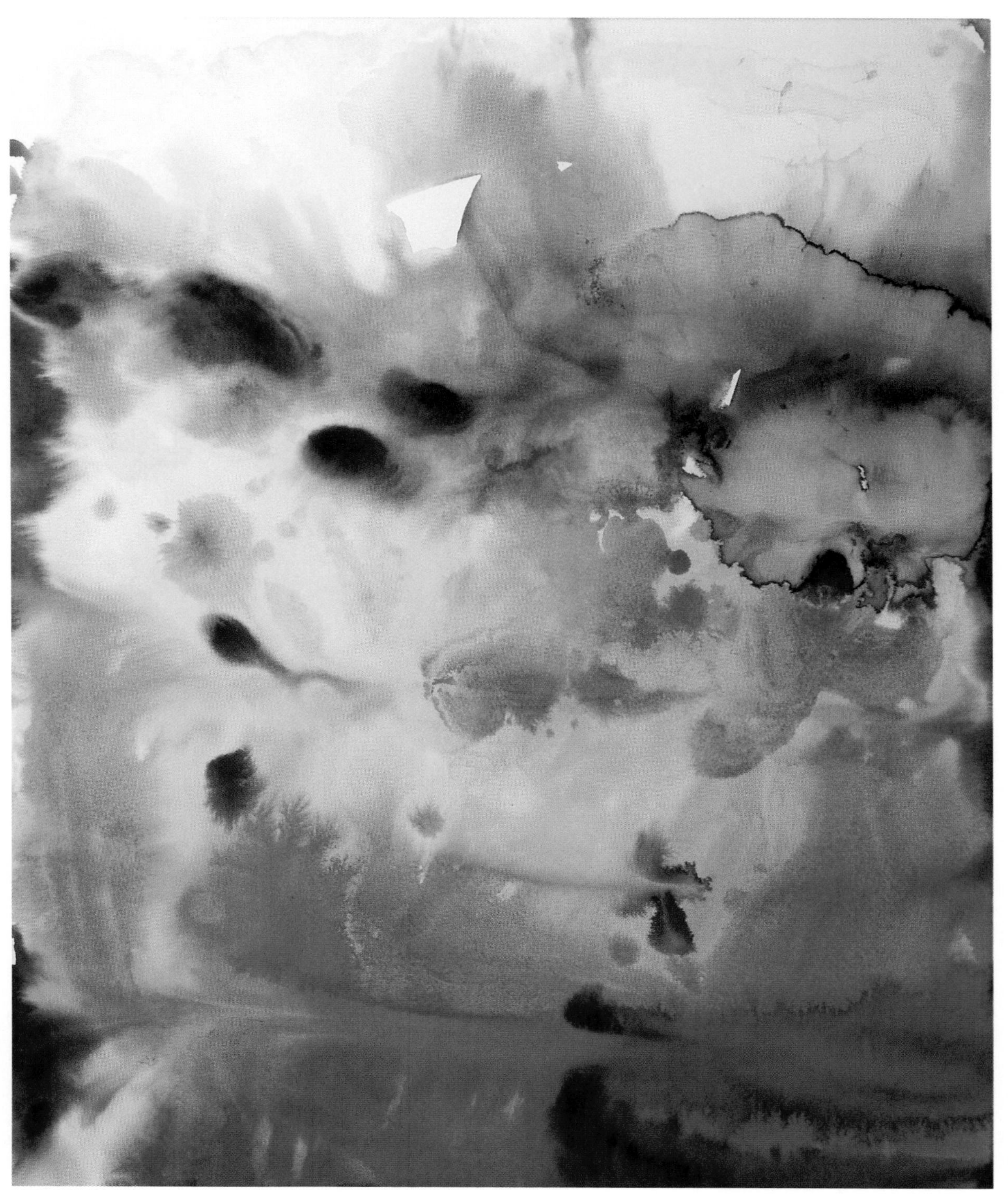

# OUR MAGICAL NERVOUS SYSTEM

The nervous system might in some ways be interpreted as a physiological map of an ancient Eastern philosphy of energy, in that it provides a pathway for communication – relaying messages that coordinate the body's functions.

*Our senses receive the world; they might see something that initiates a cognitive reaction to then spark a physiological reaction.*

An enormous amount of our personality is shaped by our nervous system. It and our mind dictate the way our body reads and reacts to life. Our body is an antenna, receiving signals from the surrounding world. We gather information through the senses, and our brain then internalizes this through a complex network of electrochemical signals that trigger psychological and physical processes in all our cells.

Once we understand how this works, we are better placed to choose how to behave, regardless of how our body intuitively responds. Our senses receive the world; they might see something that initiates a cognitive reaction to then spark a physiological reaction. Just understanding this process is a step toward being more in control of yourself and your own energy.

The autonomic nervous system (ANS) commands all the functions and systems within the body that are generally not consciously directed. It conducts the functioning of our internal organs – heart, liver, kidneys and so on. It dictates our respiratory rate, heart rate, digestion, pupil dilation and sexual arousal. We have two divisions in our autonomic nervous system – the sympathetic and the parasympathetic. The sympathetic is the alarm system that triggers the body's stress response, often known as "fight or flight". The parasympathetic, which is the division we'd like to be dominant, has the "rest and restore" role, putting on the brakes to slow us down.

As primates, we evolved to navigate our way safely through jungles and savanna. Our nervous systems developed to protect us by activating the alarm system in moments of danger, like when we were attacked by a predator. When the sympathetic is activated, a cascade of hormones, the best known of which are adrenaline and cortisol, floods our body. The release of these hormones triggers a number of physiological responses. A faster heart rate pumps blood around the body faster, directing it into major muscle groups. Adrenaline also heightens muscle power, and you may find it causes a dry mouth, shallow breathing and/or pupil dilation. You may also sweat, shake, experience tunnel vision or loss of hearing, flush or turn pale.

All these reactions are intended to prepare the body either to engage in fight, or flee in flight. Sometimes people access the third response, which is to freeze. This can be accompanied by disassociation, perhaps when a traumatic experience is inevitable and

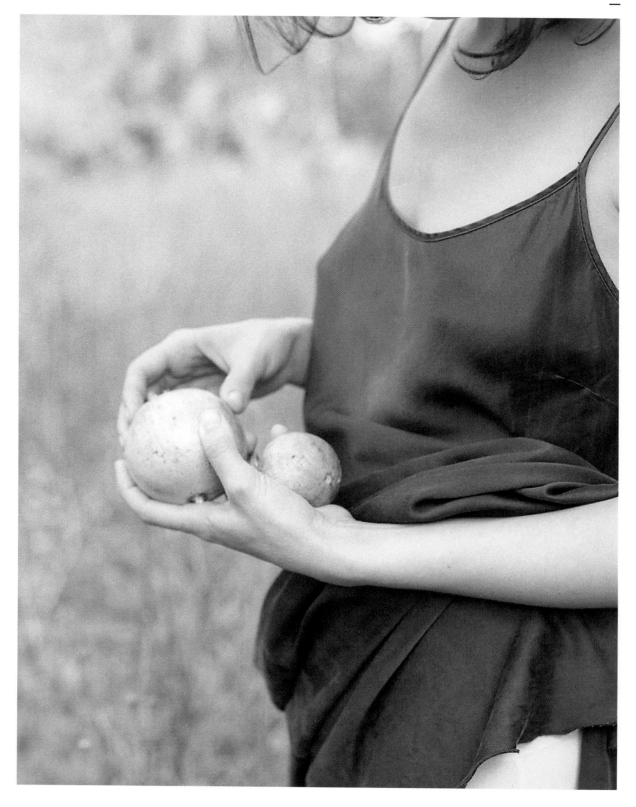

it's too terrifying for us to be present within the mind and body. Dissociation enables us to remove our consciousness from our body in order to tolerate a stressful, painful or even boring experience. There's a broad spectrum: even daydreaming is considered to be a form of dissociation.

Modern life can be so bright, loud, busy and generally overstimulated that our nervous systems malfunction and it becomes difficult for us to move fluidly between our sympathetic and our parasympathetic. We become trapped in a sympathetic dominance, which is stressful and exhausting, and we have no time to recover.

The body and the mind work in a constant feedback loop. When the mind perceives a situation to be stressful, it sets off the sympathetic. This causes the body to be flooded with the chemicals that create an avalanche of sensations, such as those listed above. Despite what the senses perceive and the mind understands, the body sometimes doesn't know the difference between a threatening predator, like a tiger, and a challenging experience at work.

Our sympathetic behaves in exactly the same way, leaving us in a edgy state of hypervigilance, or ultimately exhausting ourselves from the effort of sympathetic dominance, which is when we burn out. Either way, our body becomes a stressful

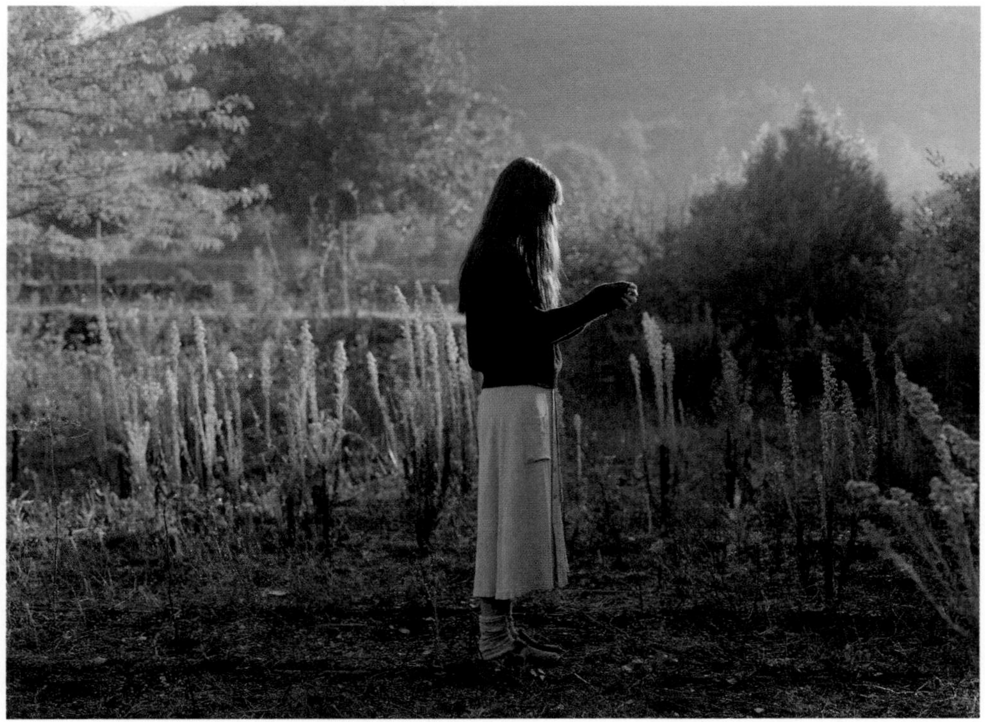

*Modern life can be so bright, loud, busy and generally over-stimulated that our nervous systems malfunction.*

place for us to inhabit. It feels unpredictable and disobedient. We lose our vitality and confidence, and can potentially become very ill. So the circle continues.

Understandably, we're much more confident with a healthy autonomic nervous system (ANS), when we can move easily between divisions. When our ANS is functioning correctly, we activate the right division to respond to the world around us appropriately. This gives us much greater confidence in ourselves and our intuition. It informs our whole life, our capacity for comfort, exploration, connection, learning and growth.

So our unconscious, visceral response essentially shapes how the world feels to us, and how comfortable or playful we are within the world. When we're functioning correctly, we're able to perform in stressful situations, we can be present and calm when we need to be, or galvanize ourselves for action. It also commands how deeply we breathe, how fast our heart beats, how easily or deeply we sleep, rest, renew and heal ourselves.

## YOGA AS A PATHWAY FOR REST

As part of my research for this chapter, I spoke with my friend Dr Sarah Wells to clarify some ideas regarding the physiological benefits of practicing yoga. For example, in order to have a pleasurable life, we need to be able to move into the parasympathetic, the "rest and digest" side of the nervous system. Yoga creates an environment that invites it to activate: we remember to breathe slowly, move with care, discipline our mind to be present, positive and supportive. To signal to the body that it is safe to slow our heart and release the good stuff, like GABA, serotonin, dopamine and melatonin – chemicals in the body that improve our mood and the functioning of our brain.

In yoga, the vagus nerve can also be stimulated (or "toned') with breath work (see page 120) – it has been suggested that slow, rhythmic deep breathing tones the nerve, and that exhaling for a longer count than the inhale can slow the heart rate and signal to the body that it is in a state of relaxation where it can rest, digest, heal and regenerate.

*Ujjayi prāṇāyāma*, the oceanic yogic breathing (see page 127) which produces a slight constriction at the back of the throat increases pressure against the closed glottis (part of the voice box) and could also bring about vagal stimulation. Inversions – head and handstands with an increase of thoracic pressure as the blood flow returns to our chest cavity – may also act on the vagus nerve in a similar way. Even Om chanting has been thought to tone the vagus nerve through vibrational excitation.

Heart-opening exercises can gently stimulate the vagus nerve with their subtle mechanical stretch of the thorax – for example when you inhale and expand across the front of the chest, lift your chin with your hands on your shoulders, opening the elbows wide, then exhale as you bring them together in front of your heart and tuck in your chin.

The Cat/Cow posture – inhaling into your belly, arching your back with your sacrum tilting up, face facing up, then rounding the back with your pelvis and chin tilted down (see page 84) – softly massages your belly and spine, which could also softly tone the vagus nerve as it passes through the abdomen.

*Yoga nidra* is an ancient technique that is a guided process of visualization, that takes you on a journey to withdraw the sense from the external world and explore the richness of the inner realm. It's a very deep form of relaxation that creates a liminal state of consciousness between wakefulness and sleep. It is deeply soothing for the nervous system.

More generally speaking, the simple act of taking time to relax and slow down during a meditation or yoga practice can help your body to access that parasympathetic response, reminding it how it feels to return to a deeply relaxed and restorative state – to counteract the heightening effects of physical and emotional stresses we encounter in our daily lives, ensuring that our bodies don't hold on to the downstream effects of these stressors.

After all, even the more subtle and silent systems that govern our bodies need to be exercised if they are to grow in strength like a muscle. The more we "tone" and tap into our intrinsic functions, the more we may be able to identify and move from a stressed to a relaxed state when we need to do so.

## TRAUMA IN THE BODY

Understanding the autonomic nervous system is a great help when we consider working on trauma in the body. Now that we know what happens when we feel a huge rush of stress – we are flooded with hormones that create emotional and physiological responses – it's easy to understand that these hormones should be spent or released in some way; otherwise they will block up or continue to fizz around, messing with our equilibrium. A movement practice like yoga, dance or shaking creates a slow release to neutralize the body, without causing a giant explosion.

The American therapist Peter Levine is known for his groundbreaking work on healing trauma and stress through working on the body. He describes how, in traumatic situations, we experience an extreme state of hyperarousal, and our whole being is consumed with this energy. He uses the example of anger, which is one we can all recognize. We feel a huge, fiery charge of emotion. If we deny ourselves an outlet, we push it deeper into our body. It lies there, dormant and unpredictable, rebelling every once in a while in a burst of road rage or an uncontrolled argument with our family.

Emotions like anger or fear are so deeply intense that we can become overwhelmed. So the energy locks into our body and our nervous system. When we don't release this power, it manifests in many different ways, such as PTSD, nightmares or more physical

*A movement practice like yoga, dance or shaking creates a slow release to neutralize the body, without causing a giant explosion.*

symptoms like pain, stiffness or migraines. It can be triggered to surface with scenarios that spark a memory – a sound, a smell or a group of people. Who knows?

Pivotal to Levine's method, called "somatic experiencing", is an understanding that, after a traumatic experience, the central nervous system should be reset through movement. If it isn't reset, stress and trauma will build up, lock in the body and prolong, or even prevent, the healing process.

If we look at animals in the wild, they regularly undergo traumatic experiences when they are threatened by predators. They have a natural way of processing and neutralizing their bodies' reactions to this: they stand up and shake, until they have discharged whatever energy is in their system that has caused them to feel fear. They allow the body to work through its natural mechanism to resolve trauma and regain its equilibrium.

This is why, when we are feeling stressed, moving and body work can allow the body to work out energy that could become corrosive and unhealthy.

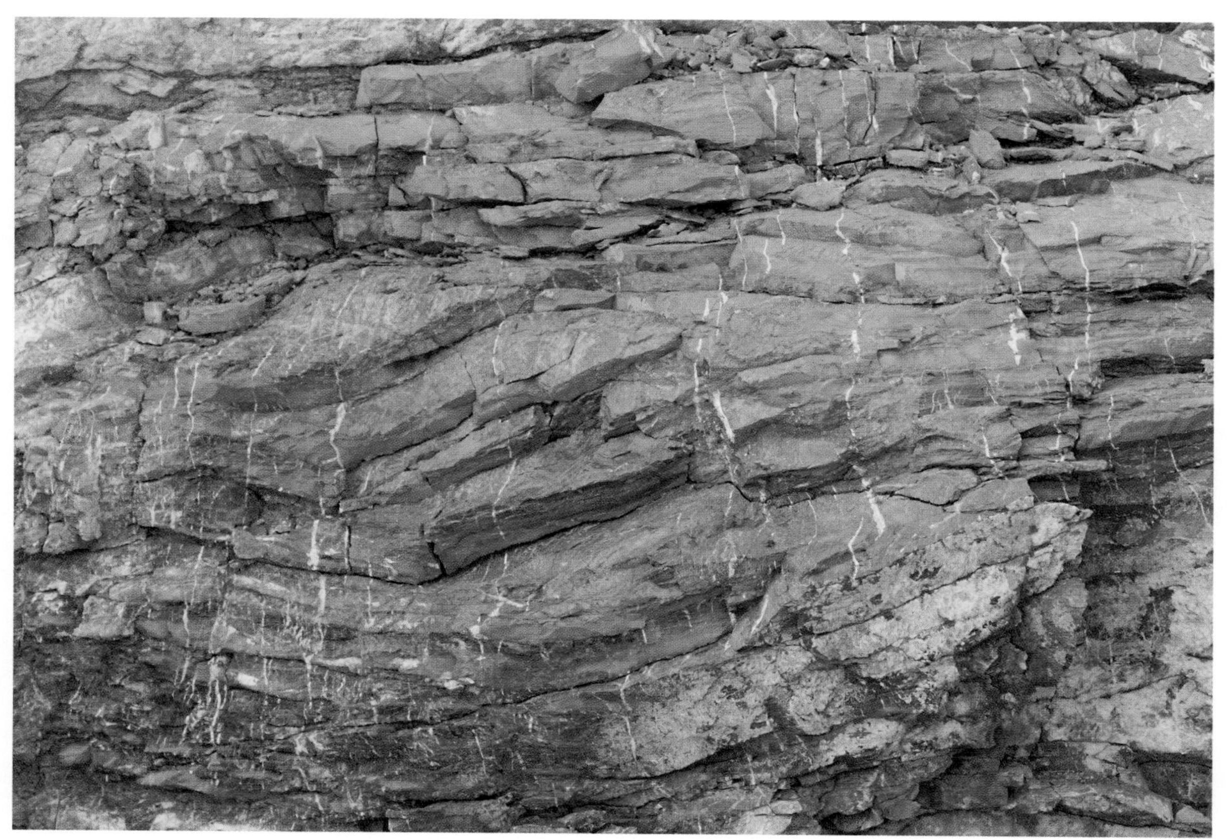

# THE EMOTIONAL BODY

What has always fascinated me about moving is how we can dislodge pockets of emotions that have crystallized in our cells. We're able to access and release trauma indirectly, through working on the body instead of the mind.

There are two people who have been pivotal in researching how we can use psychosomatic healing to identify, release and heal from suppressed trauma. The first of these, Dr Candace Pert, was an influential neuroscientist and pharmacologist. In the 1970s, she discovered the receptor in the brain that opiates fit into, like a key in a lock, allowing endorphins to work on the brain. Her research is pivotal in understanding how we can release emotions that have wedged themselves into our cells.

The other key figure in this field is Dr John Upledger, the American osteopath who developed craniosacral therapy. He calls these hidden pockets of crystallized energy "somato-emotional cysts", and they can be understood as emotions imprinted in our

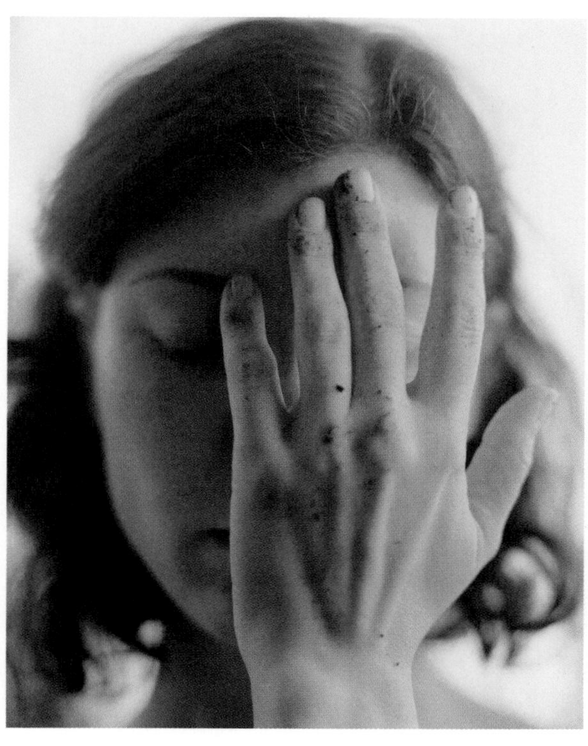

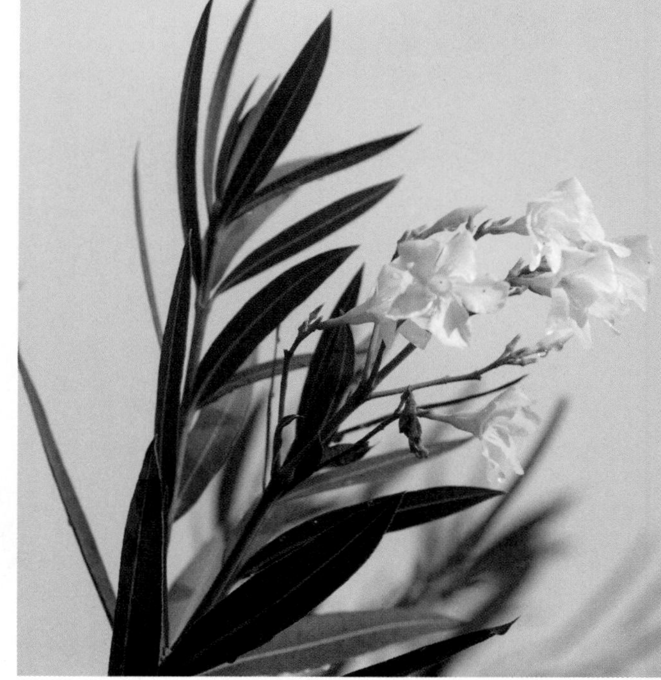

*There are practices – shapes or sounds that we make – that dislodge something energetically, so we find ourself engulfed in a deep swell of unfathomable emotion.*

body. Dr Pert believed that "your body is your subconscious mind. Our physical body can be changed by the emotions we experience". There is a constant feedback loop, body to brain, brain to body. If we work on our body, we can change our psychological, energetic and emotional landscape and access memories that our brain was unable to process because it was too painful at the time.

So these "molecules of emotions" lie tucked into our tissues, trapped in our organs and hidden in our glands. We wall them up and trick ourselves into disassociation, until one day we do something to set them free or even "let off some steam", so that we can process and heal.

Experientially, we all know this is true. There are practices – shapes or sounds that we make – that dislodge something energetically, so we find ourself engulfed in a deep swell of unfathomable emotion: a teary backbend, a surge of grief in a hip opener, laughter during orgasm, the thrill of hidden power when you go running. This release is deeply cathartic and it elicits a sense of relief, lightness and freedom. It's only accessed through the physical plane.

So movement is just such a lot of things. It's the joy of freeing your body, the delicious relief of a stretch. It's the delight in practising for the sake of it, an exploration of pure sensation. It's a process of rewilding, a reminder of our innate wisdom through allowing our body the dignity of its natural inclinations. It's the discovery of our abundant power source, how to stoke and shape and harness our *prāṇā* . It's where we can amaze ourselves by learning to retrain our body and its functions in ways we thought were out of our control. It's a safe place for us to spill out our secret sadness so we are free, strong, vibrant and able to make intelligent decisions for our lives.

Different practices in this book create the space for us to feel into ourselves and allow our emotions to unveil. Over time, we can identify their source and make the necessary life changes. For while emotions are real, they can also be dishonest, or disproportionate. They are a visceral reaction to something we perceive, but our perception can deceive us. Sometimes, we see what we want to, or what we expect to, rather than what is there.

So when we find a space of quiet through meditation, breath work or movement, we cleave our mind from the churn and witness our stories unfold. This cultivates objectivity, an effortless space for the veils to drop so that our perception is purified and our emotional world becomes truer.

We also discover a gap between our emotions and our reaction to them. Feelings mist through and we learn to be with them in a way that is more comfortable. They colour our mind and body for a while, then we take helpful steps to send them on their way, actively kindling positive experiences and emotions to fill their space.

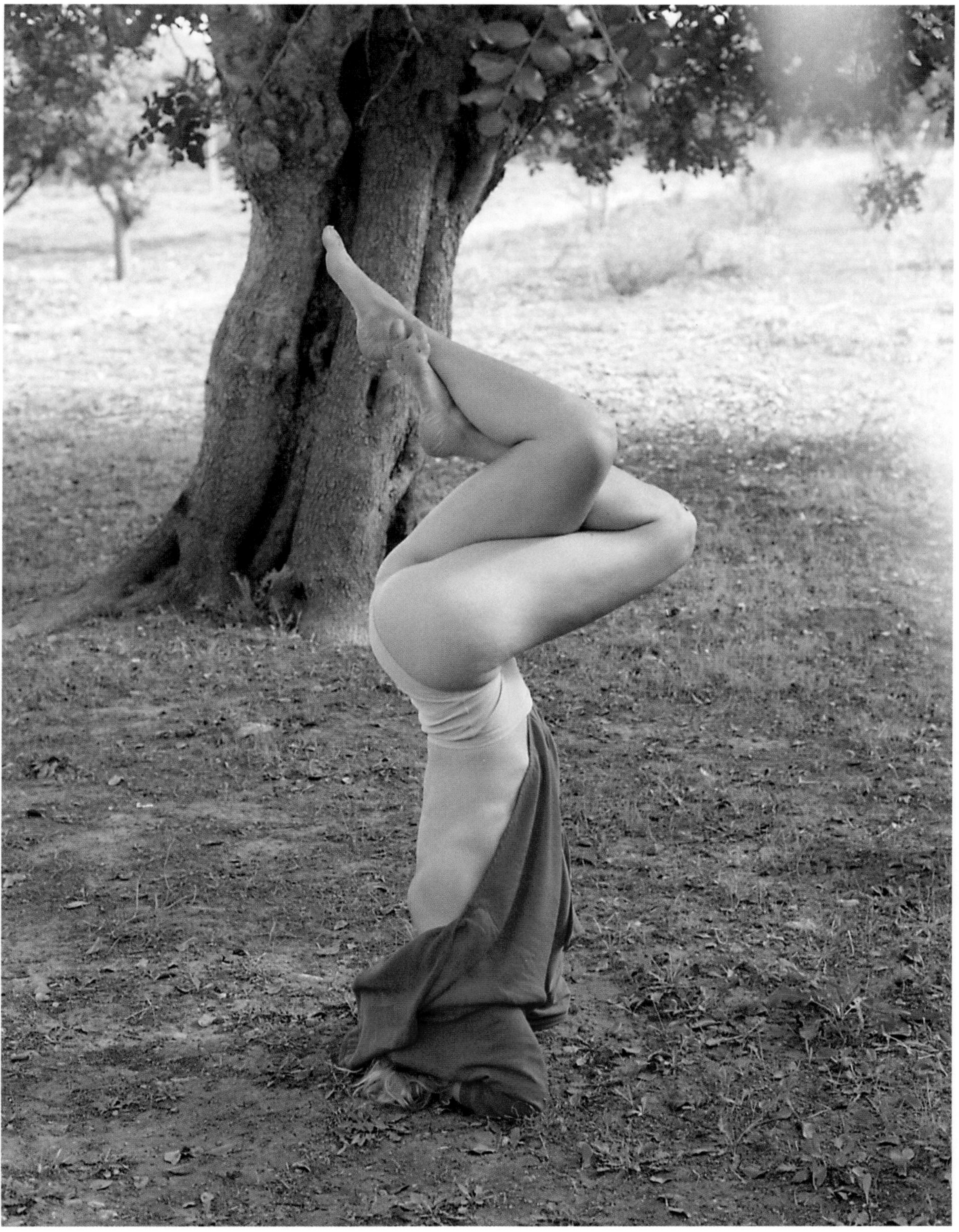

3

# PRACTICAL MAGIC

*"As is your will, so is your thought; as is your thought, so is your deed; as is your deed, so is your life."*

BRIHADARANYAKA UPANISHAD

# MOVEMENT

*If we want to live a pleasurable life, our body is where we begin our work.*

Your body is the mystery of the universe incarnate. You are a wondrous and cosmic being, made of remnants of stars and massive explosions in the galaxies. You are living evidence of the miraculous point at which all kinds of unseen forces aligned and were made manifest.

The universe conducted the meeting of two humans, with the right concoction of chemicals to heat a moment of passion that brought about your conception. You began to grow, within the belly of your mother. Each one of your cells divided intuitively, one becoming two, two becoming four and so on, to develop the incredibly complex, beautiful structure that you are. Each cell knew, and still knows, its individual purpose within the complex orchestra of your being.

We are all a never-ending process, a shape-shifting vessel of blood and bones bathed in electrochemicals. We are a laboratory and an experiment, an ongoing exploration of energy in motion, a dynamic enquiry and a source of endless fascination. There is absolutely nothing ordinary about our bodies: everything about them is fascinating, if we really choose to notice and examine our ever-shifting landscape.

Beyond this fleshy, biochemical, physiological miracle, we also developed different levels of consciousness, ranging from primal to highly sophisticated forms of intelligence that mean we can learn intricate new skills, solve problems and analyse ourselves. All of which most of us do so much that we tend to neglect our precious body by dwelling too much in the past and projecting into the future.

We need to be more in the present, with our own body; we need to take time with ourselves and learn to understand our own visceral intelligence. We experience everything on the field of our body: all there is that is seen, and the many unseen mysterious forces driving our existence. The senses are our windows into this world and other realms. Our flesh is the catalogue of all our life; it remembers each experience, even if the mind keeps secrets.

It's crucial that we create the best environment in which our body can function. It has self-healing superpowers – it is endlessly renewing. We just need be still and soften, or sleep long enough and deeply enough to let our cells do their regenerative thing. We all have a miraculous inbuilt relaxation system. We can't really force ourselves to relax: it's more a question of just surrendering into ourselves, and this is what we practise on the yoga mat. We need to make changes in our lives that facilitate healing, rather than fighting our fleshy intuition and getting stuck in a corrosive state of stress.

In yoga practice, we can begin to view the body as a miraculous whole, rather than separating and anatomizing bits, isolating individual organs, muscles or actions. Our constellations of movement teach us to understand the intricate web of muscles and fascia that link together to make the whole. As we begin to appreciate the continuity and connections within ourselves, this awareness will segue into our perception of the world around us. If we explore the connections within, we will have a deeper appreciation of how we are connected to the natural world and all its beautiful animal and human creatures.

Movement is the language of the body. It is poetry. When we move through space with total presence and absorption, we experience this perfect grace and allow our body to tell its own story. Our instinctive ways of being, our primal ways of moving and our visceral intelligence are infinitely wise and nutritious.

If we want to live a pleasurable life, our body is where we begin our work.

We can learn, heal and grow through movement practices. We become stronger and more comfortable, and therefore confident in our own skin. We can find cathartic practices that create energetic release, to heal past trauma and be free of old wounds. We develop movement patterns that help us live longer. As well as all these beautiful health benefits, when we move in flow, we create a spool of time where we leave behind the many different voices of our mind, to check into an effortless space of nuanced awareness. We fall back into our own rhythm and find a renewed sense of ease that we will carry with us throughout the day.

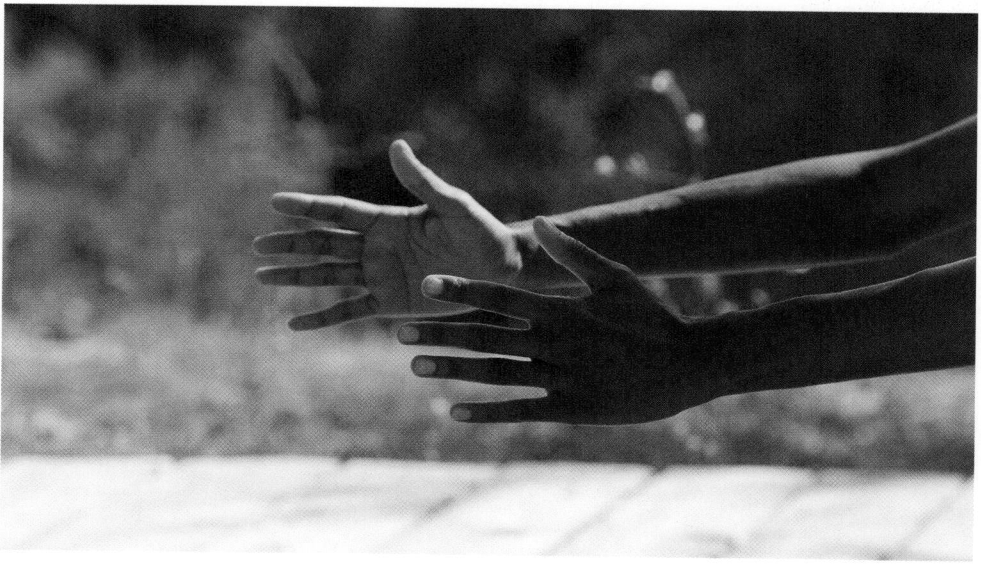

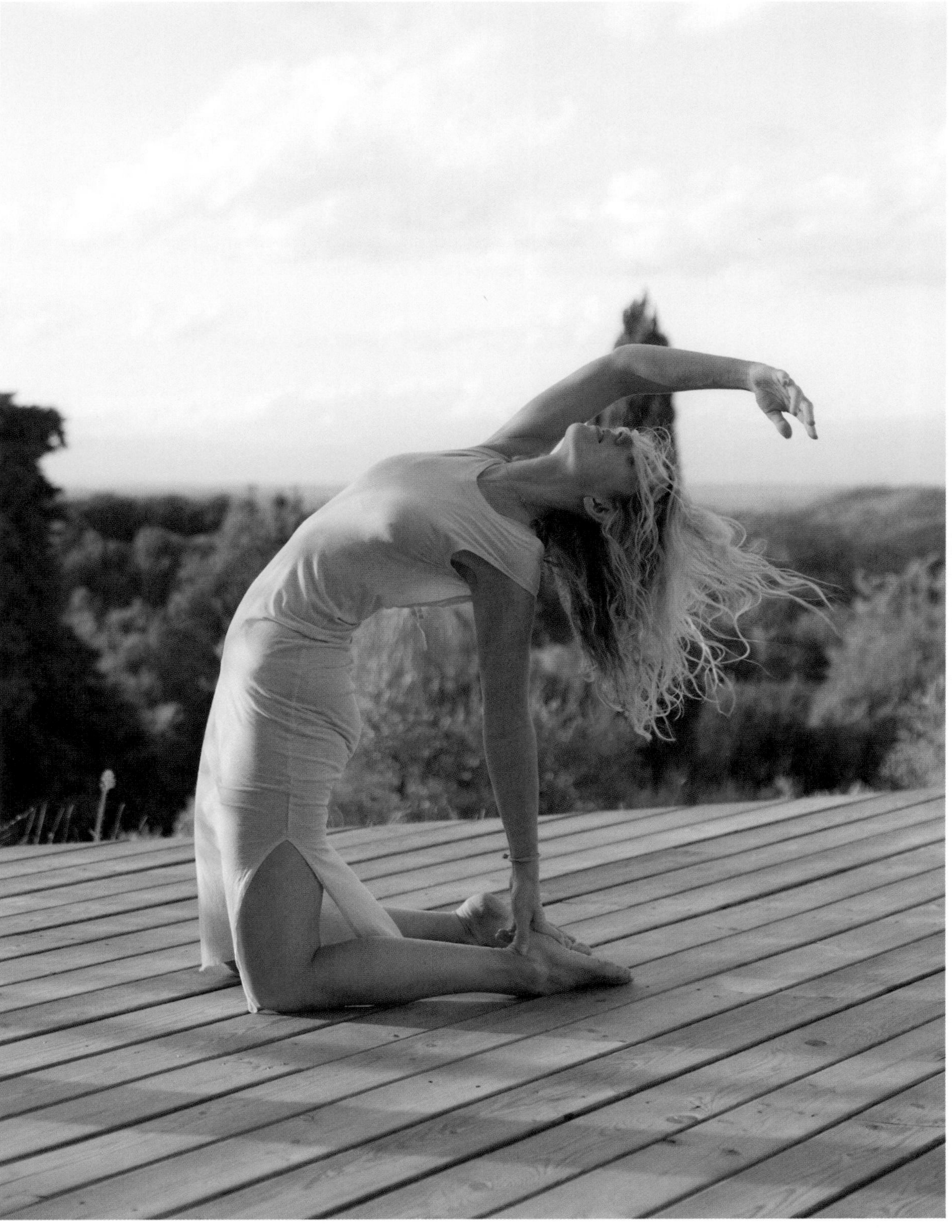

# NOTICING

*We're able to identify what will serve us most at any given moment: whether we need to push ourselves into class, go for a run or languish in bed.*

We cultivate a sense of wondrous curiosity about ourselves and the world within and without. As we develop our awareness, we both realize the depth of our own mysterious nature and develop a much clearer understanding of ourselves, discovering the extent of our conditioning and lifting the veils of perception.

Yoga – movement in particular – is a very tangible way for us to train ourselves to notice our mental and visceral landscape. It's the chance for our body to be heard, for us to be aware of who we are at that particular point in time, noting how we are feeling by exploring the weight of our flesh and bones, the depth and length of our breath, the clarity of our minds and the atmosphere of our full being.

When we begin to notice this more, we observe the people, places and situations in which we naturally thrive, and those that we find unsettling. We develop a sharper sense of ourselves and begin to recognize the moments of discomfort that we should lean into and move through, and those situations and people that are better left behind, so we can curate a lifestyle that is supportive and nourishing.

*Svādhyāya* – the study of self – through moving the body is deeply empowering. It's thrilling to learn new things and see what the body is capable of. Physical strength translates into how we hold ourselves, how we move through a room and generally how we respect our body. It gives us confidence.

It also liberates us to tailor our practices. We're able to identify what will serve us most at any given moment: whether we need to push ourselves in class, go for a run or languish in bed. As we gain confidence we might become more creative. We learn to be happy with an unfamiliar sequence, more relaxed about not being "good" at one prescribed way of moving, because we are aware that there are many. We become less attached to mastering the pose than to discovering how to embody it and immerse ourselves in the experience. We reclaim the full spectrum of our movement, overriding limiting patterns of movement brought about by sedentary lifestyles or stress.

### SEDENTARY LIFESTYLES

Our natural way is literally to move through life – our body longs for it. It's also essential to our health. It's not a luxury. We're essentially animals, and there are some very basic things that we human creatures need to do:

- relieve tension, strengthen our bones by loading our body weight onto them in different ways, build muscular strength and create ease and flexibility;

- ○ protect ourselves from the dangers of a modern, sedentary life;
- ○ remind our body of the various ways we were made to move;
- ○ keep our vital energy flowing freely;
- ○ manage stress indirectly through the body by understanding our autonomic nervous system; and
- ○ work through any old trauma that may be lodged within.

## MOVEMENT ISSUES

Sitting for days on end in an office chair was not in our plan. As a culture, we have movement issues, and the risks of our sedentary lifestyles are quite shocking – they include higher risk of cancer, diabetes, poor circulation, memory loss or Alzheimer's and weak bones. So, particularly if we are desk-bound, we need to factor in movement throughout the day to protect our health. It's not enough to frame eight hours of stasis with a burst of activity – we need regular movement punctuating the day.

Creating little movement snacks every 30 minutes is ideal. Just standing up and making an excuse to have a walk around, taking a little wiggle on your chair, stretching your arms in the air and doing a side bend are good – anything that stretches the body and shifts your weight around your bones. Make it as varied as possible.

## REWILDING

We need to recreate a healthy movement portfolio by changing our environment and moving in varied ways, just as our ancestors did out in the wild. This is where a creative movement practice is so important. It's not just moving more, repetitively and habitually, but moving in different ways.

Katy Bowman is a biomechanist and a pioneer in the world of movement. If we're not careful, she says, we become "animals in our own cage...But there's no lock, we can let ourselves out". Bowman talks about how we are formed by our environment: our bodies adapt to fit the shapes we put them in, and the loads we place on them through our orientation in space, the force of gravity pulling us down, as well as any extra weight we may be carrying, like bags on our shoulder, for example.

Our loads are all unique. Bowman uses the metaphor of the wind rushing through the branches of a tree – no two trees will have the same experience of its force, because each tree has different branches and its own particular portfolio of leaves. We humans also have different shapes, weights and alignments. We have our own style of movement, and our bodies bear the load in their own way. What is right for one person will not necessarily be helpful for another.

If we use our body in varied ways, we can gently help re-establish equilibrium, instead of further encoding small idiosyncrasies into habitual movement maps. Repeating

*Each tree is individual, has different arms, a varied reach and its own particular portfolio of leaves.*

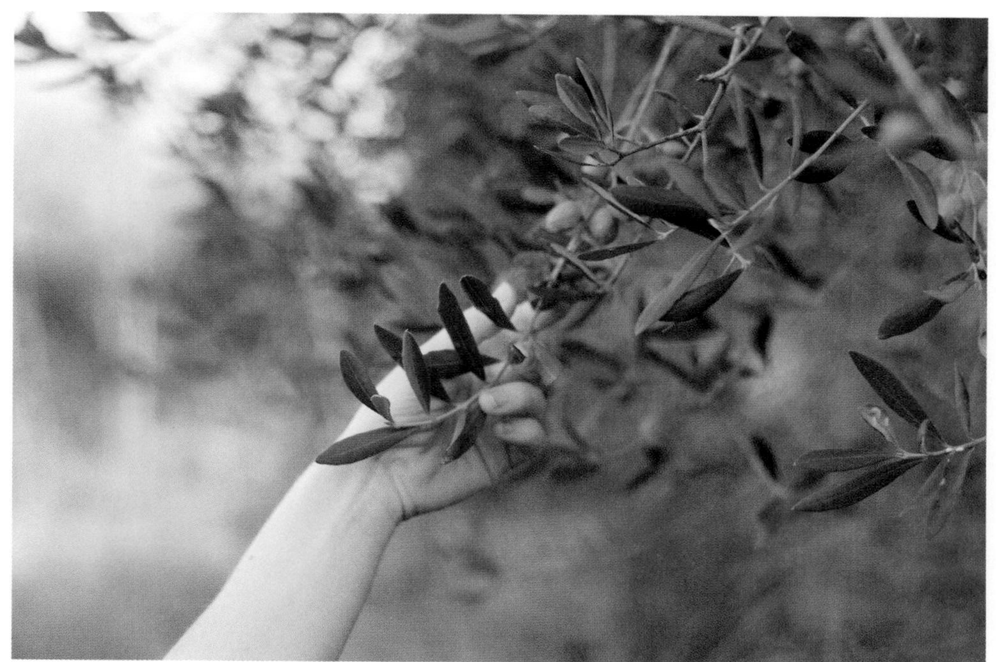

a selection of movement patterns (sit, walk, run, carry bag, type on laptop, slouch on sofa) creates a restrictive cognitive and physical map of movement that is self-perpetuating and mutes our natural mobility. We should always be trying varied ways of moving, so that our body can remember.

### FIND YOUR TEACHERS

We all require different methods of movement at different stages in our life. As the wonderful Peter Blackaby, creator of the concept he calls "intelligent yoga", says, there's no perfect or "prescriptive" way for us to move. If you're new to postural yoga, try lots of different classes. There are plenty of offerings online, but it's always best to go to a studio for the attention of a teacher and the energy of practising in a group. Ask the receptionist for help choosing the right class for you. It may sound obvious, but beginners is a safe place to start. If you don't take the time to find a good first experience, you could end up being intimidated or frustrated and put off for life. Choose wisely.

When you first begin to practise, it will be difficult. You'll find your body stiff and clumsy. But persevere. You'll feel alive and spacious afterward. Be patient, talk to your body kindly. Literally repeat positive mantras in your head to stop any negativity and judgment from circling round your mind and discouraging your body. This is what mantras are for!

If you're perpetually restless and struggle to sit still, initially a flow practice is a good way to catch your own attention. Once you've established some discipline and you're able to siphon your mind into your body, try to move on to something more therapeutic. A fast body-mind often needs the nourishment of rest and stillness.

It can also be useful to practise a more traditional school of modern postural yoga for a time: a practice that calls itself Hatha or Iyengar. This allows you get to know some of the traditional poses so that you understand basic alignment and create a stable foundation from which to explore.

I practise with a number of wonderful and very different teachers. They all have a profound respect for their own body and empower their students to listen to and honour theirs. Each teacher has a different knowledge and use of language. But they all have an inclusive, non-dogmatic approach that teaches you to enjoy your body, challenge it appropriately and be sympathetic to your own limitations. The kindness they foster in class transcends the mat and percolates into the surrounding community.

## DISCOVER YOUR OWN RHYTHM

You can use your *āsana* practice in many different ways, and you'll find that it will shift and evolve throughout your life. I used to push my body much harder than I do now. I needed the challenge, and the feeling of accomplishment that followed. More recently, I've approached my body gently on the mat. I was curious to notice that during the period of writing this book, my movement practice became therapeutic, a space for me to relieve my body from the aches and dormancy of sitting for days. I sought an energetic release elsewhere. I danced and went outside more: running, walking and swimming. I craved a nature fix and variety to my routine.

My *āsana* practice and teaching are breath-centred. In creating a sense of intimacy with our breath, we begin to discover an organic way to move. The breath guides and shapes the body into a chain of movement. It becomes easier and more natural. We layer sequences and find we slip easily into shapes that used to require more force, contraction or an effortful launch.

Of course, practice isn't always seamless and graceful, even for the most dedicated yogis. There will always be times when your body feels locked and sticky. At the beginning, it takes discipline, grit and trust to get going. You have to back yourself. The more time you put in at the beginning, the faster you'll reap the rewards and the easier the practice becomes.

Always remind yourself to focus on your breath. It will anchor your mind, ease your body by creating a natural surrender and softness. It harnesses your internal power and helps you notice your natural dynamic. Slow your breath, slow your body and your nervous system will also steady itself.

*Always remind yourself to focus on your breath. It will anchor your mind, ease your body by creating a natural surrender and softness.*

A slow stream of movement means there is actually time to drink in the poetry, to be observant of your own precious nuances. Moving quickly and trammelling the body through poses bypasses the opportunity to feel everything and cultivate deeper awareness, which is the point of the practice: training yourself to notice so you can have more clarity and make intelligent decisions for yourself.

If you go to a flow class, notice that in repeating a simple, layered sequence again and again, you find that the same series of movements begins to feel very different. There is an alchemic quality in repetition. Your mind melts, and you drop into the rhythm of your own bones. *Ṛta* is the Vedic principle of the natural order of the universe and its innate rhythm. It's *Ṛta* that guides the days, the seasons, the moon and the tides. It also vibrates in our bones, and a graceful flow steeped with awareness will transport you into a different state of consciousness. You'll begin to float effortlessly through space and reconnect to your own pulse, so you notice a deeper sense of your own harmony within the world around you.

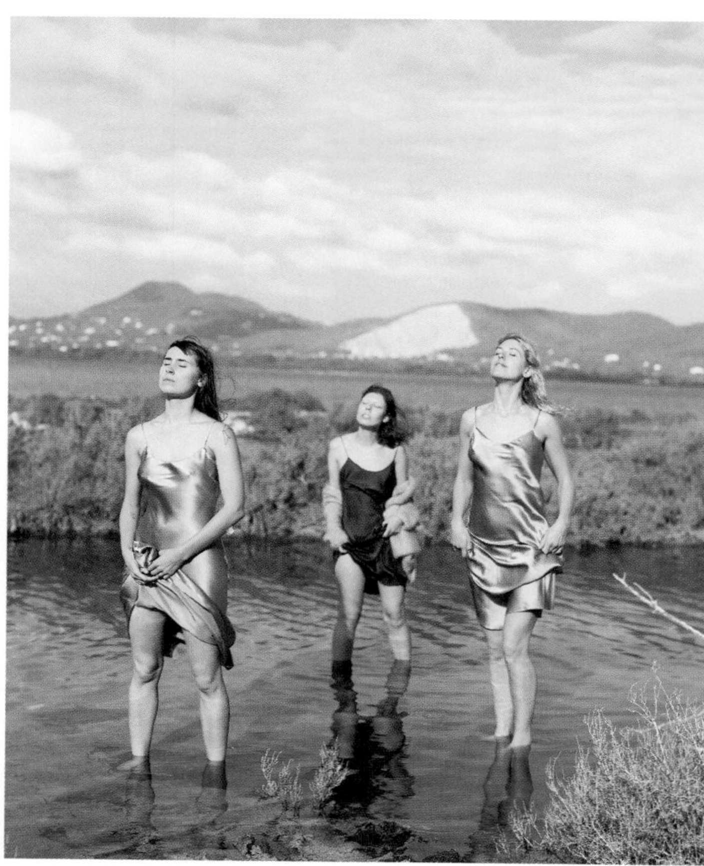

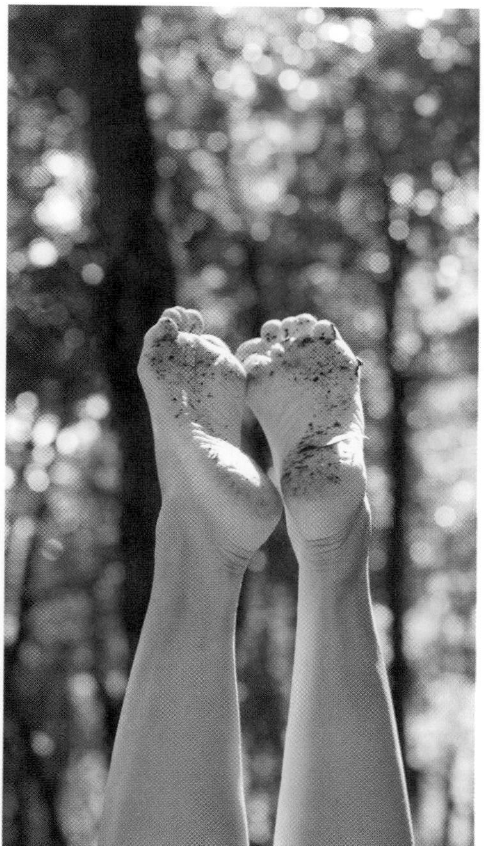

## TREASURE YOUR VESSEL

If we choose to submit our sacred vessels to the same sequence of postures for an extended period of time, we stress our bodies in the same places every day, and often don't explore our full range of muscles and their spectrum of movement. We risk injuring ourselves by eternally repeating the exact same sequence, or pursuing the glory of a pose. These sneaky injuries of overuse build up over time, and sometimes never fully heal. For example, too many *chaturangas* can lead to shoulder injuries. A pulled hamstring is also common in a competitive practice. Forceful teachers with heavy-handed assists have been known to crack ribs and cause slipped discs.

These dangers are real, and yoga injuries normally come about when a practice is goal-oriented or a teacher is charged with ego. Ironically, it's the more intensely dynamic practices seeking to transcend the body and the ego that often lead to injuries. Always be observant of your body and respect its boundaries. The best openings come naturally, with surrender. Not through force.

With this in mind, I love this quote from movement artist Bonnie Bainbridge Cohen:

> *What I learned from yoga is that it's not about the form and posture. It's how you engage in the posture. When you engage in the posture instead of trying to create a form, you are free to be where you are.*

It doesn't matter how "advanced" your practice is. It's the purity of presence in that moment, exploring the pose through your breath and awareness.

Movement keeps me together. I'm always learning how to work with my mind to create more comfort, exploring power or softness with my breath. I break a sweat and feel strong. But I don't dance that knife edge every practice. I'm not looking to dominate my body, to train it to push through pain and to deafen myself to its signals. I'm here to awaken, to heal and to explore my inner world.

I challenge myself enough to build the heat, to feel a level of discomfort so that I have a sensation to work through and I can learn something about myself. It's often said that you are your own best teacher. If you practise with curiosity, you will discover things for yourself, about yourself. You don't always need to be guided by someone else, you just need to be observant and responsive.

I practise meeting the feelings in my body, and being present through them, whether they are just physical tension or whether a pose has spilled another emotion out of my cells. I cultivate my inner witness: I just observe and things come up. It's always interesting to see where the mind wants to go to distract itself. When that happens, the best thing to do is to bring it back using the breath and just be there with the

*I'm here to awaken, to heal and to explore my inner world.*

emotions as they arise, noticing how they move and change shape, texture and temperature.

Initially, it can be scary to meet yourself on the mat. You feel almost naked, vulnerable and tender, because you've been groomed not to feel, in order to deal with the strain of modern life or to hide an emotion that is painful or inconvenient. But the mat is a safe place for you to recreate stressful sensations, so that you can teach yourself how to control your mind and train your body to deal with them more comfortably, so you can process them quickly and move forward.

Yoga practice for the sake of it, for the pure experience that will be different every single time, and the self-knowledge that will settle into you and guide you through the rest of your life. What a beautiful thing ...

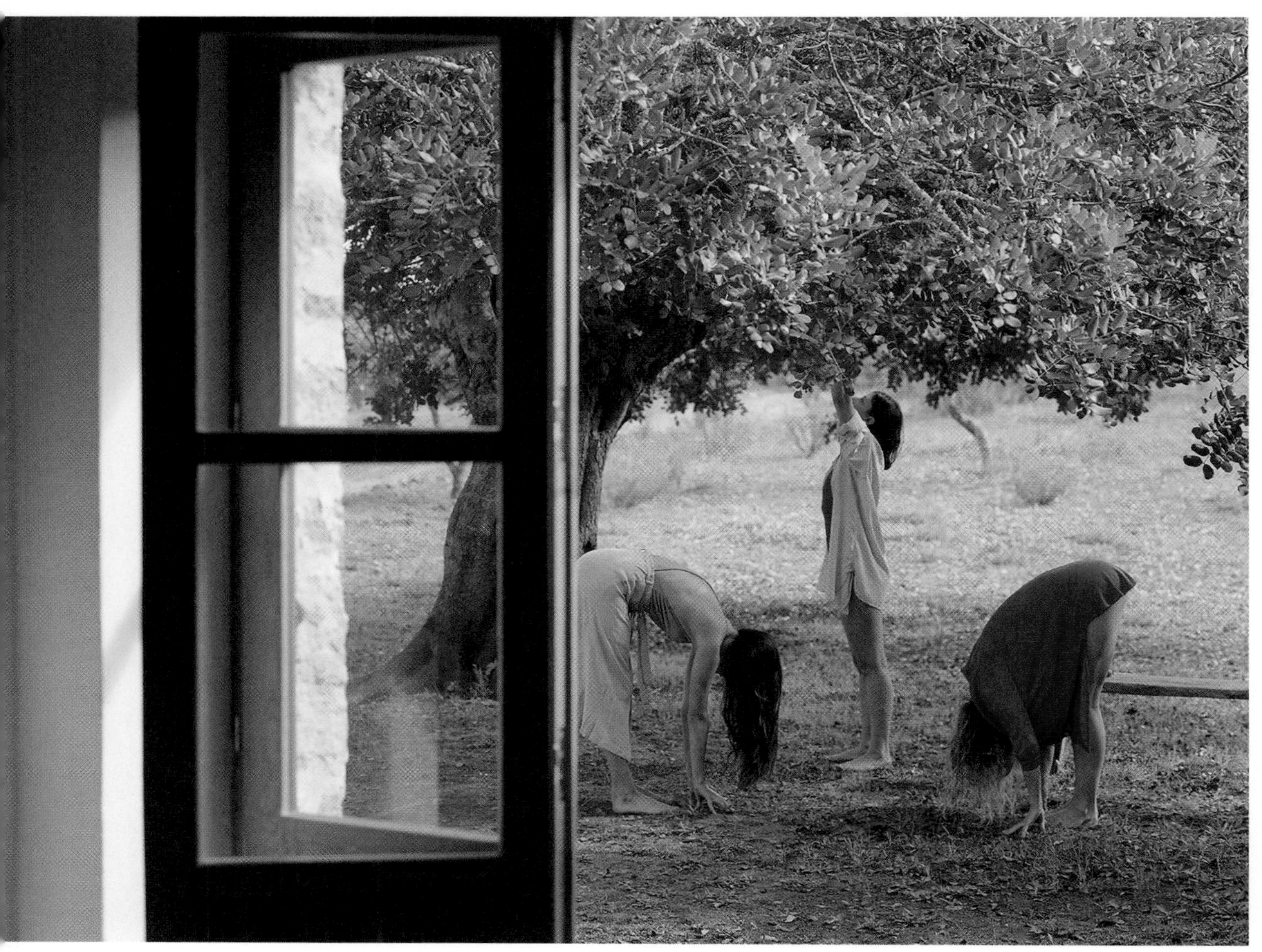

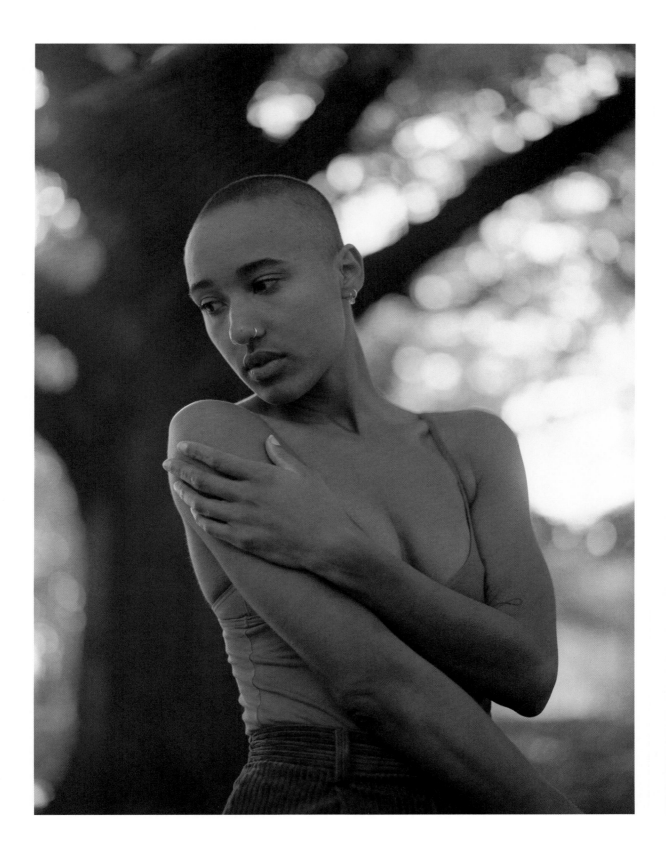

Tāḍāsana: Root to Rise 72
Tāḍāsana: Breathe to Move 74
Sukhāsana: Pleasant Pose 74
Kinetic Poetry 76
Half Sūrya Namaskār 78
Sūrya Namaskār: Sun Salutation 80
Stoke Your Fire 84
Free Movement: Electric Body 91
Mystic Moon 92
Fertile Ground 96
Jessi Sequence 98
Your Heart is Ancient 100
Remember the Sky 102
Human Ocean 106
Back to the Source 108
Earthly Constellations 110
Rock & Roll 112
Sun in My Heart 114
Ṣavāsana 118

# POSES & PRACTICES

## TĀḌĀSANA: ROOT TO RISE

*Tāḍāsana* means "mountain posture" in Sanskrit. It's a conscious standing posture, with the focus on distributing the weight of the body evenly and working with the architecture of your bones to light up your muscles. *Tāḍāsana* is the foundation for all standing postures, so always take time to set yourself up and sink in at the beginning of a practice.

The simplicity of *Tāḍāsana* feels nuanced and nutritious. Look for the points of contact with the earth, really feel into the feet. Only through fully grounding are we able to rise and feel strong and spacious. If you give yourself a foot massage before your practice, your soles will be more responsive to the surface on which you stand.

Stand with your feet hip distance apart, placing the outer edges of the feet parallel.

Keep the feet on floor and pulse gently up and down, bending the knees. Observe the natural undulations of the body.

Transfer your weight forward and back over the toes and heels.

Explore shifting your weight from side to side, circling your body around the feet and distributing your weight evenly from right to left foot.

Peel your toes away from mat.

Feel the ball of your foot, the little toe mound and centre of your heel. Spread and lengthen your toes and then release them back onto the floor.

Bend your knees slightly and feel your weight drop.

Bend your knees further and allow your feet to feel weightier.

Find your plumb line. First rock subtly forward and back before finding stillness, then move from side to side and find a place where you feel absolutely perfectly aligned.

Spiral your knees slightly away from each other, then counteract this movement by corkscrewing your feet into ground.

Press your feet firmly down to stretch your legs, without locking out your knees.

Energize your legs by engaging your muscles.

Weight your tailbone to the floor.

Breathe in, and squeeze your shoulders right up to your ears.

Exhale and draw shoulders down, as if lower points of the blades are sliding down your back in a deep V.

Lift your breastbone.

Absorb your lower ribs into your body, so that they're not jutting out.

Spiral your palms slightly forward, energizing your fingers, letting the energy travel all the way down to heavy fingertips.

Float your head higher, and let your lower jaw soften away from your upper jaw.

Feel the vitality of your feet and legs pushing down and into floor.

Explore the difference in your *Tāḍāsana* at the end of practice, once you have opened the hamstrings and can stand absolutely rooted.

**Breathing**

Once you've settled into your *Tāḍāsana*, begin to focus your attention on your breathing. Invite your breath to explore the back of the lungs and spread to the front. Maintain your awareness on the back of your body as you breathe.

**Inhale**, imagine the breath travelling down your body, into your feet. Allow them to soften and receive the ground.

**Exhale**, carry the breath from the feet up through the body, as you then stand taller.

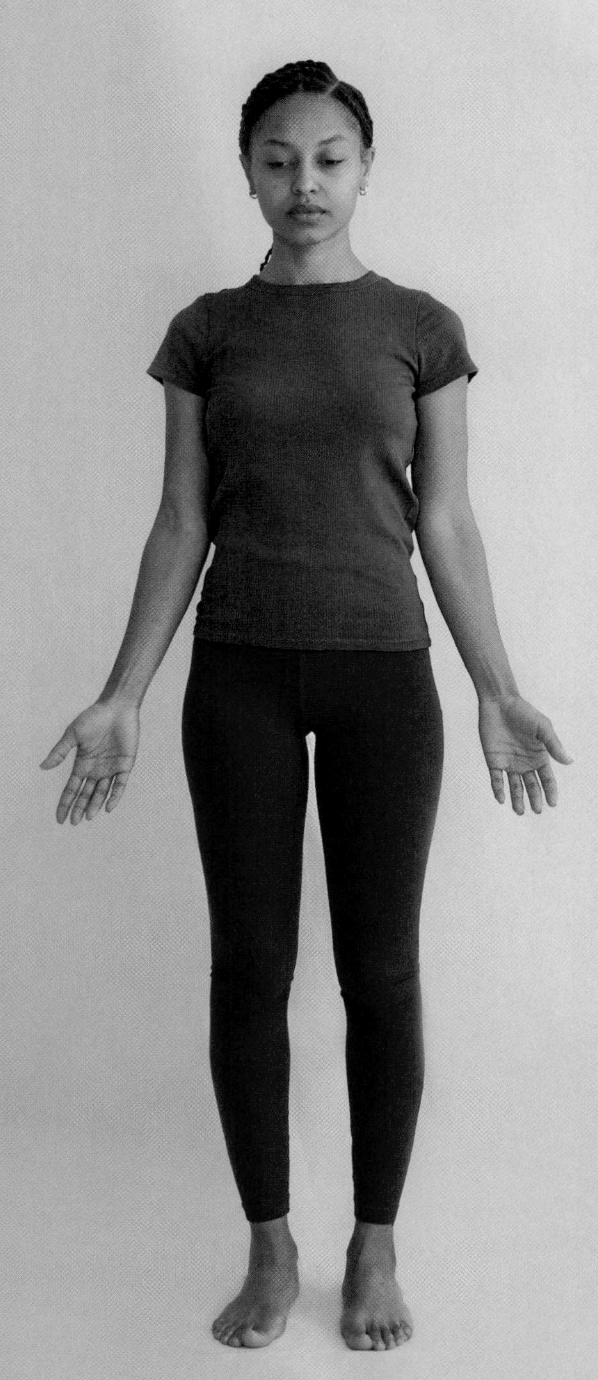

## TĀḌĀSANA: BREATHE TO MOVE

Explore how the breath can lead the movement with this sequence.

**1**

Find your way into *Tāḍāsana*, as described on the previous page.

**2**

**Inhale** deeply into belly, ground through feet, float your arms lightly to the sky on the breath, keeping your wrists and shoulders soft.

**Exhale**, swim your arms to your sides and stand taller, lengthening through the spine and levitating your skull skywards. Feel your energy expanding within you.

Repeat five times. Try it with your eyes closed and see if you can further refine your experience of shifting energetic and physical sensations. For example, if you really settle into the breath, do the arms feel lighter and the movement more organic?

## SUKHĀSANA: PLEASANT POSE

This is the normal sitting position for meditation and *prāṇāyāma*.

Place a block or a few blocks under your bottom. The more height you have in your support, the gentler the pose is on a stiff body. If your hips and your knees feel tight, stack a few blocks on top of each other and prop yourself up comfortably.

Bend your knees and cross your shins, one in front of the other, with each foot placed under the opposite knee. Your legs should look like a triangle. Hands rest on knees or in a *mudra* (hand gesture, see page 136).

Make any adjustments you need to, moving your seat around until you feel the pelvis neutralize on the blocks.

Ground through the weight of your legs and articulate length through spine.

Soften your shoulders, lift your sternum. Keep your neck long, broaden the back of your skull, lift through the roof of your mouth and the crown of your head.

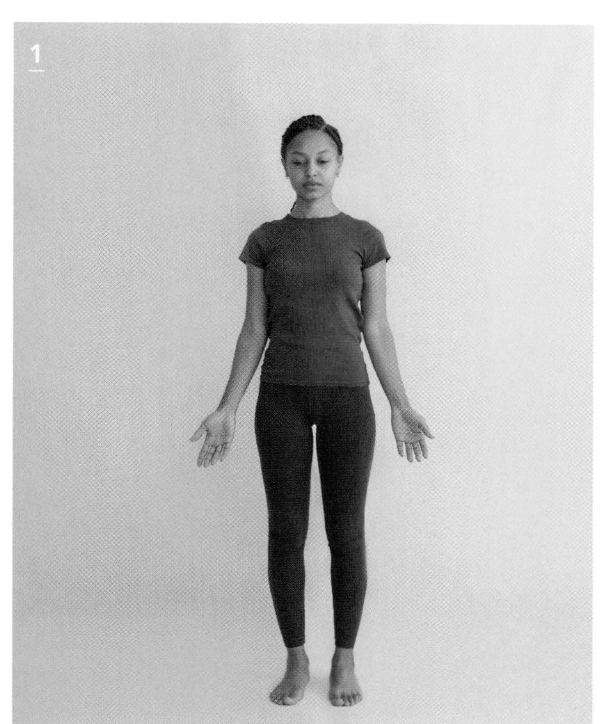
1

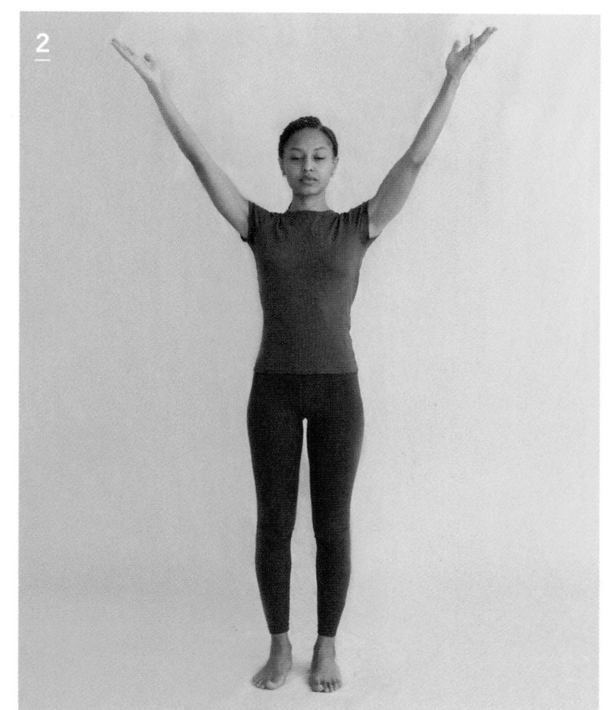
2

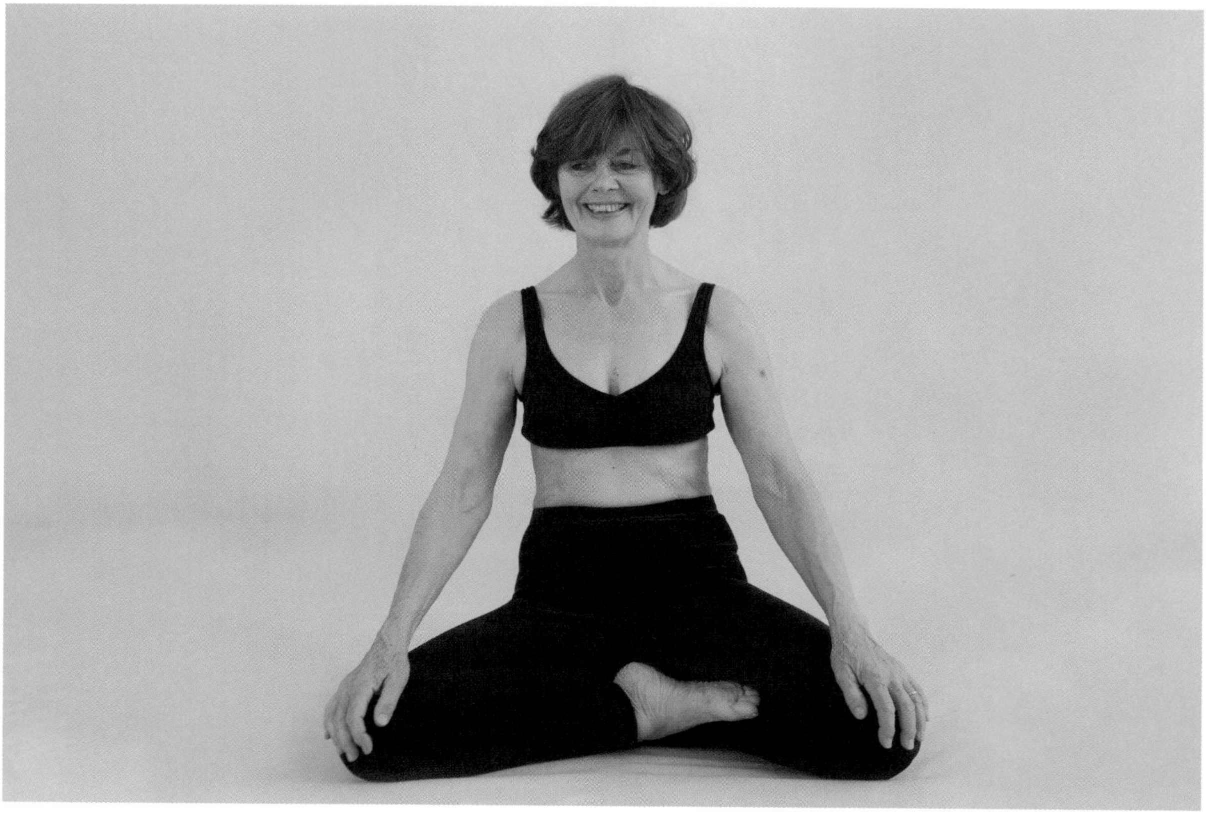

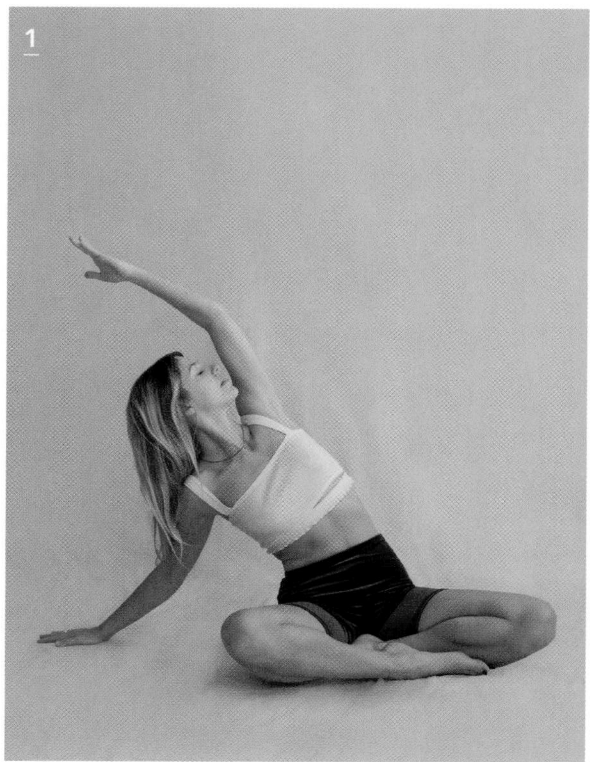
1

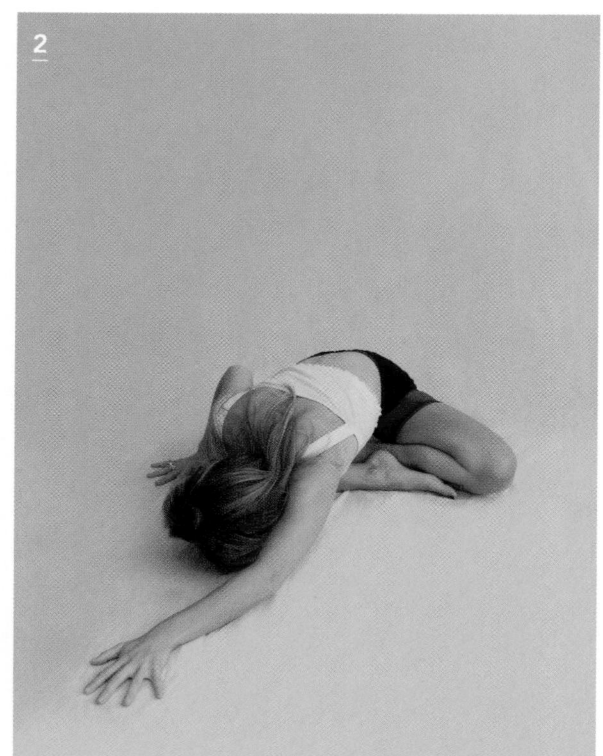
2

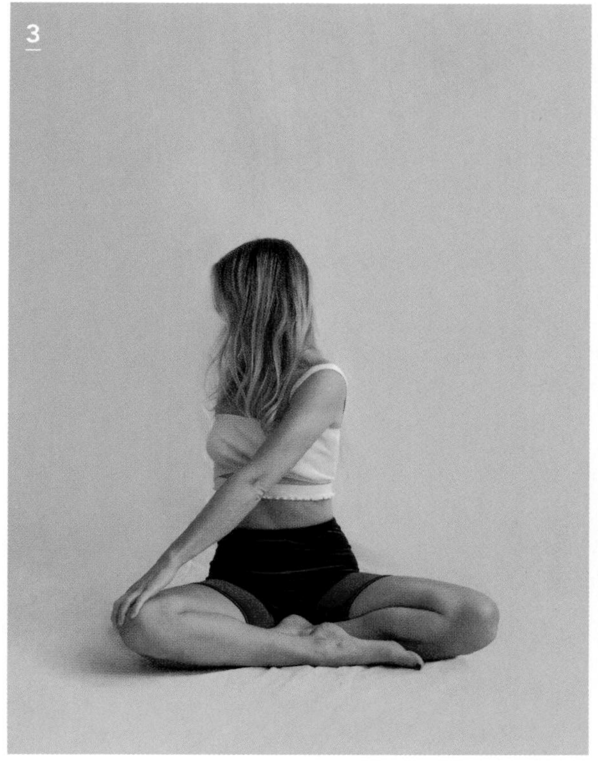
3

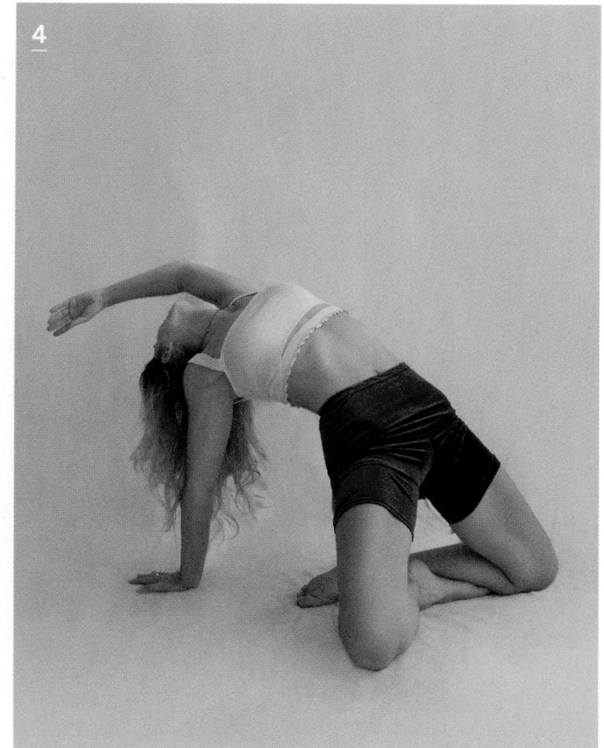
4

## KINETIC POETRY

I love this little sequence as an opener. It's influenced by the wonderful David Kam, and I sometimes preface it with a decadent sufi grind, rotating the hips, then a seated Cat and Cow, with the hands resting on the knees, pausing to drink in the poetry of the spine and magnetic stillness. I like to explore each shape for ten deep breaths, then thread poses 1, 3 and 4 together into a delicious flow. I practice coasting on the waves of the inhale and exhale, until the sequence hypnotizes my restless mind.

**1**

Find a steady seat, where you feel rooted and tall.

Lean towards the right and place your hand or fingertips on the floor behind you, rooting your left hip to the floor.

Roll your left shoulder back, stretch your left arm away from your body and circle it skywards, as you soften your right elbow and side-bend to the right.

Draw the left arm bone into the shoulder socket and rotate the left ribs and the sternum skywards.

Keep the neck long, the chin gently tucked in and the shoulders relaxed. Explore the natural trajectory of the stretch on the pattern of the breath.

**2**

Transition into this pose directly from pose 1.

**Exhale,** rotate the ribcage to the left as you bend your right elbow. Bow down and lower your torso towards the floor as you stretch your left arm diagonally towards your right knee, reaching the hand towards the ground as you direct your sternum towards your knee.

**3**

**Inhale,** sitting tall.

**Exhale,** placing your right hand on the ground behind your spine and your left hand on your right knee.

**Inhale** deeply and hook your left hip back in space.

**Exhale** and scoop up the back of the heart, meet that resistance and slowly begin to twist to the right, maintaining the lift of the sternum and length of the neck. Roll the right shoulder firmly back and notice the breath is somewhat restricted. Then curve the shoulder slightly forward to find better access and space to breathe.

Breathe deep, global breaths into the side ribs and the back.

Return to centre as you inhale and unwind on the axis of your spine around to the left.

**4**

**Exhale,** plant the heel of your hand behind your spine and begin to arch your lower back, lifting your chest.

**Inhale,** press into your hand to lift your hips and press them forwards, at the same time sweeping your right hand across your body, up and back behind you.

If you are warm and it feels accessible to you, you can play with this pose, activating the back body by pressing it forwards into your front body and keeping the heart high.

On an exhale, return to the seat, and begin the sequence on the other side.

## HALF SŪRYA NAMASKĀR

This is a lovely way to open the body, particularly if you are new to the practice and are building up strength for more weight-bearing sequences, such as the full *Sūrya Namaskār* on page 80. Try to follow the breath during this sequence. Once your body knows what shapes it is making, you will see how the breath begins to guide the movement organically. When you fall into your rhythm, the experience takes on a hypnotic quality that transforms it into a moving meditation.

**1**

Begin with *Tāḍāsana* (see page 72).

**2**

**Inhale**, ground your feet, relax your shoulders and float hands to sky, bring palms together.

**3**

**Exhale**, carry palms down through midline of body. Draw navel to spine, fold forward over legs, placing fingertips or palms flat to floor under shoulders. Bend knees, or use blocks under hands, to raise the floor to you.

**4**

**Inhale**, breathe from belly to heart to lift torso to halfway, fingertips on floor with bent or straight legs. For tight hamstrings, bend knees and cup shins with palms. Keep spine and neck long, shoulders soft.

**5**

**Exhale**, empty your breath and bow forward again, letting your sit bones broaden and your thighs rotate inward.

**6**

**Inhale**, soften knees, root feet, rise to stand as you swim arms back up toward the sky, shoulders soft. forward, to create space in the shoulders.

**7**

**Exhale**, bring your arms alongside your body to make your way back to *Tāḍāsana*. Stand tall, raise crown of head, keeping heart lifted, shoulders soft, fingertips heavy.

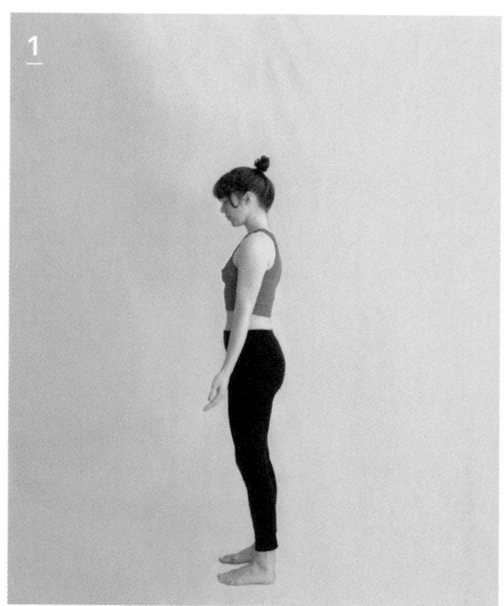
1

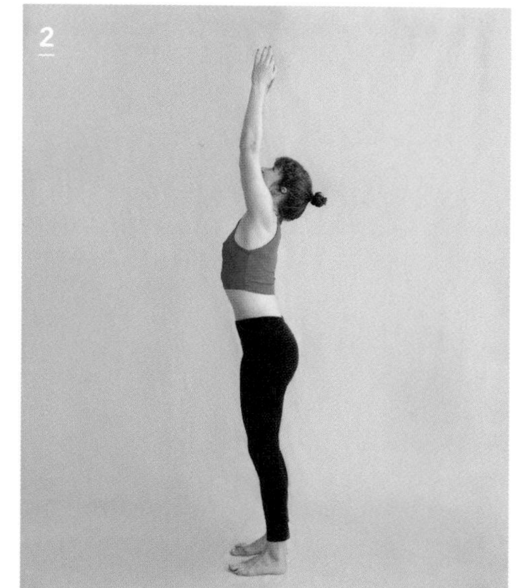
2

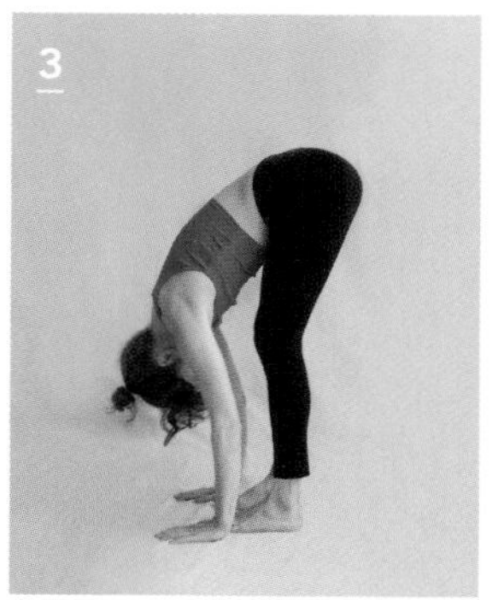
3

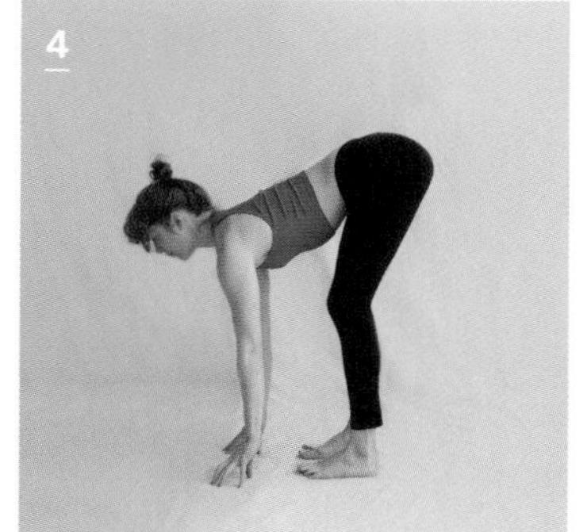
4

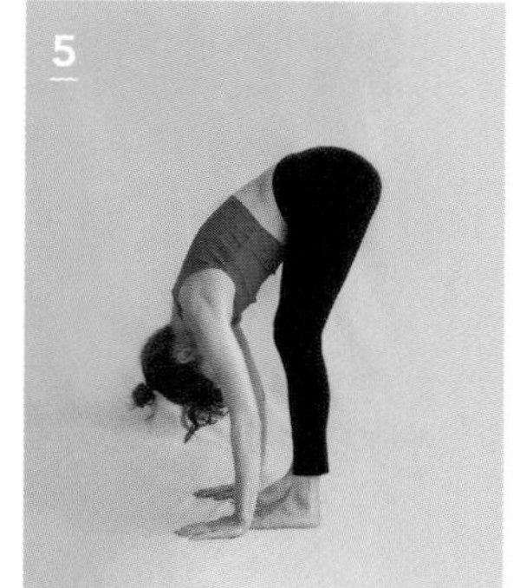
5

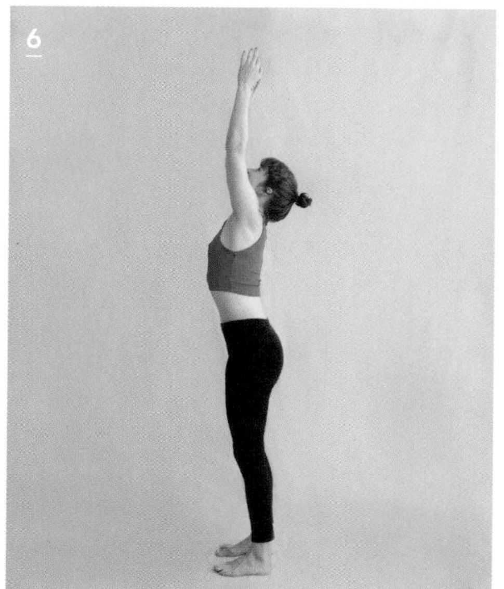
6

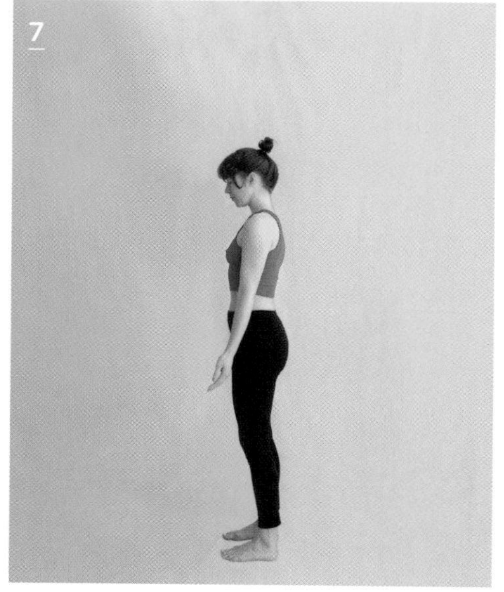
7

## SŪRYA NAMASKĀR: SUN SALUTATION

A traditional prayer of gratitude to greet each day and bring warmth into the body. You move the body between reaching up to the heavens and bowing into the earth. This is a poignant gesture to honour the skies and the land, gathering energy into the body and offering thanks back to the earth.

Begin in *Tāḍāsana* (see page 72).

1

**Ūrdhva Hāstāsana**

**Inhale**. Float your arms up to the sky on your breath, bringing the palms to meet.

2

**Uttānāsana**

**Exhale**. As the breath empties out of your lungs, fold forward and bend your knees to bow over your legs, lifting your sit bones high, bringing your fingertips to touch the floor.

**Modification**: If you're new to yoga, it will take time for your hamstrings to open. Keep your back long and either bend your knees deeply, place blocks under the palms or cup your shins with your hands.

3

**Inhale**, breathing deeply into the belly and up to the chest while lifting halfway and lengthening from the sit bones to the crown of the head.

4

**Kumbhakāsana**

**Exhale**. Bend your knees and release your palms to floor, step back into Plank, making a straight line from shoulder through hips to heels, keeping your navel tucked in and your sternum pressing through into the chest to dome the upper back. Reach through the crown and the heels, flexing your feet.

**Inhale**, stay here for one breath.

5

**Exhale**. Lower slowly to the floor, palms under shoulders, bringing your knees to the ground first if you need to.

6

**Bhujaṅgāsana**

**Inhale**. Stretch and activate the legs, point your toes and press them into the ground. Roll your shoulders back and down, finding length in your neck. Lightly imprint palms into mat and float chest away from floor into Cobra.

7

**Exhale**. Lower yourself slowly to the floor.

**Inhale**. Press the floor away from you, stretch your arms and press your knees into the floor to bring your seat towards your heels. Keep the torso, your spine and your arms long.

8

**Adho Mukha Śvānāsana**

**Exhale**. Retaining length in the upper body, stretch your legs into Downward-Facing Dog, hooking the hips high. As you plug the palms into the ground, externally rotate the upper arms, spiralling the eyes of the elbows outwards. Soften the lower ribs into the belly. Internally rotate the thighs. If your spine and hamstrings are open, you can begin to sink your heels towards the earth. Stay here for five slow, mindful breaths.

**Modification:** If the spine begins to round, bend your knees. Never sacrifice the spine for the perceived glory of the pose.

9

**Inhale**. Bend your knees deeply, keep your arms long and your hips and sitting bones high.

**Exhale**. The end of the exhale is where you have most power. At this point, step one foot to the front of the mat, followed by the other.

*continues >*

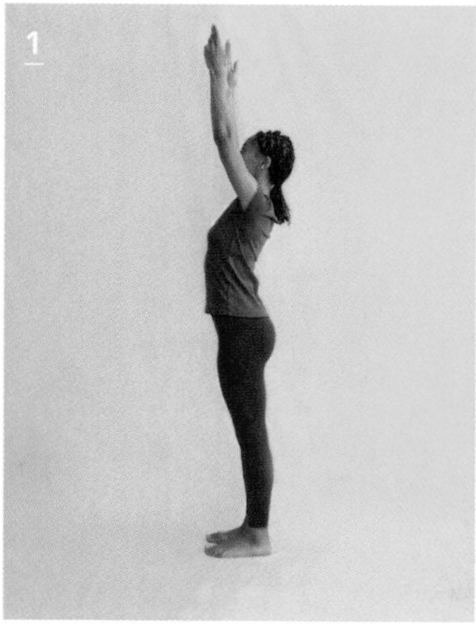

1

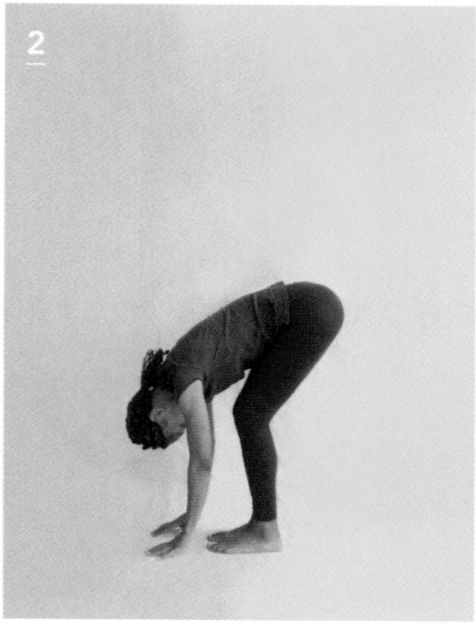

2

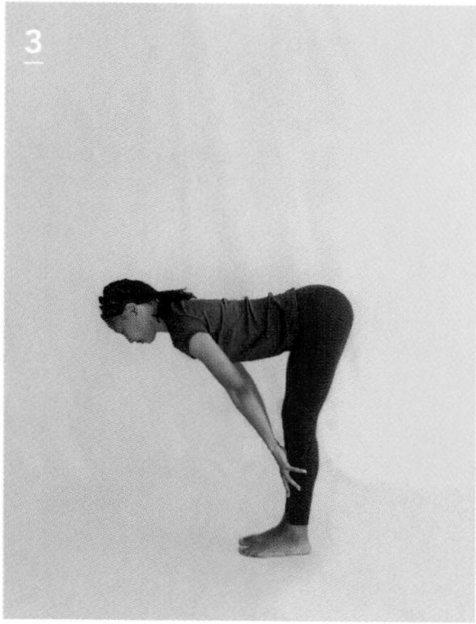

3

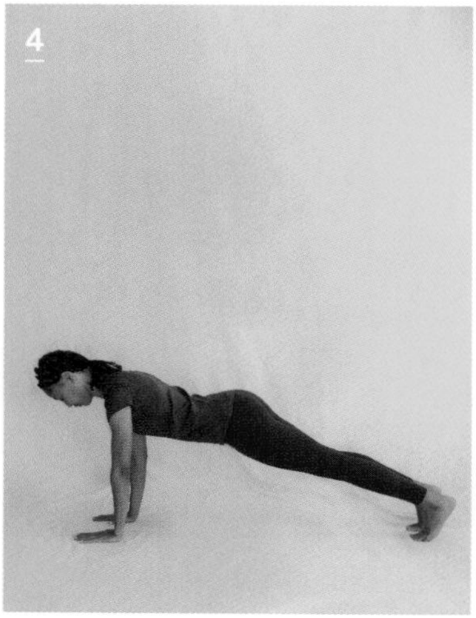

4

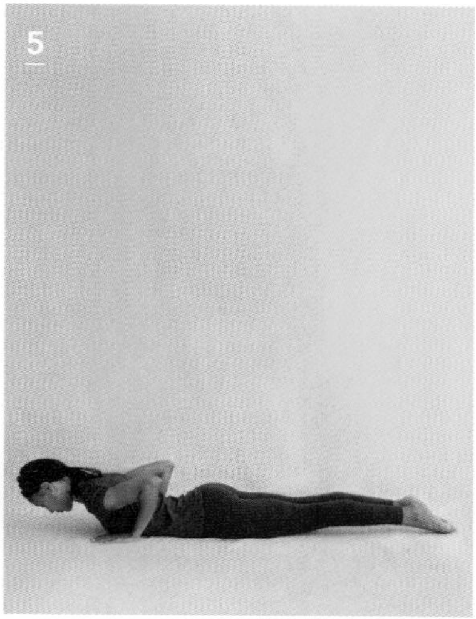

5

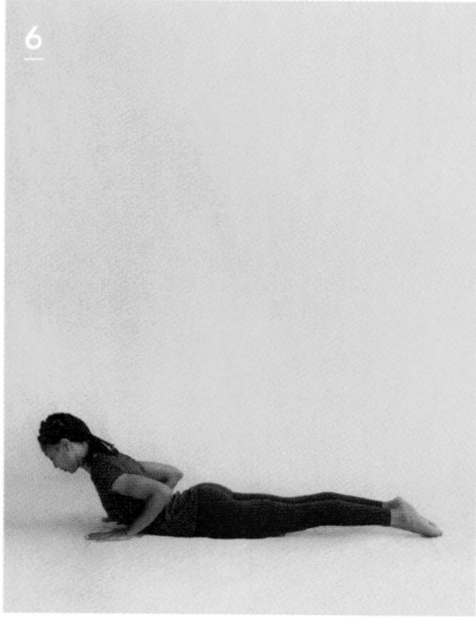

6

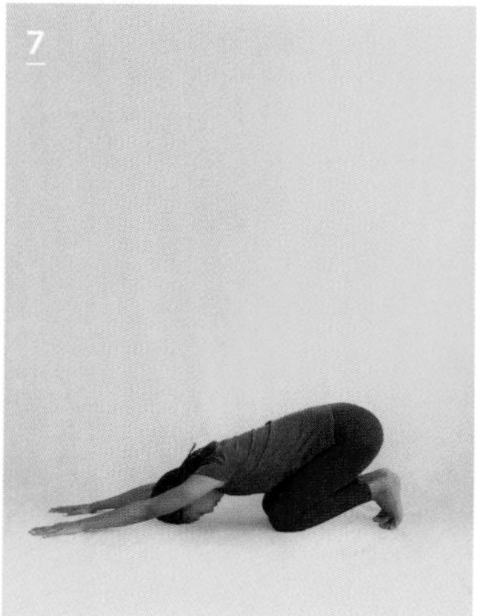

7

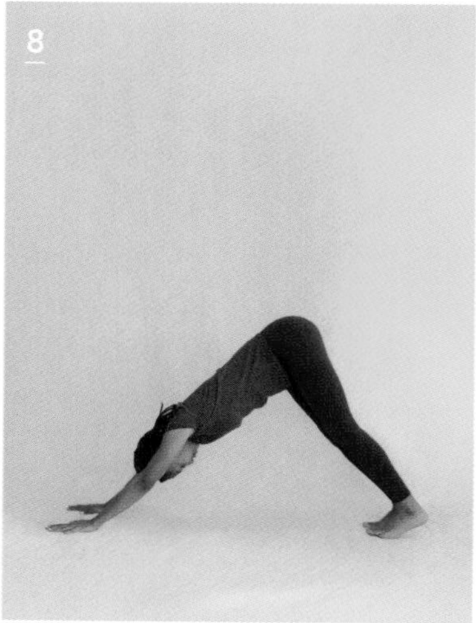

8

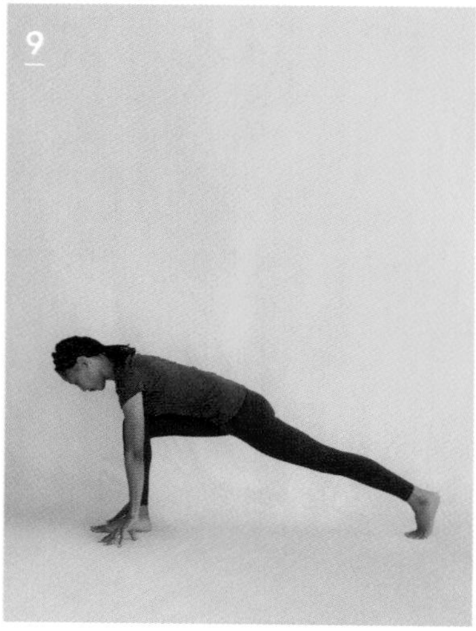

9

## SŪRYA NAMASKĀR *continued*

**10**

**Inhale**. Lengthen the spine to lift halfway, keeping the neck long.

**11**

**Exhale**. Bow forwards, empty the breath and use the space to fold over the legs.

**12**

**Inhale**. Soften the knees and lift up to stand, floating the arms as high as they will go. Keep your feet planted and your shoulders soft.

**Exhale**. Bring your arms alongside your body to make your way back to *Tāḍāsana*. Stand tall.

### Optional Extras

Here are some additional positions that you can build into your sequence to make it more interesting and juicy.

**1**

Instead of stepping straight back to Plank, lunge one leg back and release the knee onto the floor. Ground through foot and knee as you reach your arms to the sky, lifting your lower ribs away from the hips. Then plant your hands back on the floor and step into Plank and continue the sequence as before, transitioning from Cobra into Downward-Facing Dog. To return to the top of the mat, lunge the other foot forward and then fold in *uttānasanā*. Both sides should now feel even.

### Adho Mukha Śvānāsana variations:

**2**

Lift heels high, press into toes, bend knees, pull pelvic floor back. Release and repeat.

Plug toes into floor, soften knees and slowly move heels from side to side.

**3**

Alternate bending knees.

Lift one palm and thread underneath body to cup outer seam of opposite leg, just above ankle. Bend knees if necessary.

### Bhujaṅgāsana variations:

Lift up and down in Cobra a few times, circling shoulders as you go.

Tuck the chin to the chest, soften the neck and allow the head to be heavy. Slowly roll the head from side to side. As you turn to one side, pull the opposite shoulder back and breathe there deeply before moving on.

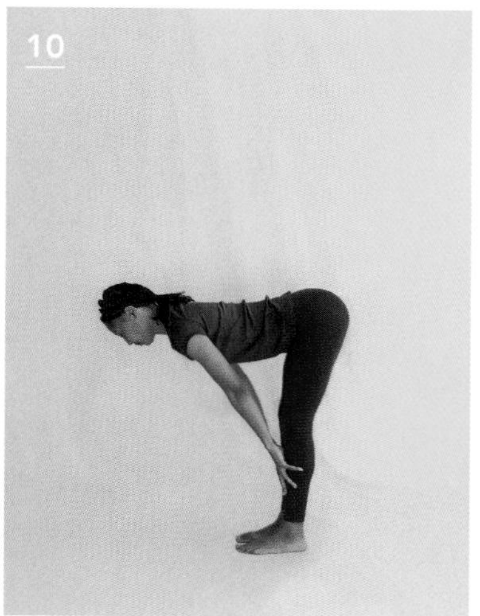
10

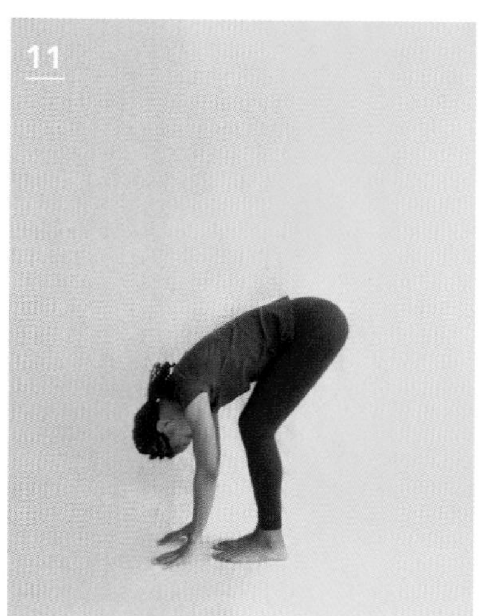
11

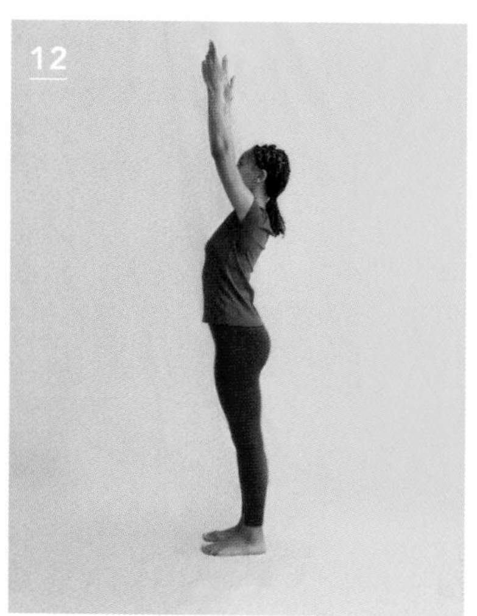
12

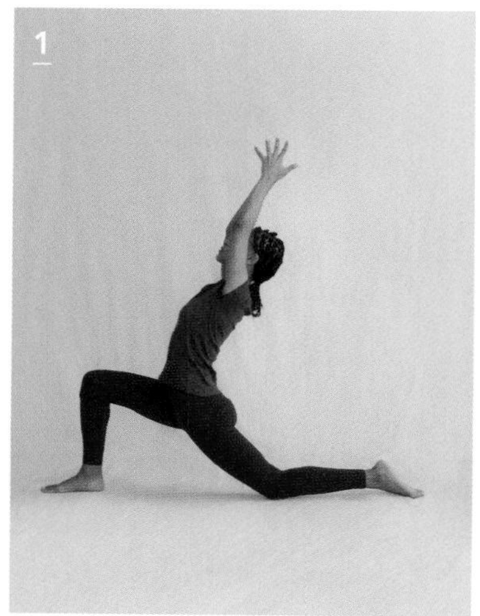
1

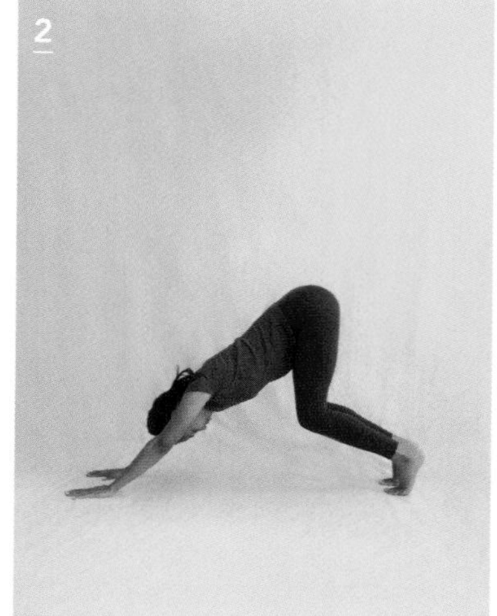
2

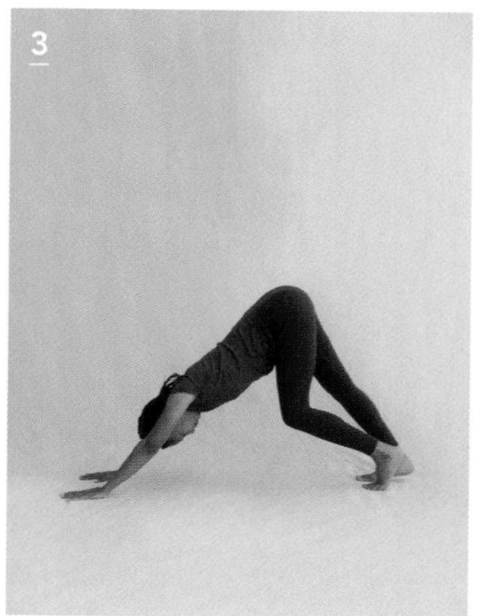
3

## STOKE YOUR FIRE

Core work is not the most exciting or delicious aspect of a practice. But if you're feeling low on power, learning to breathe through the heat will create discipline and self-control, and will rekindle your inner fire. The abdominal muscles give the spine essential support. Strengthening these muscles tones your pelvic floor and creates a container for your energy. When you are connected from your centre, your outer layers can soften. Energetically, core work creates power, motivation, action and strength, and can result in confidence. You can use the following sequence, co-created with Jessi Brown, at the beginning of your practice, adding steps to make it more challenging. Always warm up your body with a few sun salutations (see page 80) first.

### 1

Sitting in *Sukhāsana* (see page 74), cup your hands on the shelf of the crest of your hips.

**Inhale**. Puff up your chest, breathing into your upper lungs. Lift your ribs away from your hips, and squeeze your shoulders up to your ears, creating awareness in your core muscles.

**Exhale**. Slide your shoulders down your back as you exhale. Pull in your waist but continue to lift your breastbone. Draw your belly button back, scoop your heart up and beam it forward. You should feel the muscles in the upper back awaken as the shoulder blades project into the chest. Maintain this shape to turn on your core. This will train your body to understand the sensation of deep abdominal awakening so you can translate it into other poses.

### 2

Prepare for Cat and Cow: settle onto your hands and knees, spreading your palms under your shoulders and making sure your knees are under your hips.

**Inhale**. Direct your breath into the pit of your belly as you tilt the pelvic bowl forwards and begin a slow chain of movement through the spine on the crest of the breath. Lift your chest forward between your hands and slide the lower ribs away from hips. Carry this arching action down through the spine until your pelvic bowl tilts back and up, and you create the sensation of spreading your sit bones. Accentuate this action by creating the sensation of energetically drawing your hands back toward your knees.

### 3

**Exhale**. Plug your knees and hands into the floor. Lower chin to chest to start a chain-like curve of movement pressing the chest into the upper back, drawing the navel to the spine and knitting your lower ribs toward your hip points. Your front body contracts as your back body opens, hollowing out the belly. Your hips curve under and around.

**Inhale**. Sit bones lift and the wave ascends again.

Repeat 5–10 times. Close your eyes and see if you can refine the sensation of movement through each vertebra, extending the breath with the movement.

#### Optional Extra

Here is an additional position you can build into your sequence at this point to make it more juicy.

**Exhale.** Curl your toes under and lift your knees a few inches from the ground, drawing your thigh bones into your pelvis. Your hip points head towards your lower ribs. Press into your palms and energetically push your arm bones away from each other. Pull your shoulder blades down your back and away from your ears.

**Inhale**. Release your knees to the earth again, and as you inhale, balloon your belly and arch your back as you lift your head and sit bone.

Repeat five to ten times.

*continues >*

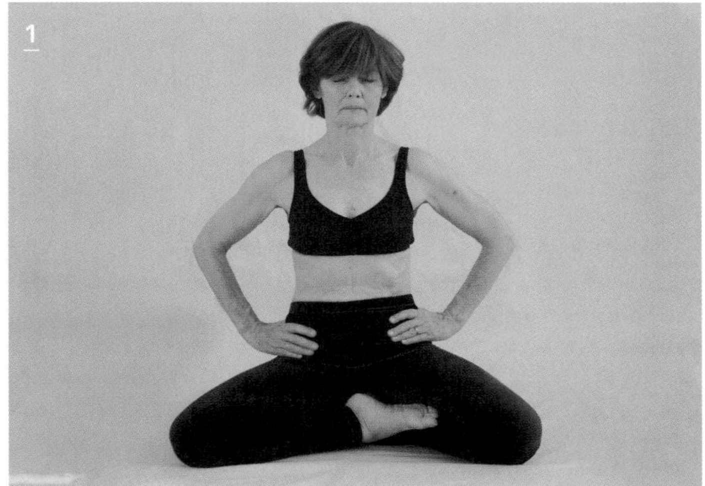
1

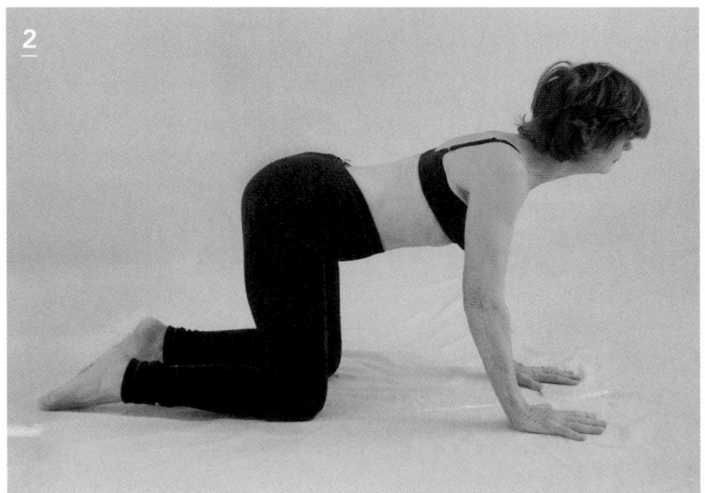
2

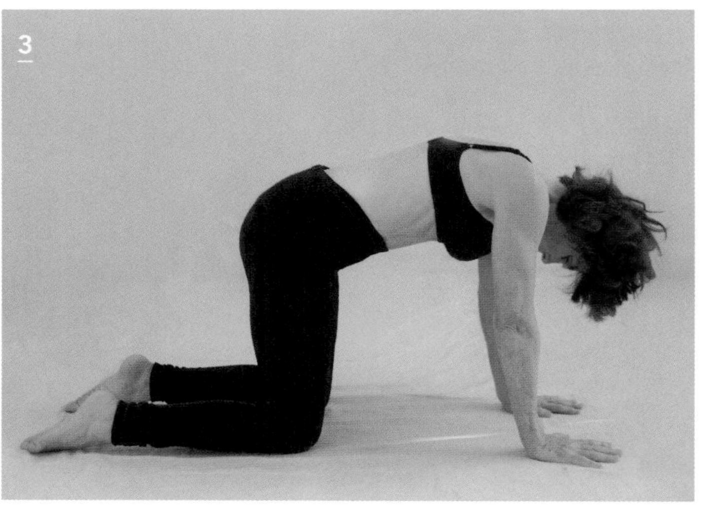
3

**STOKE YOUR FIRE** *continued*

4

Come back to a neutral tabletop position.

**Inhale**. Peel your left foot and right hand off the mat. Slowly stretch them away from each other, feeling a diagonal pull across the navel.

5

**Exhale**, use the breath to pull your belly back towards your spine, bend your arm and knee and navigate your knee to your elbow. Round your back and draw your pubic bone towards your sternum, and your hips towards your lower ribs. Draw your sit bones together, tailbone and pubic bone together – four points drawing to the centre and up. Repeat five times on each side.

For a variation, try starting on your hands and knees, then stretch your right arm forward and left leg back. Draw your left knee to your nose and reach your right arm back alongside the body, fingertips pointing to the back of the mat. If this feels too unstable, place your right hand on the ground and squeeze your knee towards your nose, as shown here. Hollow your belly to connect to your midline.

Work into the hips and glutes. Begin on all fours, with the weight distributed equally between hands and feet. Circle your right knee out to the side and slowly paint a huge circle with the knee, five times in one direction. Return to centre, repeat in the other direction, then repeat on the other side.

6

**Plank pose**

Place your palms under your shoulders and broaden across your collarbones. Your body should forms a straight line from the crown of your head through your shoulders to your hips and your heels. Engage and firm your leg muscles.

Keeping your hands where they are, give your legs a different workout by placing your heel on top of ball of your foot. Amplify and stabilize the engagement of the legs by energetically magnetizing the feet towards each other, though they remain where they are on the mat.

You can create a sequence with Plank pose, echoing the templates of movement above, on all fours. Work with the breath to guide the movement.

**Inhale**. Expand the energy of the body into the pose.

**Exhale**. Draw your right knee towards your right elbow.

**Inhale**. Straighten your right leg.

**Exhale**. Squeeze your left knee towards your elbow.

Alternate sides and repeat ten times.

*continues* >

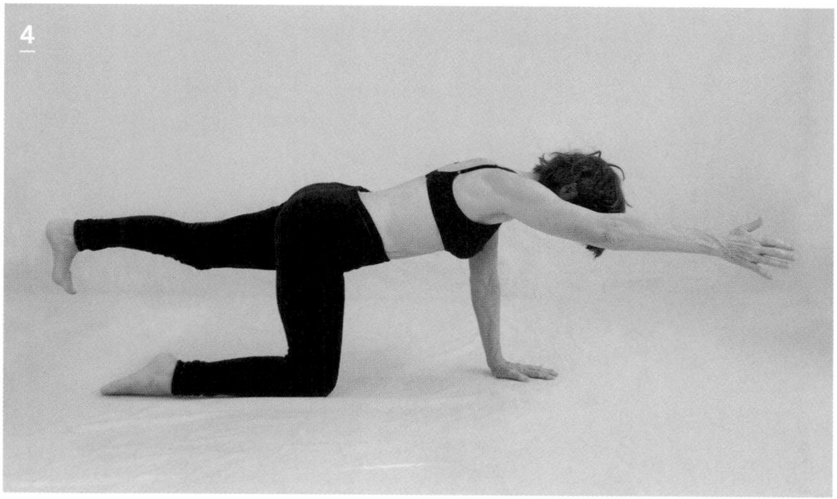

4

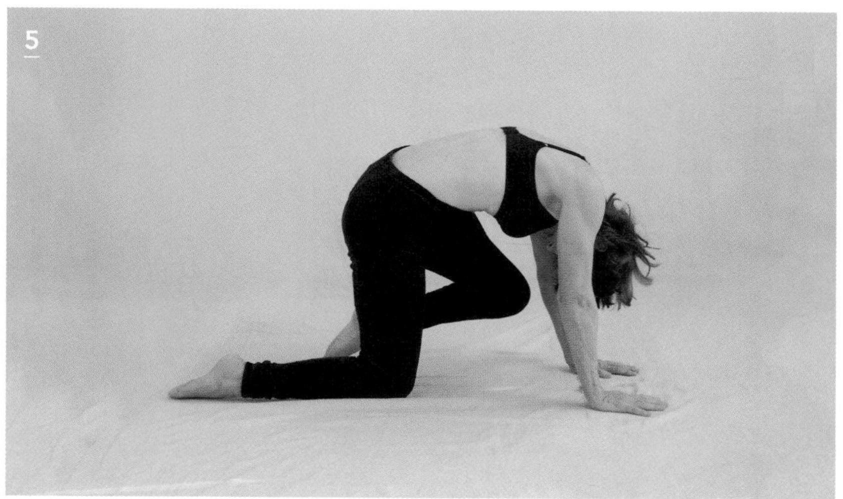


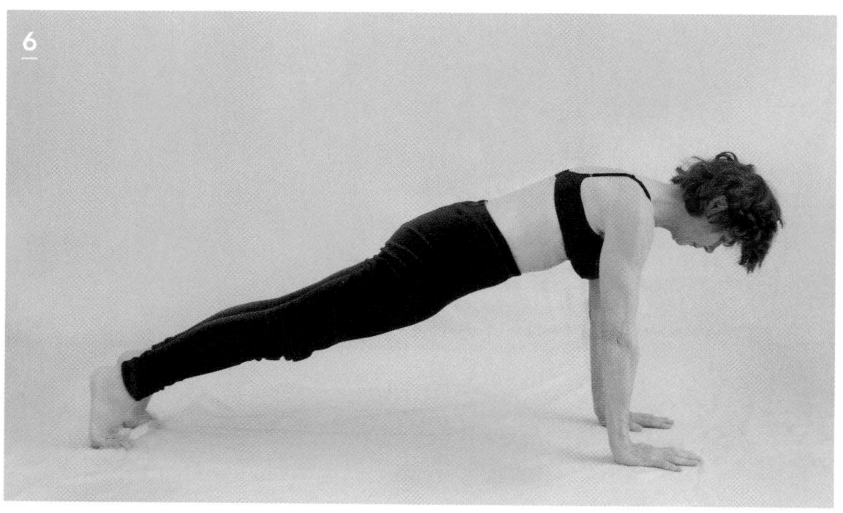

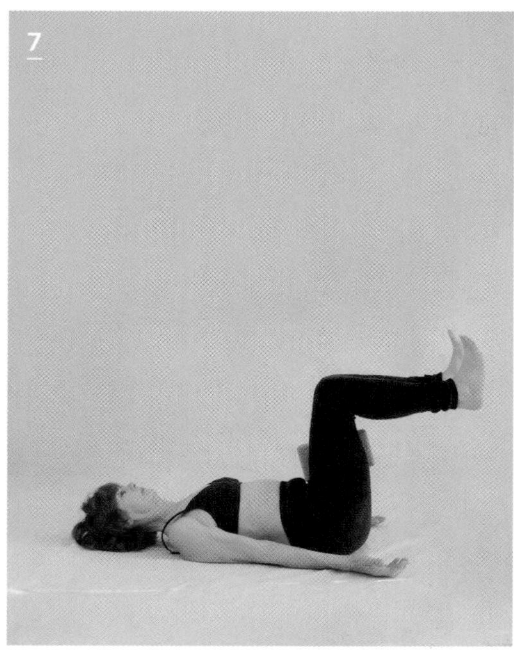
7

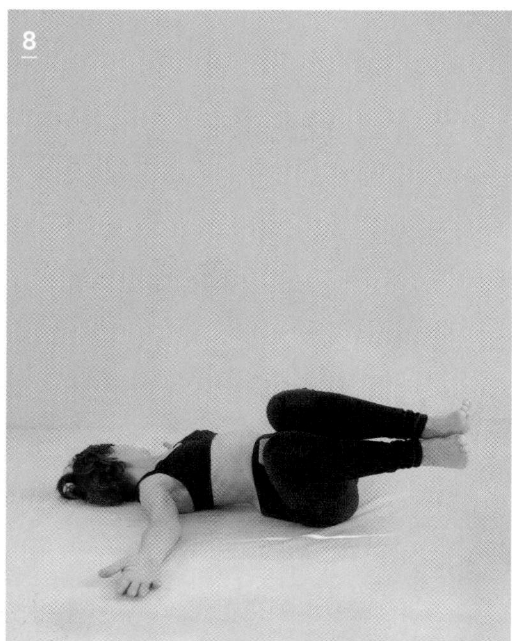
8

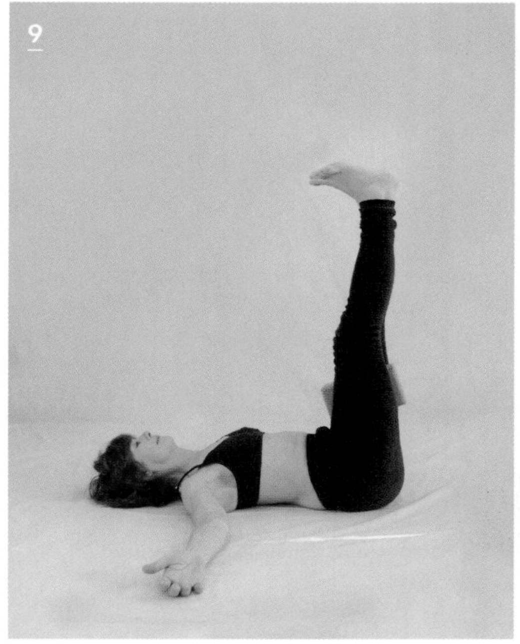
9

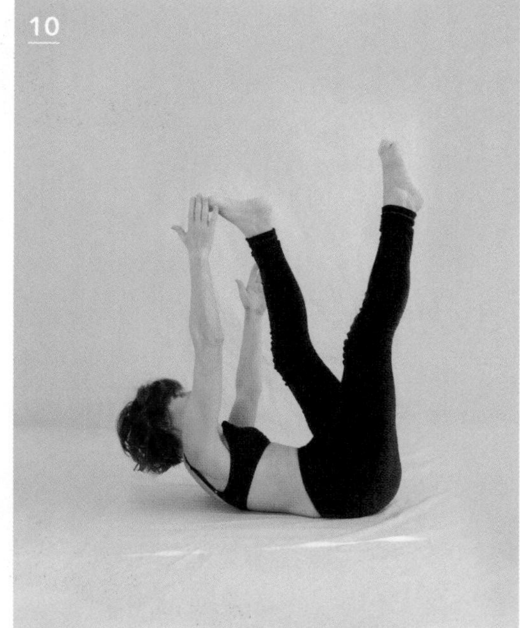
10

## STOKE YOUR FIRE *continued*

### 7

**Practice for a deep pelvic floor connection**

Lie on your back. Place a block widthways between your thighs, above your knees – when you squeeze it you will energize the muscles that connect to the midline and light up your core.

Your upper body remains stable and your lower body moves as a unit. Only go as far as you can maintain control in the upper body – your shoulders should remain flat on the ground. If your lower back is feeling tender, bring your feet to the floor. At end of an exhale, you receive the most energy and stability for effort. Explore the practice by only moving on the exhale. Observe the nuances of these practices: imagine the air is thick like treacle and move slowly. If you speed up, you will lose the connection and the effort will go into the hip flexors rather than the core.

Raise your legs and bend your knees into a right angle as you exhale.

**Inhale**, squeeze the block.

### 8

**Exhale**, feel your pelvic floor lift. Move your knees slowly to one side and hover them over the floor.

Inhale, remain here.

**Exhale actively through mouth**. At the end of the exhale, drag your knees slowly back to the centre to hover above your hips.

### 9

For a challenge, straighten your legs. Float your legs above your hips. Practise with your legs straight and glued together. Lengthen your legs and reach them out of the hip joint, which will create the sensation of space. Squeeze the inside of your toe mounds to light up the inner seam of your legs. Keep your arms by your side in a T shape, palms up, to avoid your shoulders rolling. Move your legs move from side to side, as above.

### 10

Hover your legs in the air, above your hips. Anchor your belly button down, towards your spine. Hover your arms in the air, above your shoulders.

Reach one leg and the opposite arm up toward the sky. Stretch through the big toe mound, feel the inner line of the leg energize.

Repeat five times on each side.

To develop this action further, lift your head off the mat as you reach your arm up and try to touch the toes on your opposite foot.

Repeat five times on each side.

**To cool down**, counter deep core work with some sweet abdominal stretches. Cobra (see page 80), Upward-Facing Dog or Bow Pose are nice ways to soften the abs. It's also lovely to lie on your front, with a block or towel rolled up and placed under your belly. Soften into the ground and focus on relaxing and melting the belly over the towel.

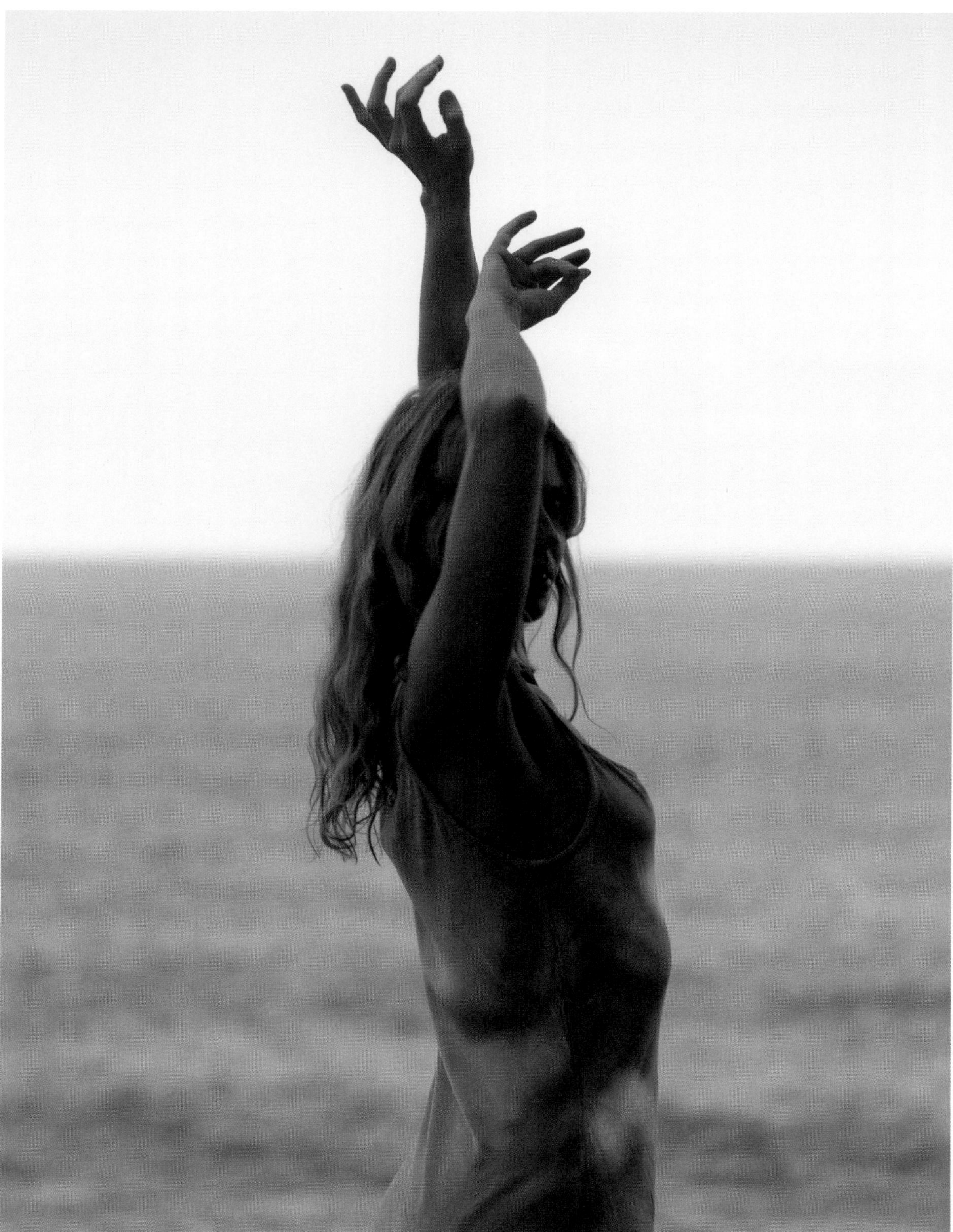

## FREE MOVEMENT: ELECTRIC BODY

A glorious practice for any time. It's my favourite thing to do in the morning – it starts the day off in celebration, with a sense of energy and *prānā* (life force) permeating your whole being.

I often teach this practice at the beginning of events or retreats. Sometimes people need to move immediately, to physically shake out their day before they're able to drop into a place of stillness. If you're teaching, it's a fantastic way to illustrate the concept of *prāṇā* to people who have never considered it before.

You need music, because you're going to shake and recruit every part of your body, so you'll want something primal and rhythmic, probably with drums. A song that makes you move your hips and shake your ass, with something slower for later on (see below). I often then lead into more floaty and ethereal music, before slowing down to sit and take in the fizz of energy, and then beginning to move again.

Start your playlist. Stand with your feet hip-distance apart, with your knees soft.

Close your eyes and gently begin to shake. Take your time for the body to accept the movement, then begin to bounce up and down.

Tuck your chin in slightly, shake and soften the shoulders. Allow the movement to travel down from your shoulders to your arms. Spend a while noticing this sensation. We hold so much in the neck and shoulders, so allow for this tension to be dispelled from the body.

Feel the heat stoke the body from the inside out.

Begin to shake your arms, your wrists and hands. Really, really shake them, as if you are flicking the unwanted energy out, shedding the unproductive and unwelcome. Flick and shake your hands, raise them over your head – the more you move and shake, the more vibrant you will feel, so you want to give it everything for at least five minutes (about ten is perfect).

When your chosen songs have come to an end, or you feel tired, stop. Pause the music. Stand completely still. Close your eyes and feel your own electricity. Experience the tingle of life, the spark of *prāṇā* throughout your whole body. Feel the little bird in your chest and the pace of your breathing. Be with yourself.

Sometimes I stop here, if I am continuing with another practice. Otherwise, when the poignancy begins to evaporate, I turn the music back on and begin dancing again.

Start to move more creatively, dancing around the room. Imagine infusing your movement with some words suggested by my friend Fern Trelfa, and see how this influences the shape your body takes: rolling, spirals, rushing, honeyed, jagged, robotic, abrupt, watery, slippery, floaty, ethereal.

Let your hips roll. Tune into the music and see if you can be moved from within. No one is watching – this is for you. Be creative. Feel the shapes and the rhythm move organically from within. You will soon see that the body wants to make shapes of its own and, if you are open, you will let it find them.

Dance like this until the slower, floaty track arrives. If you have been dancing fully, intensely, slow down and begin to move fluidly, floating through space. The air will feel more tangible. See if you can move in circles. Let the head find the spiral and translate it through the body. Duck and dive, swirl and be carried on musical spirals.

Finally, come to rest. Either sit on the floor to meditate, or make your way to lie down for a *Śavāsana* and witness the bright stillness of your electric body.

## MYSTIC MOON

Here's a gentle practice for when you'd like to soothe your body. This is good during your moontime (when you are menstruating), or when you're tired to your bones and you need to give yourself some TLC. If your sleep times are short and thin, bring this practice into your life regularly, to train your body to slow down and surrender. It will remember.

You will need some props to support the body so that your bones can release into the earth more easily. A block, a bolster or some pillows are perfect.

Start off with some gentle *prāṇāyāma*. This signals to your autonomic nervous system that it's time to put the brakes on and allow the parasympathetic ("rest and digest") to do its work.

**1**

Make your way into *Sukhāsana* (see page 74).

Bring your palms to meet and slowly slide your hands down from your heart to your womb. As you do so, peel the heels of your hands away from each other until only your thumbs and index fingers are touching, creating a little triangle. Slide your hands down your body until your thumbs cover your navel and your fingertips point to your pubic bone. This gesture, known as *yoni mudra*, is said to channel your feminine, creative energy – your *shakti*. It is deeply grounding and soothing: a perfect stilling for the waters of your womb. Breathe here for five minutes, taking the time to withdraw the senses within and begin to come home to yourself.

**2**

Softly open your eyes, interlink your fingers and reach your arms to the sky. Take a few deep breaths here, reaching high as you inhale, and allowing body to soften into itself as you exhale, releasing your arms.

**3**

Reach your arms forward and make your way into *malasana*, Garland posture, to squat. Make sure your heels are on the floor, or bring the floor to you by placing a block under each heel. Bring the palms to meet and, if possible, nestle your arms inside your thighs. Allow the hips to sink and pelvis to soften as you breathe deeply, keeping your spine long and your sternum lifted. Stay here and explore sensation for a few minutes, using the exhalation to evoke softness and space.

Then release your hands onto the floor and stretch your arms out in front of you, palms facing up. Bow into yourself in a gesture of surrender. Stay here for five breaths.

**4**

Bring your fingertips onto the floor and slowly stretch your legs to make your way into *Uttānāsana*, a forward bend. Place your feet hip-distance apart, with the outer edges of your feet in line and your thighs rolling inward, and cup your elbows with your hands. Allow your head to be heavy and your neck long. Stay here, breathing deeply for a few minutes, exploring how it feels to allow gravity to do its work to open the body. Stay present with the breath. Witness a sense of calm percolating into the mind and subduing your mental circus.

*continues* >

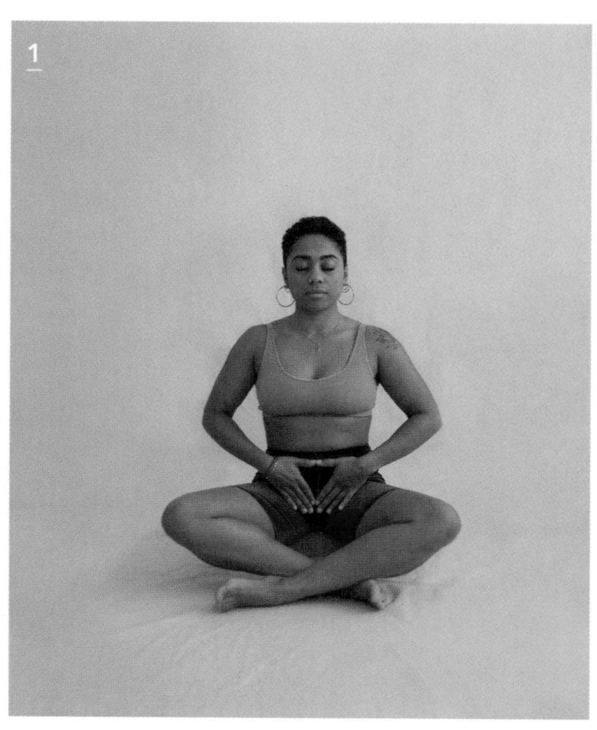
1

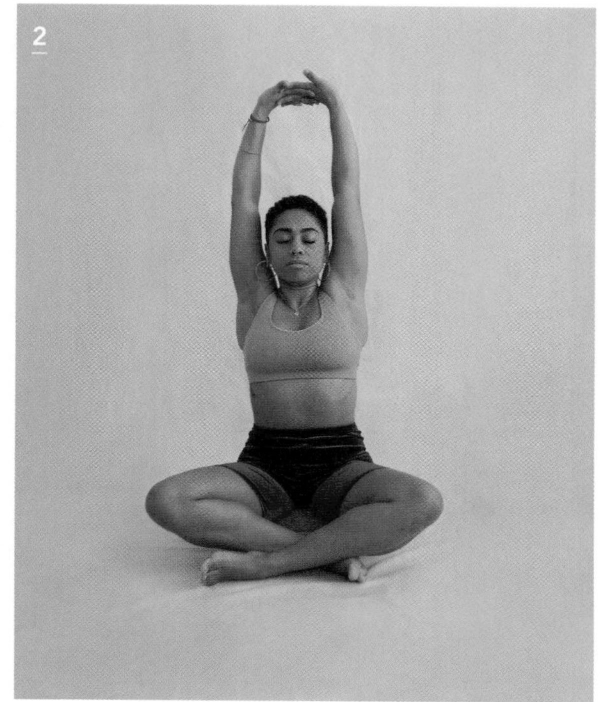
2

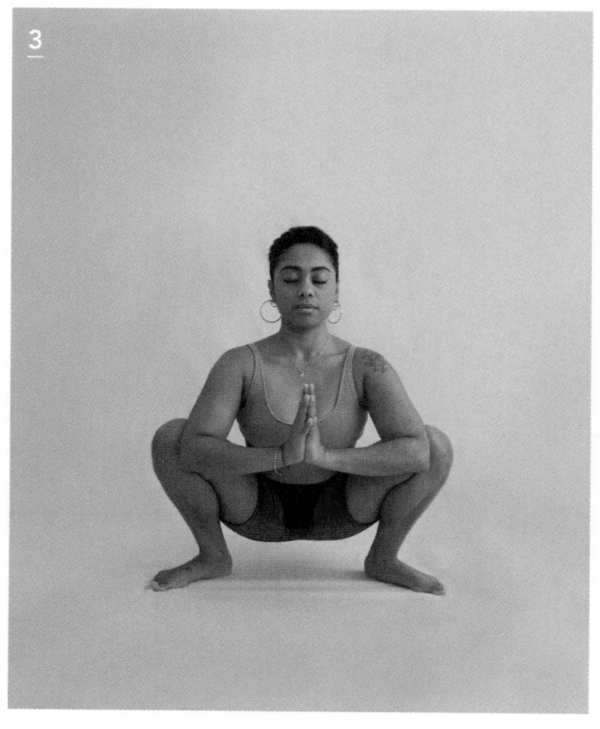
3

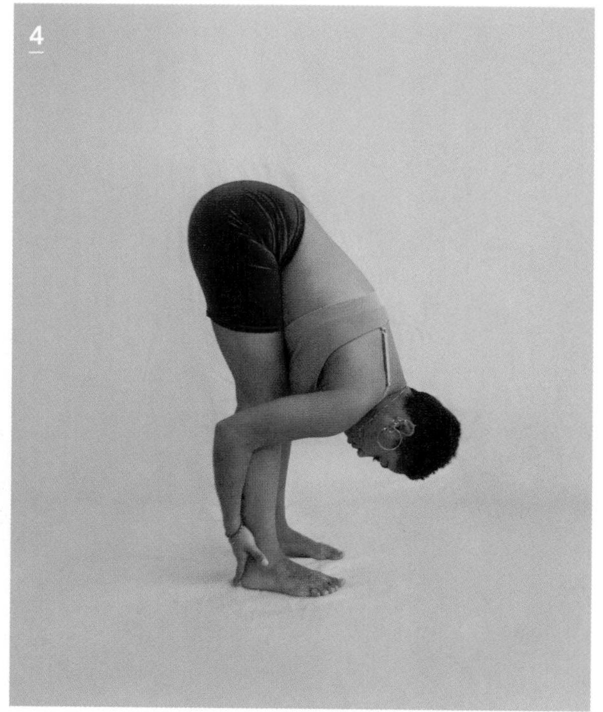
4

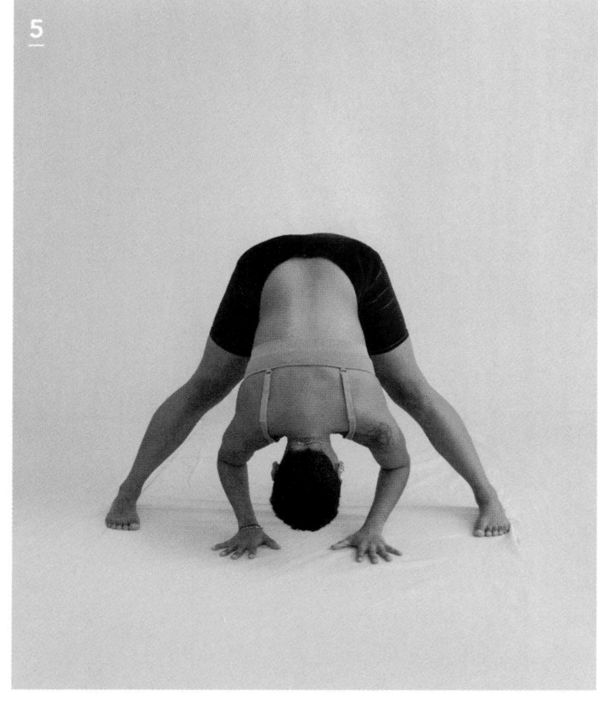
5

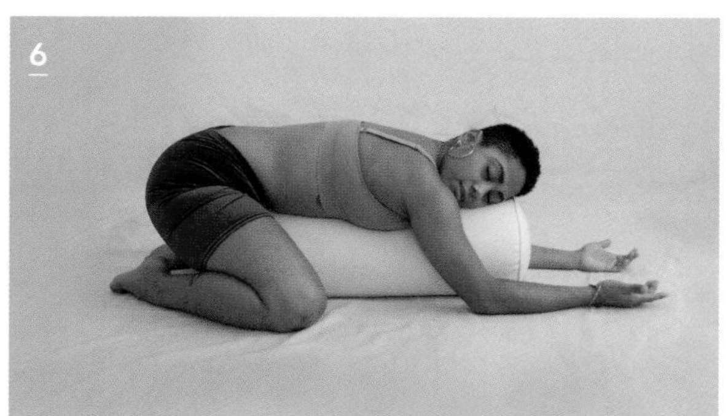
6

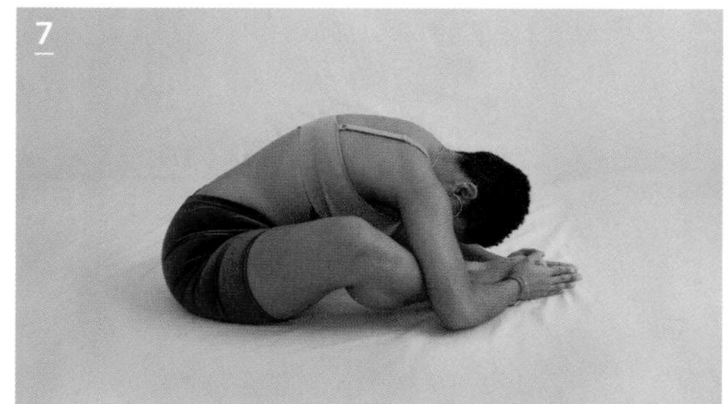
7

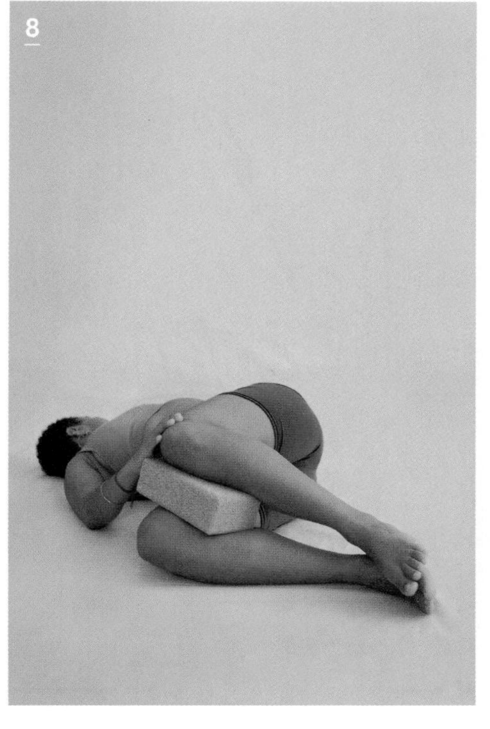
8

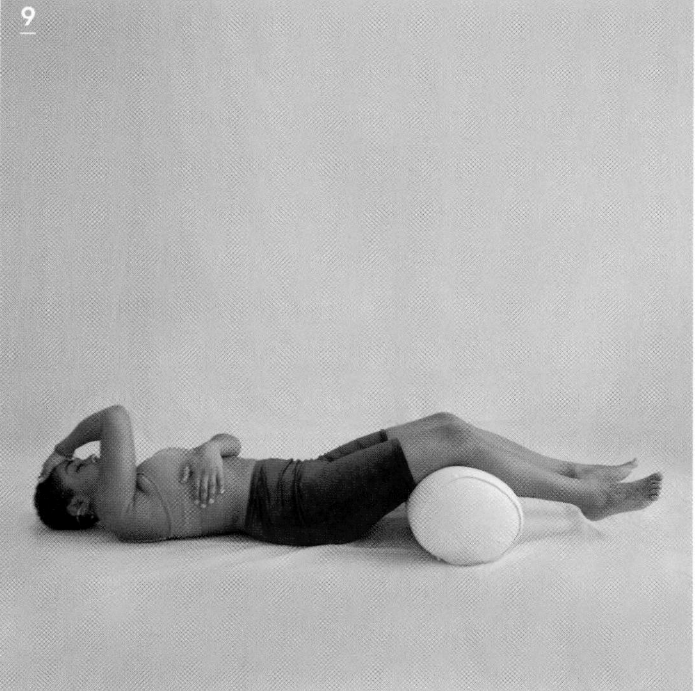
9

## MYSTIC MOON *continued*

### 5

Step your feet into a wide-legged forward bend, *Prasārita Pādottānāsana.* Make sure the outer edges of the feet are in line, with an internal rotation of the thigh bones and broadening of the sit bones. Keep your knees bent as you fold forward, as it allows the spine to lengthen and the top of the skull to slowly release towards the floor. Either keep your hands on the floor for support, or cup your elbows with your hands and hang out.

### 6

Walk your hands around to the top of mat and slowly make your way back to *Adho Mukha Śvānāsana*, Downward-Facing Dog. Linger for a few breaths, if your body would like to.

Then bring your knees onto the mat, placing them hip-distance apart, in preparation for a supported child's pose, *Bālāsana.* Place a bolster between your legs and drape your body over the support, resting your elbows on the floor and turning your palms skyward and your head to one side.

As you breathe here, work on the idea of letting go, of surrendering. Feel your tissues ungrip and release. Sink into the grounding quality of the pose. Lie here for a few minutes, then turn your head to the other side for a few minutes.

### 7

Inhale and slowly push up, then move the bolster out of the way and make your way to sit. Bend your legs and bring the soles of your feet together, as close to your seat as is comfortable. Melt your upper body forwards, keeping your shoulders soft and your head heavy. Stay here for three to five minutes.

### 8

Slowly peel up and make your way to lie down on the mat. Go into a reclining twist by bending your knees and bringing the feet onto the floor. Place a brick or a bolster between your thighs and slowly release your knees to the right. The closer you draw the knees to your navel, the more pronounced the twist will be. You want it to be comfortable enough for you to soften into and let the weight of the legs inform the release. Hold for three to five minutes, then slowly make your way back to centre and repeat on the other side.

### 9

Unravel into *Śavāsana*, the Corpse pose. Place the bolster under your knees. Bring your feet as wide as the mat. Adjust your body, so that your back feels broad, your shoulders soft and your neck long. Place the heel of your right hand to your forehead and bring your left hand to the right side of your torso. Lie here for a few minutes, feeling held and contained, noticing if your mind begins to still. Then release your arms and bring them alongside you, about 30cm (12in) away from your body, with your palms facing up. Feel the weight of your skull. Allow your bones to deepen into the earth and let your heart slowly sink into the bed of the lungs. Invite the body to continue to surrender and open.

## FERTILE GROUND

These empowering, grounding sequences will help you root yourself by nourishing your hips, glutes and psoas. You can bookend these practices with some gentle openers, such as dancing or salutations, and a nice slow floor sequence to cool down before *Śavāsana*. Make sure to breathe mindfully, deeply and slowly.

Often underused in our sedentary lifestyles, the gluteal muscles need some love to keep them strong. Peachy glutes will stabilize your pelvis and create more support for the spine, lower back and knees. Like core practices, glute work can be fiery and uncomfortable. But your booty – and its lovers – will thank you for it.

**1**

**Opener: Bridge**

Lie on your back.

Bend your legs, placing your heels on the floor under your knees.

Push your feet into the earth and lift your hips.

Melt your upper back into the ground, soften your lower ribs into your body, draw your hip points up.

Slide your sit bones towards the back of your knees, creating space in your lower back.

Press the balls of your feet into the earth to activate your adductor muscles through the inner seam of your leg. Plug in your heel to activate the glutes.

Notice how subtle movements can shift the landscape of a pose. Press the heel of your left foot and ball of left foot – don't peel anything off the ground. Just press deeper into the ground, and observe how your glutes engage.

Release to the floor.

**Inhale**, lift your toes.

**Exhale,** squeeze your glutes, reach your knees forwards, away from your hips and slowly peel the spine away from the floor as you lift your hips, squeezing the glutes as you reach the maximum point of incline.

Inhale, slowly release back down onto the floor.

Repeat twenty times.

**2**

**Juicy Grape (Zephyr) Glutes**

Fully root your feet into the earth. Find the four-point connection: two on the back of the heel, one each on the ball and the outer edge of the foot.

Push the left foot into the mat and float the right heel.

**Inhale**, feel the connection through your left leg.

**Exhale**, float your right leg up towards the sky.

**Inhale**, while the left leg stays up, slowly lower your bottom to the floor.

**Exhale**, emphasizing the connection of left heel, push the ground away and lift your bottom.

**Inhale**, lower your bottom to the floor.

Repeat five to ten times and then swap legs.

**3**

Lie on your front, with your hands underneath your forehead, palms down. Press your right foot into the floor to activate your leg. Root your pubic bone and the top of your thigh down.

**Inhale**, squeeze your glutes.

**4**

**Exhale**, float your left leg away from the ground. Focus on carrying the weight from your glute, not the hamstring.

**Inhale**, slowly release your leg.

Repeat five to ten times and then swap legs.

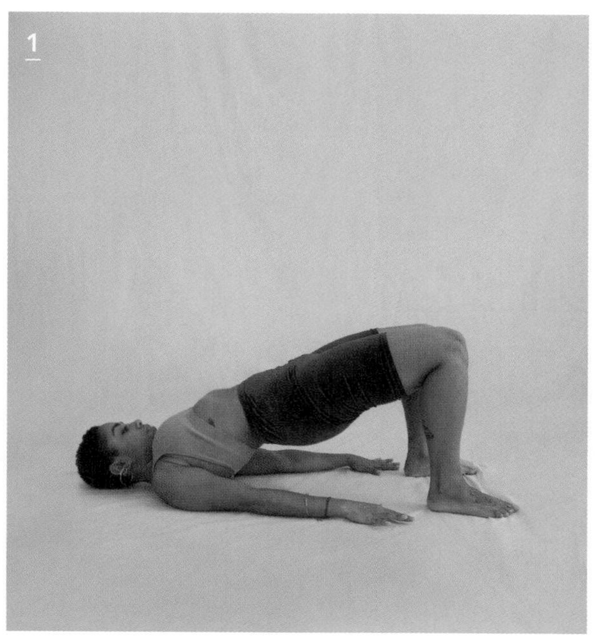
1

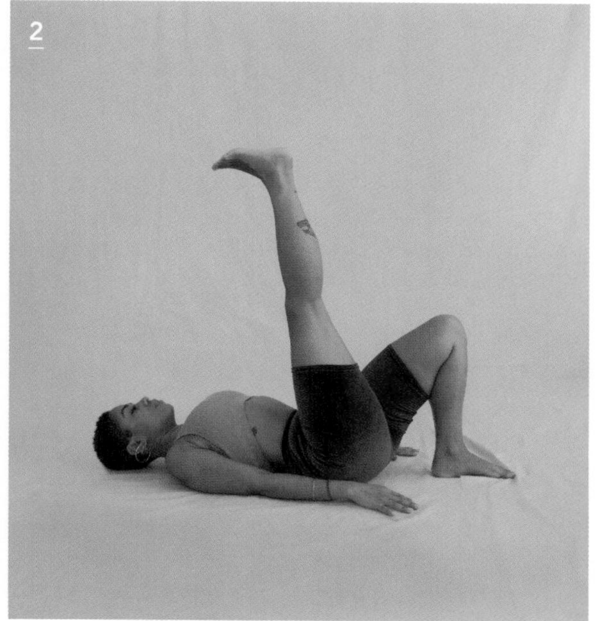
2

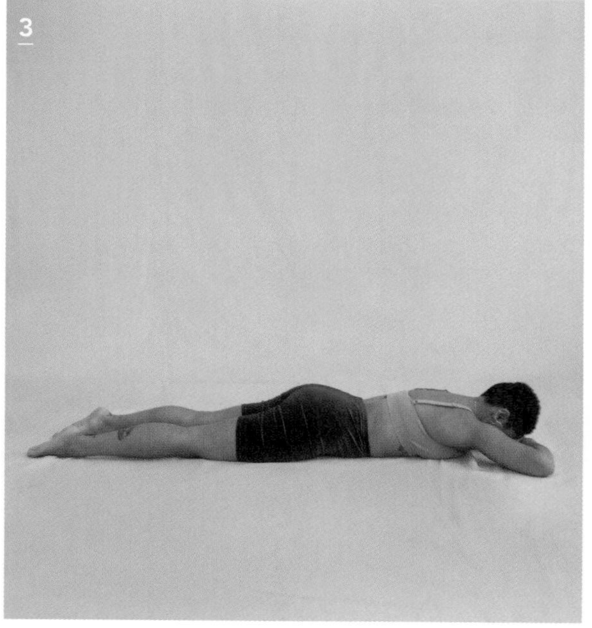
3

4

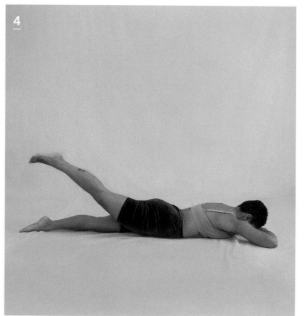

## JESSI SEQUENCE

Created with Jessica Brown, this is a slinky, snaky flow to oil up the hips and juice up the spine.

### 1

Begin on all fours and stretch your right leg behind you, parallel to the floor. Bend your knee at a right angle and open through the front of your right hip. Bend your knee toward your right shoulder.

### 2

Stretch your right leg in line with your hip and flex your foot. Slowly turn your head to gaze at your bent knee.

### 3

Bend your right leg, point your foot behind you and across to the left. Your leg should be hip height or above. Allow the movement of your leg to initiate a curving chain of movement through the spine. As your leg moves, your head turns organically.

Continue snaking leg back and forth five times.

### 4

**Utthan Pristhāsana: Lizard pose**

Step your right foot forward.

Place both your palms to the inside of your foot towards the centre of the mat.

Press your foot onto the floor and circle the knee and hips.

### 5

Peel the inner seam of your right foot from the floor, push down onto the outer edge of the foot. Circle and oil up your hips.

You can moderate the pose by bringing your forearms to rest on the floor, lifting up onto your fingertips, or straightening and bending the leg.

### 6

Wiggle your front foot into the centre, frame it with your hands.

Pivot on your back knee, with your back shin parallel to the top of the mat.

Place your right hand on the inside of the front foot.

Stretch your left arm towards the sky.

Cup the back of your head with your left hand.

Rotate the left ribs up to the sky.

Push your knee into your arm and your arm into your knee to establish a firm hip connection.

Use the floor to connect into the body – tuning in to these points of contact creates stability.

### 7

**Camatkarāsana: Modified Wild Thing**

Press into your front foot and start stretching your leg as you lift your heel and turn your toes forwards while raising your torso to upright.

Circle your right arm skywards and reach your left hand to the floor beneath your shoulder. Your right arm is in line with your right leg as your fingertips stretch away from the outer edge of your right foot.

Press your hips forward as you turn your sternum to the sky, beaming your heart open.

Repeat steps 1–7 on the other side.

### 8

**Counterpose to wind down**

Lie on your back, placing a block under pelvis.

Stretch one leg out, flexing the foot.

Squeeze the other knee into your chest.

Repeat on the other side, then prepare for *Śavāsana* (see page 118).

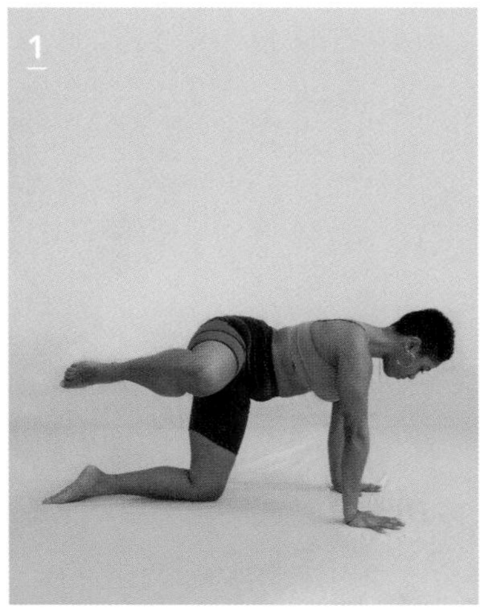
1

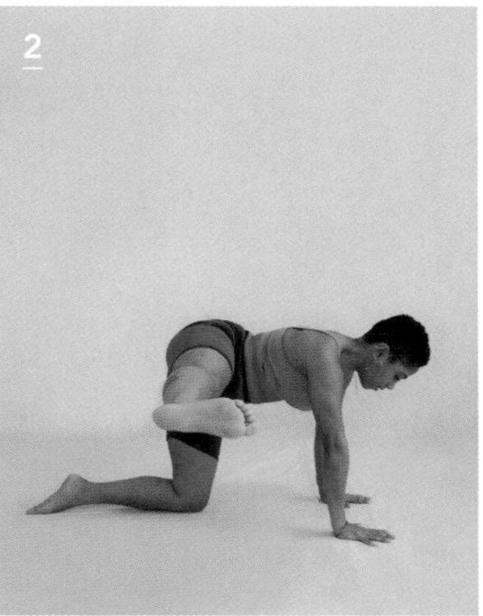
2

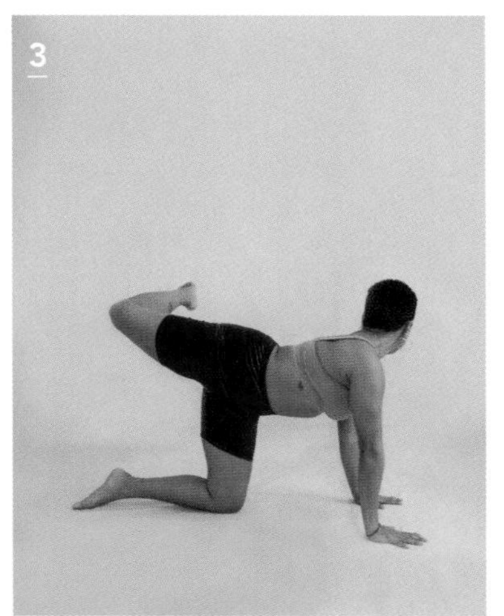
3

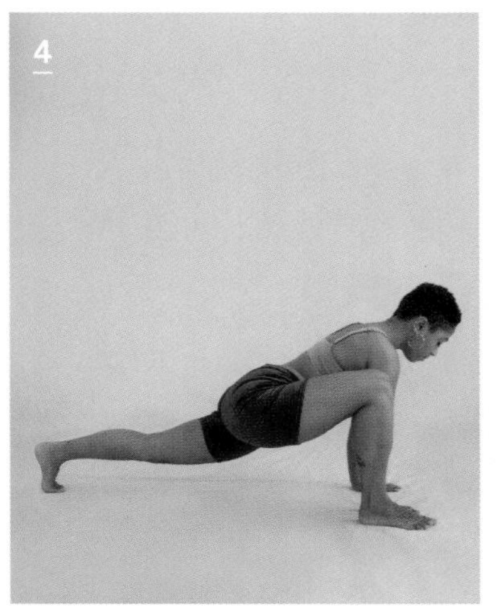
4

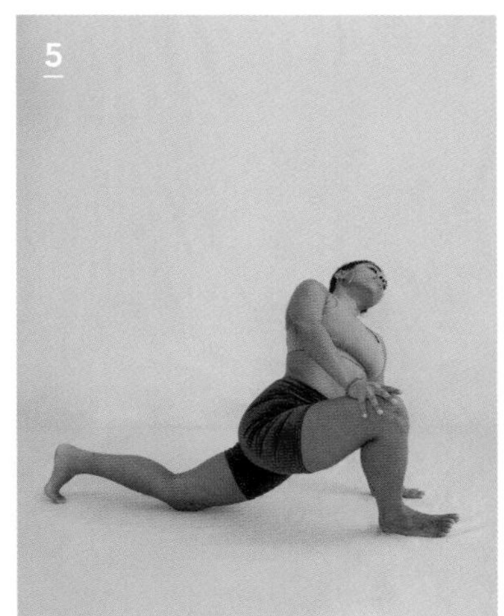
5

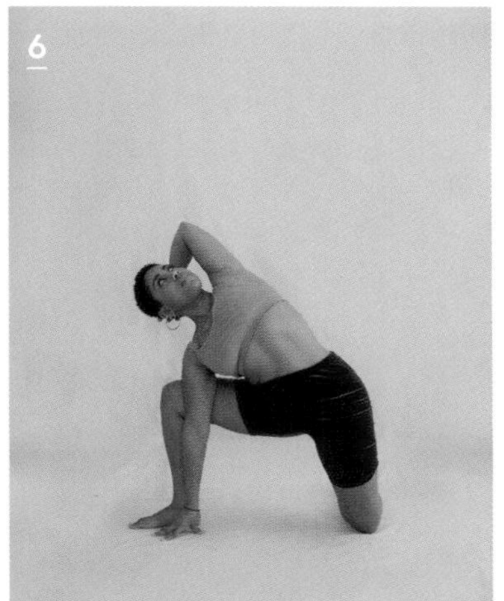
6

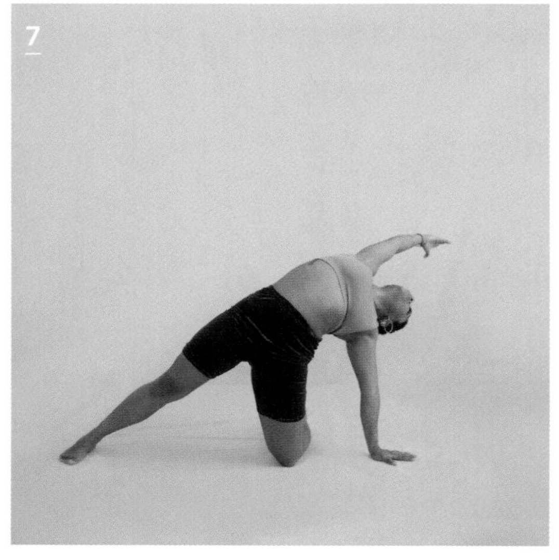
7

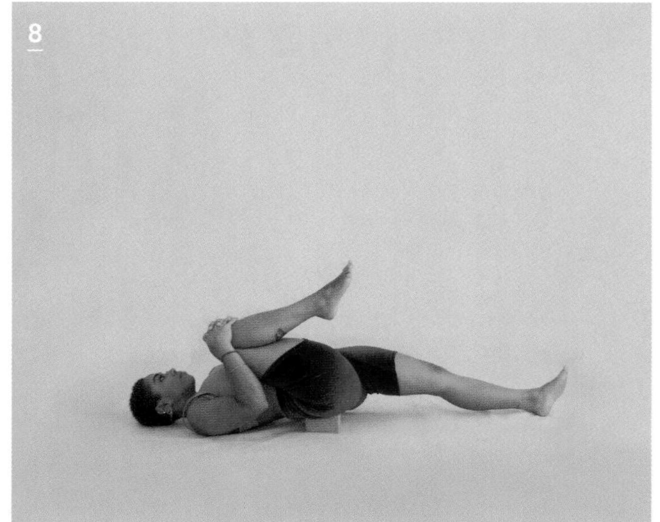
8

## YOUR HEART IS ANCIENT

Backbends as heart openers – mysterious ways to crack you open. Most people leak a tear or two, at some point during their practice. "Heart openers" like the following poses are often responsible for these swells of emotions that leave us feeling more open and receptive.

1

**Passive heart opener**

Lie on a bolster as if for *Śavāsana* (see page 118). Lengthen your neck, soften your shoulders and let your arms roll away, palms up. Breathe.

2

**Gentle Opener**

Sit in *Sukhāsana* (see page 74).

**Inhale** Reach back, with your fingertips facing forward. Push down and lift your heart and sternum.

3

**Exhale** Bring your hands to your knees. Round your upper chest and push your knees into your hands.

Repeat three to five times. On the last repetition, hold the two poses for five breaths each.

4

**Twist**

Return to centre and lengthen through your spine. Twist to the right, place your left hand on your right knee and your right fingertips on the floor behind you.

**Inhale** Breathe deeply into ribs, lifting the sternum.

**Exhale**, twist slowly, letting your shoulder blades slide down the back.

Hold the twist for five breaths, then return to centre and repeat on other side.

5

**Garudāsana: Eagle pose**

Bend your arms at a right angle and wrap your left arm around the right. Reach your elbows and fingertips high, drawing your shoulders away from your ears. Press your forearms away from you.

6

Open your arms wide and bend your elbows to create a cactus shape, spreading your fingers.

Hold for five breaths, then repeat *Garudāsana* on the other side.

Follow with Cat and Cow, as described on page 84.

7

**Adho Mukha Śvānāsana variation**

Begin in Downward-Facing Dog (see page 80).

8

Reach for the outside of the left ankle with your right hand, bending your knees if needed. Rotate chest and heart to the left, then return to the original pose.

9

Float your right leg high, then lunge your right foot forward, between your hands.

Float your arms toward sky, directly over your hips. Be careful not to throw your head back and block your neck. Energize the legs to create a feeling of power, allowing you to remain stable.

Bring your arms into a cactus shape (see step 6). Pull your elbows towards each other and feel the upper back project forwards. Draw your shoulder blades together and slide them down your back, lifting your sternum to the sky.

Either hold position for five to ten breaths, or alternate as described below:

**Inhale**, Reach your arms high, over your shoulders.

**Exhale**, bend them into cactus arms.

Repeat this Downward-Facing Dog variaton on the other side.

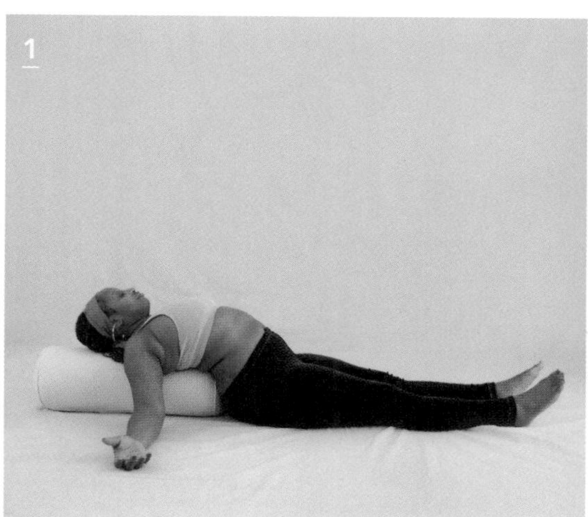
1

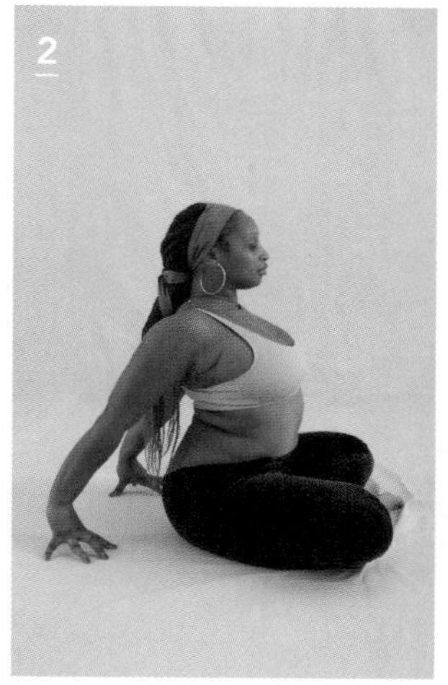
2

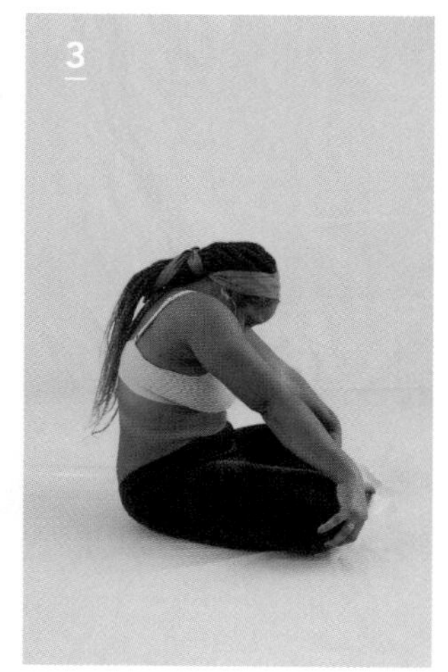
3

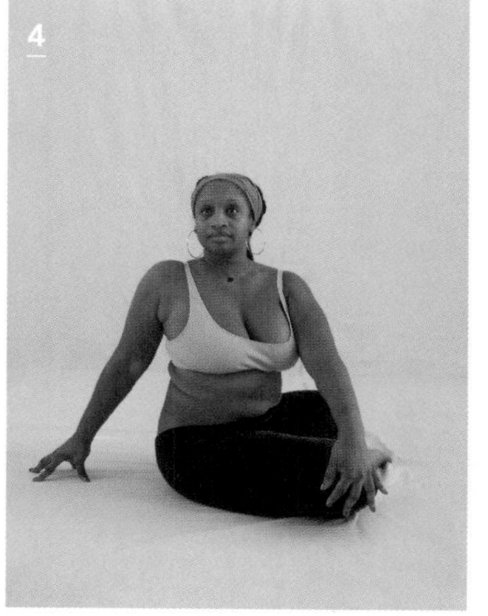
4

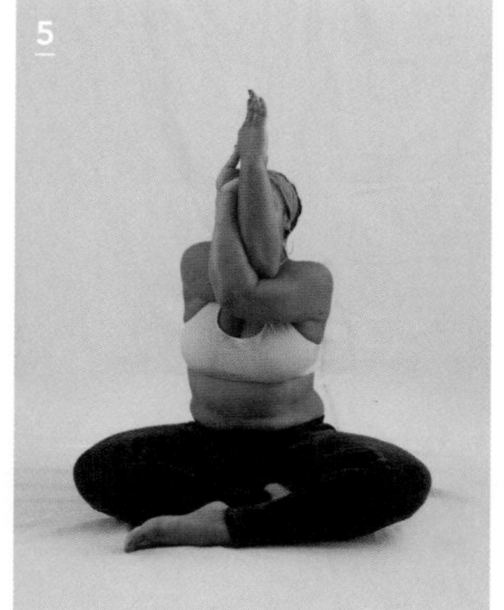
5

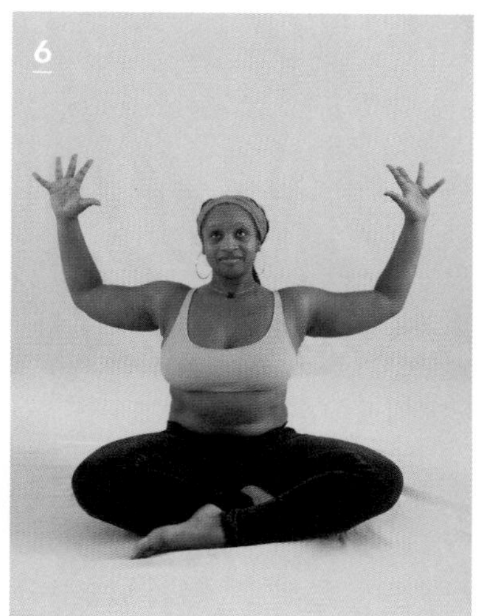
6

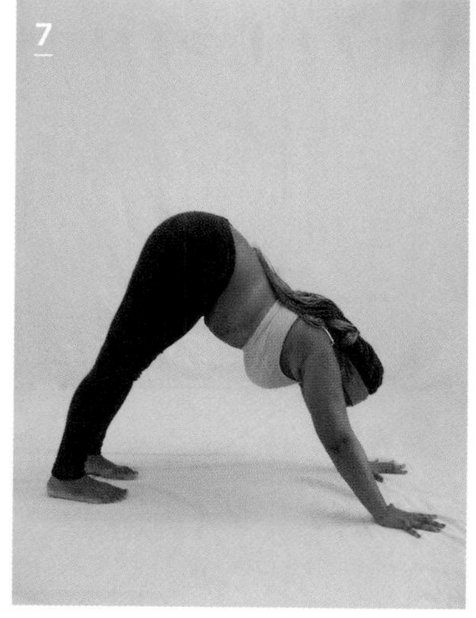
7

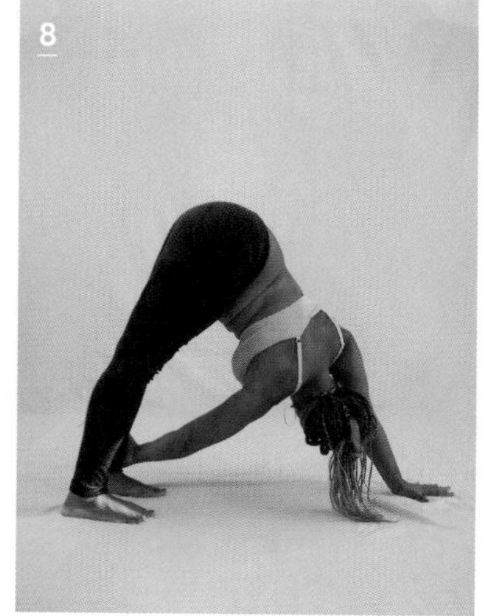
8

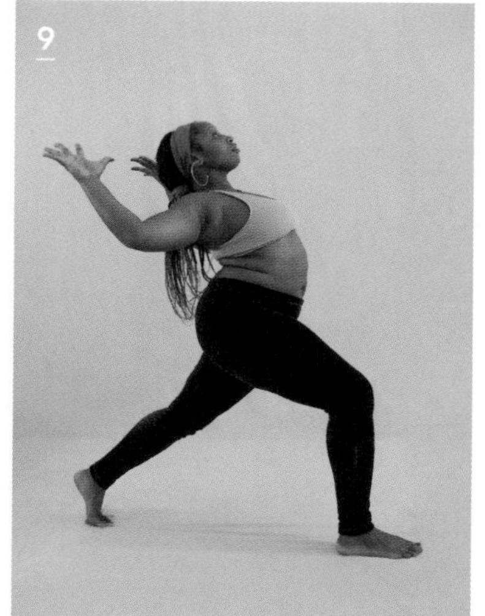
9

## REMEMBER THE SKY

A practice for freedom and relief when desk-bound.

1

Begin in *Tāḍāsana* (see page 72).

2

**Inhale**, float your arms over your head.

**Exhale**, interlink your fingers.

**Inhale,** reach your arms to the ceiling and stretch them high.

**Exhale**, bend to the right, grounding through your feet.

**Inhale**, centre.

**Exhale**, bend to left.

Repeat three times on each side.

3

Float your arms behind you, interlink your fingers and stretch your elbows. Draw your shoulder blades together and soften your lower ribs into your belly.

**Inhale** and reach your hands away from your hips.

**Exhale** and continue to breathe deeply for five to ten breaths.

4

Cup your hands at the back of your head, with your fingers interlinked.

**Inhale**, fan your elbows open, lifting your chest.

**Exhale**, tuck your chin to your chest, drawing your elbows together.

Repeat five to ten times.

5

Breathing deeply, open your elbows and slow-motion circle one elbow up and back, creating a stretch through your ribs. Then repeat with the other elbow, as if you were swimming backstroke, one arm moving at a time. Explore the movement, lingering and repeating anywhere you feel stuck.

Now reverse the direction and create circles with your elbows as if you are swimming a front stroke.

Stretch from side to side, reach diagonally, close your eyes, trying to find where the body wants you to move.

*continues >*

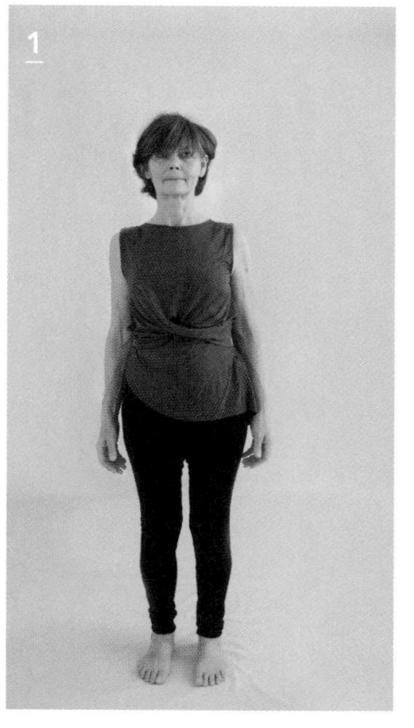
1

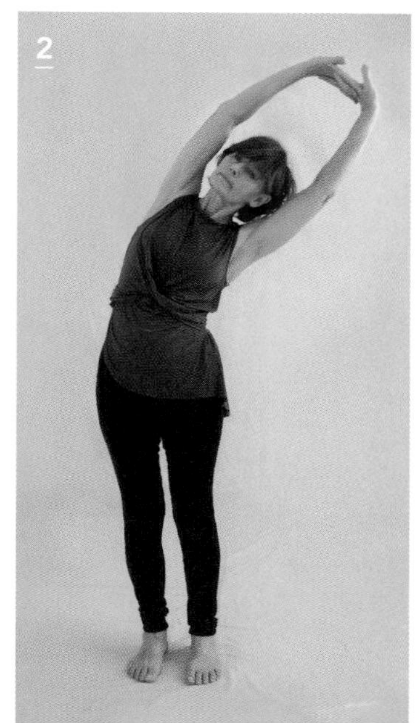
2

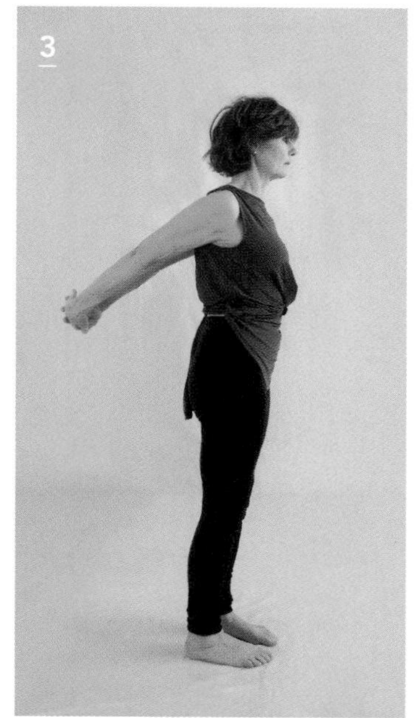
3

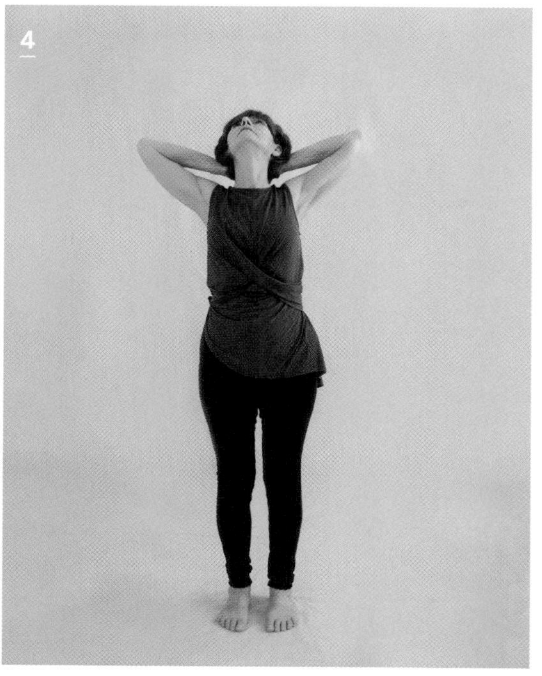
4

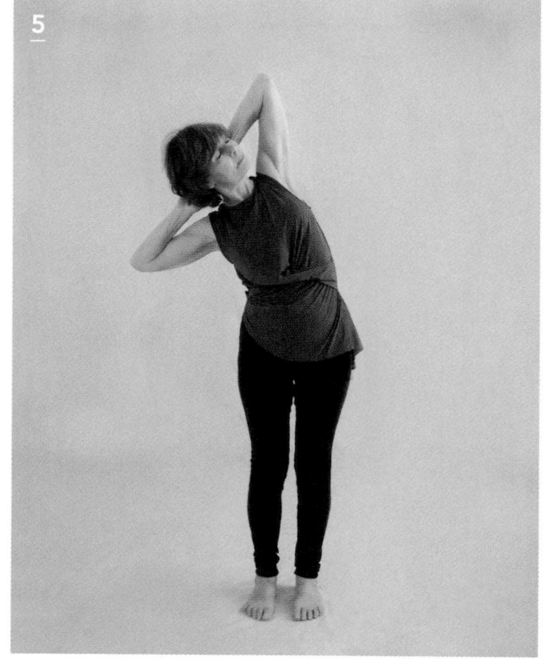
5

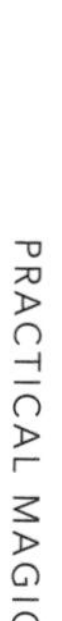

## REMEMBER THE SKY *continued*

### 6,7,8,9,10,11

Return to *Tāḍāsana.*

**Inhale**, raise your left arm high. Trace a huge circle with your fingertips, reaching across the body.

**Exhale**, bend the knees and trace your fingers to the floor.

**Inhale**, cross your right hand across your body as you stand tall, reaching right arm high.

**Exhale,** release your right arm, stand tall.

Repeat three to six times on one side, then transfer to the other. Experiment with weight and gravity, focusing more on the breath and allowing the arms to move and fall organically. Find your own rhythm.

**Optional Extra**

Begin with your feet hip-distance apart, outer edges of the feet parallel. Bow forward over your legs. Roll your inner thighs back, lifting your sit bones high and widening them.

Cup your inner arms with your hands. Keeping the spine long, bend your knees and allow gravity to soften your upper body toward the floor.

Sway your upper body from side to side. Breathe deeply here for ten to twenty breaths.

Bend your knees and, as you inhale, roll up slowly, one vertebra at a time, to stand.

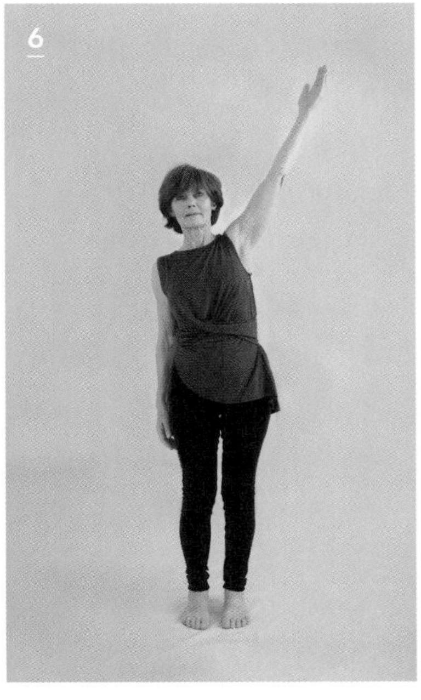
6

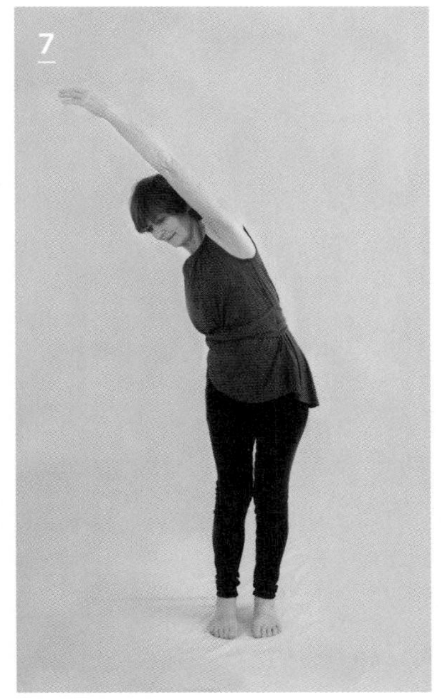
7

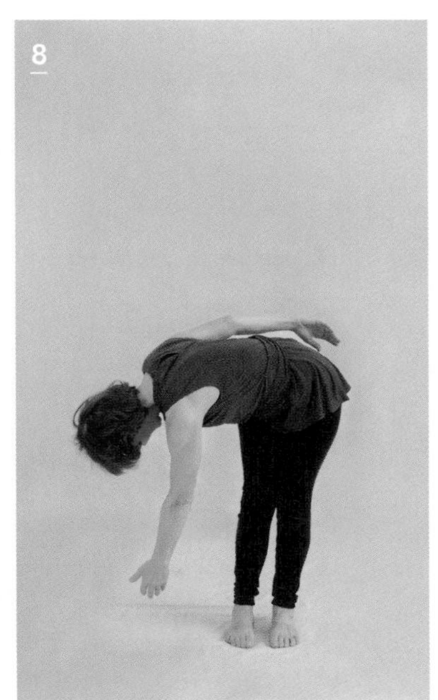
8

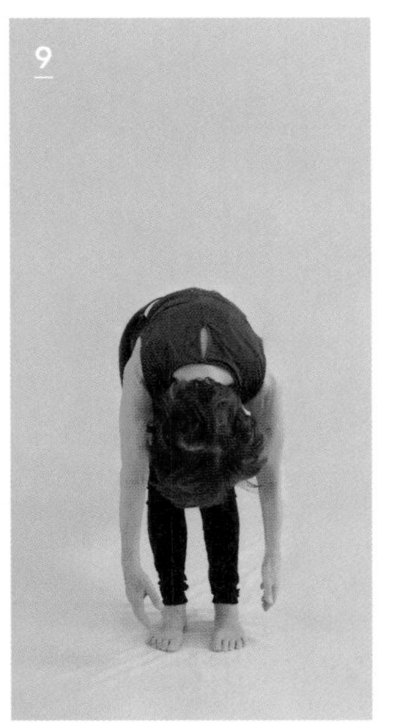
9

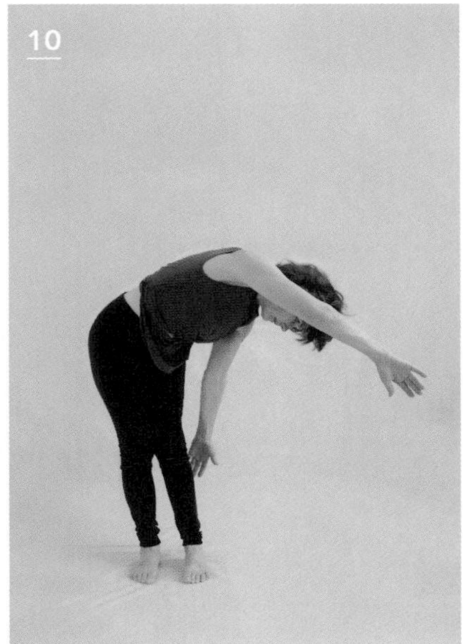
10

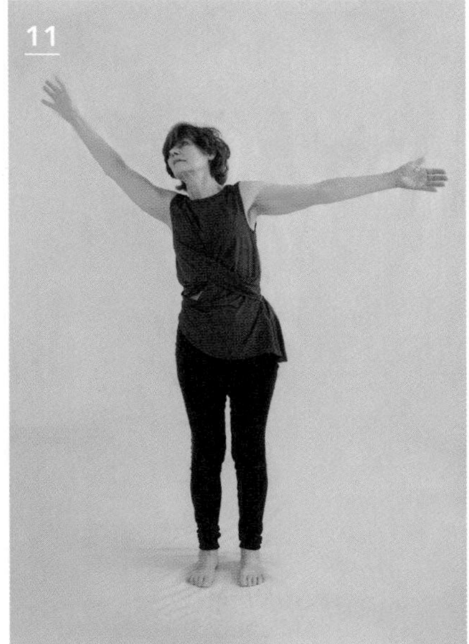
11

### HUMAN OCEAN

A luxurious, rolling way to move through the spine. Feels sensual and hypnotic. I like to explore this with my eyes closed, to feel it better.

**1**

Begin in *Bālāsana* (Child's pose), with the arms stretched out wide and energized, shoulders soft and palms facing the floor.

**2**

**Inhale**, press into the shins to raise your hips, dome the back and draw the navel in.

**3**

Allowing the kinetic chain of movement to snake through the spine, release the hips to the floor. Let the feet open wider than hip-distance apart, with all your toenails touching the mat as the heart lifts and the back bends.

Allow the head to lift as you stretch the arms.

**4**

Slowly lower yourself to the floor, from your belly to your chin.

**5**

Aim to keep your hands underneath your shoulders, then draw the elbows in, press the palms and the toes and lift up to Cobra – whether that is a low one or a high one with fully stretched arms or keeping the elbows bent.

**6, 7, 8 & 9**

Slow down if your lower back begins to feel tender. Press into your knees to lift your hips up and back, with a little arch of the back, before returning to *Bālāsana*.

Repeat slowly, working with the breath to explore the slinkiness of movement.

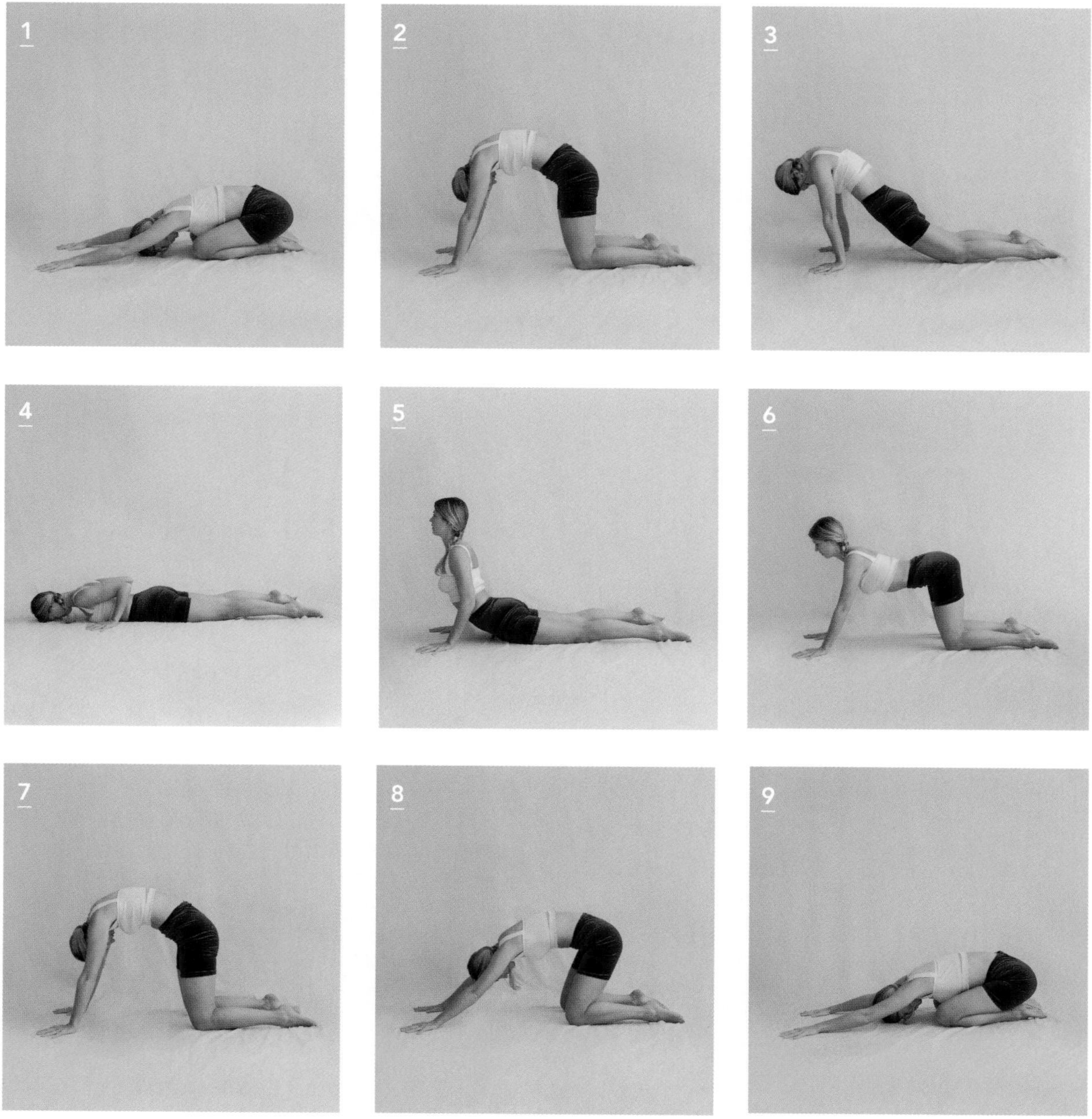
1
2
3
4
5
6
7
8
9

## BACK TO THE SOURCE

This is what I do after *prāṇāyāma*, to greet my body before asking more of it. This sequence is great for those with tight hamstrings, glutes or discomfort in the back. You will need two cork blocks and a strap or belt.

**1**

Place one brick behind you lengthways, on the thin edge. With your knees bent, slowly lie back on the block, using your elbows to support you. The block should sit between the shoulder blades, with the top resting just below the cervical spine (neck).

Place the other block widthways under the back of the skull. Bring your arms by your side, palms facing up. Allow the arm bones to roll away from the body.

Relax and breathe, feeling the chest open. This can be an intense stretch, so feel free to lower both blocks, ask a teacher to assist you or leave it out.

**2**

Remove the blocks and ease the body down onto the mat. Bend your knees and rock them from side to side, then let them settle on the right side. Draw the knees towards the navel for a deeper twist.

Reach out your arms and gaze to the left hand. Soften the shoulders. Allow the legs to be heavy. As you breathe in, feel the ribs expand. As you breathe out, invite the twist to be found.

**3**

Return to the centre. Cross the right shin over the left thigh, to create a little triangle. Interlink your fingers around the left shin or thigh.

Maintain a neutral pelvis. There should be a natural arc in the lower back. Take a deep inhale. As you exhale, squeeze the thigh or shin towards you. Breathe deeply here for a few minutes, exploring where the stretch travels through your body.

**4**

Release, then cross the right thigh over the left thigh. Reset the hips. Hold the shins or the ankles, flex the feet and bring the lower legs to a right angle. Begin to ease the feet towards you, to feel a deep opening at the back of the pelvis.

Inhale, use the hands to pull the legs towards you and resist that effort by pressing the legs into the hands. Breathe here twice. On an exhale, release the effort and gradually pull the legs towards you for a more profound stretch.

Relax, notice how your body feels, and then repeat on the other side.

**5**

Bend your legs and hook the strap just below the ball of the right foot, holding an end of the strap in each hand. Inhale and stretch the right leg, but keep the shoulders on the floor, sliding down the back so the neck is long, and keep the chin gently tucked.

Try stretching the left leg. If that is too much, keep it bent. Activate the right leg, pressing into the belt.

**6**

Hold the strap in the right hand and place your left hand on your hip to weigh it down. Slowly circle the right leg out to the side. If the left hip begins to lift, you've gone too far. Keep the left foot flexed throughout. See if you can work with the breath to ease into this position a little more.

Return the right foot skywards. Move the strap to your left hand and place your right thumb in your right hip crease to pin that hip down.

Slowly cross the right leg to the left, stopping when the right hip begins to lift. This might not be very far, but you will feel a stretch. Explore with your breath.

Return to centre, release the leg and take a few moments to drink in the difference.

Repeat on the other side.

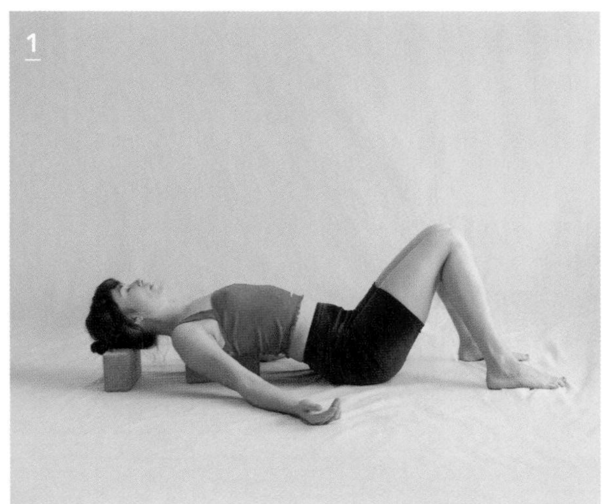
1

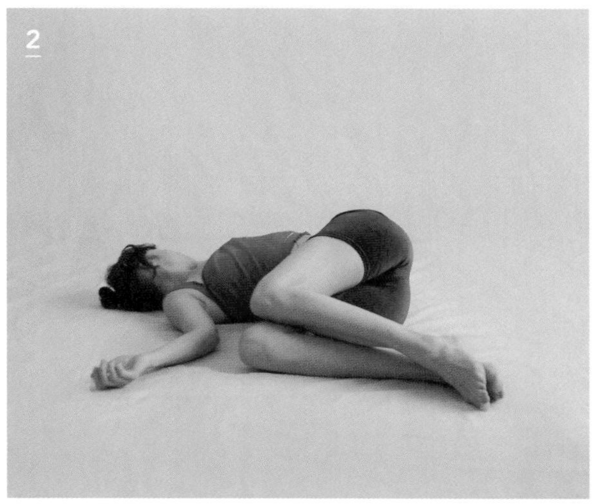
2

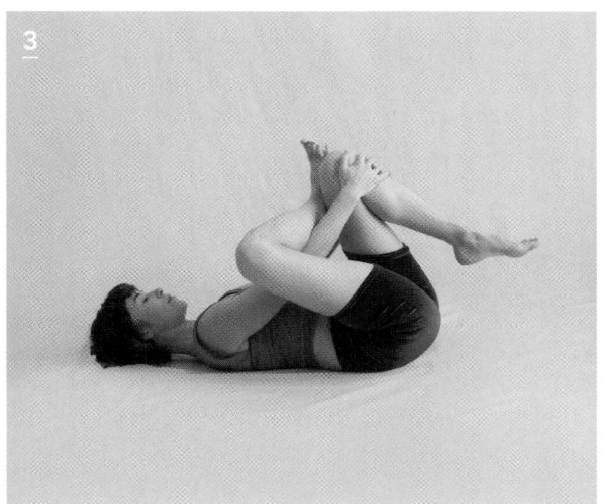
3

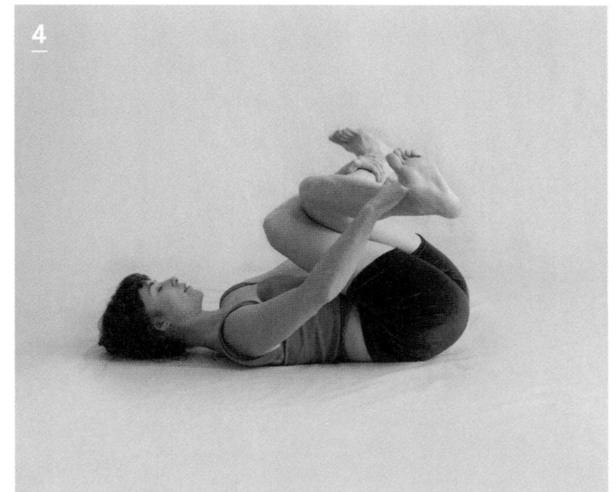
4

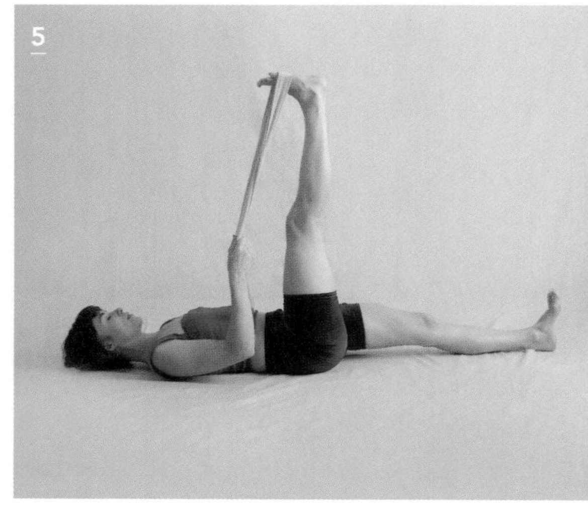
5

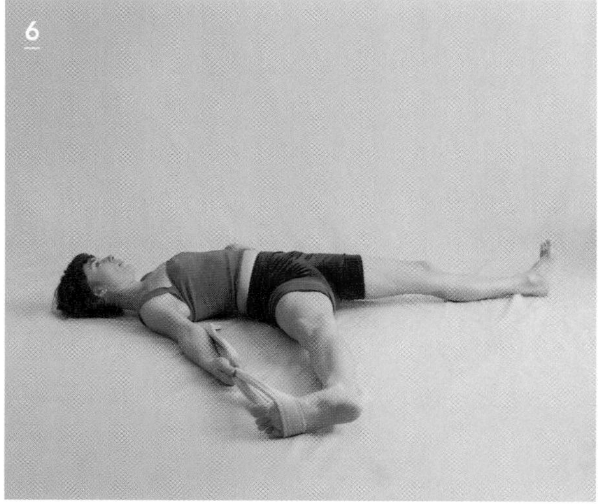
6

## EARTHLY CONSTELLATIONS

These are a few poses to slow the body down, allowing it to soothe, to fold into itself and also ease open in a deep and passive way, often surrendering into gravity to coax space and invite openings.

### 1 & 2

**Paśćimottānāsana**

Sit with your legs together, knees bent and feet flexed. Adjust yourself so you're sitting on the crest of your sit bones, with the pelvis tilted forwards, and a little internal rotation of the thighbones.

Inhale and telescope length through the spine. With the fingertips either on the floor by the legs, or lightly resting on the shin bones, begin to hinge forwards. When the spine begins to round, come back until you can keep it straight.

If you have open hamstrings, you can begin to stretch the legs as well.

Breathe here for a few minutes. Then stretch the legs and allow the spine to relax forward.

There are two ways to come out of *Paśćimottānāsana*. If your spine is straight, hinge up at the hips, retaining the length. If it is rounded, climb up slowly, one vertebra at a time.

### 3 & 4

**Jānu Śīrṣāsana**

Sitting up, squeeze the right knee in towards you. Point it out to the side with the right foot flexed, pressing onto the inner seam of the left leg. You can place a block underneath the knee for support.

Activate the left leg by flexing the foot and lighting up the thigh muscles. Retaining length through the spine, reach the fingertips on the floor.

**Inhale**, lengthen up through the spine.

**Exhale**, pivot the ribs to the left and begin to hinge at the hips and bow forwards. As before, the pose is more active if you keep the length through the back.

**Inhale** to rise and repeat on the other side.

### 5

**Upaviṣṭa Koṇāsana**

Reach your hands behind you for support as you yawn open your legs as wide as you can without it being too uncomfortable. You can bend your knees and flex the feet.

Press into your hands to lift the hips up, and replace them with the pelvis tilting forwards, so you are resting onto the edge of your sit bones.

Use your hands to rotate the thighbones inwards to create more space through your seat.

**Inhale**, let the breath thread length through the spine, with the fingertips resting on the floor.

**Exhale**, begin to fold forwards at the hips.

Lengthen with each inhale and explore a deeper fold with each exhale. As before, experiment with keeping the spine long or rounding.

Bend the knees, place the hands underneath and use them to bring the legs to the centre.

### 6

**Tarāsana**

Bring the soles of the feet together to create a diamond shape with the legs. You can place a block under each knee for support.

Use the hands to tilt the basin of the pelvis forwards, as above. Shuffle around until you feel you have the prime position.

**Inhale** deeply, sitting tall.

**Exhale** and bow forwards. Tune your consciousness into sensation. Witness every single pulse of feeling as it arises, and breathe until it falls away and another arises it its space. Feel the longing of the body to ease and softly open.

1

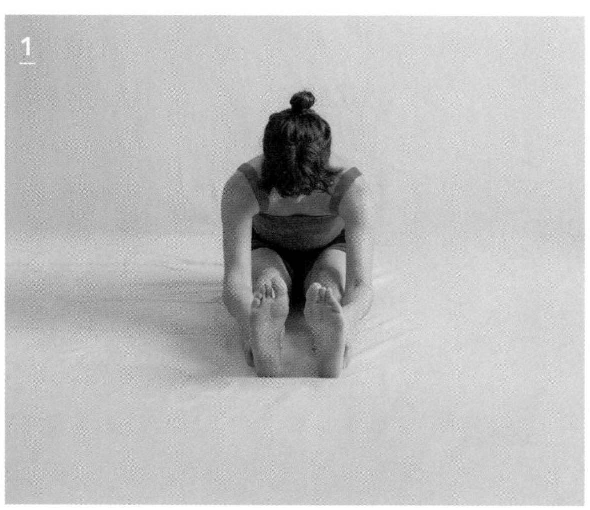

2

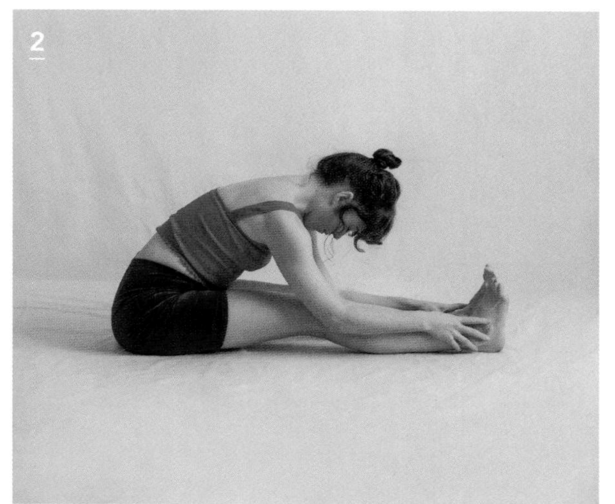

3

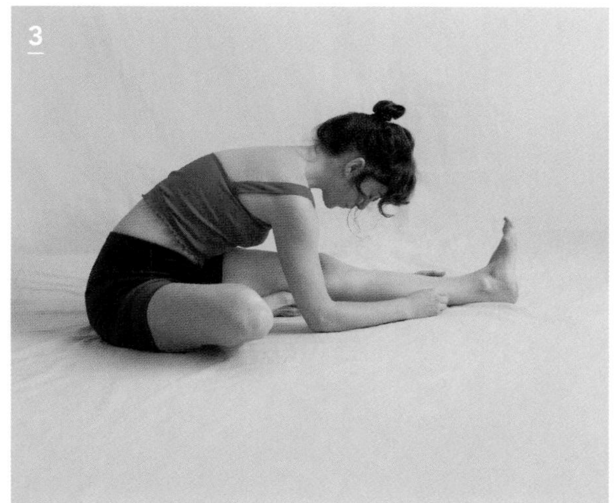

4

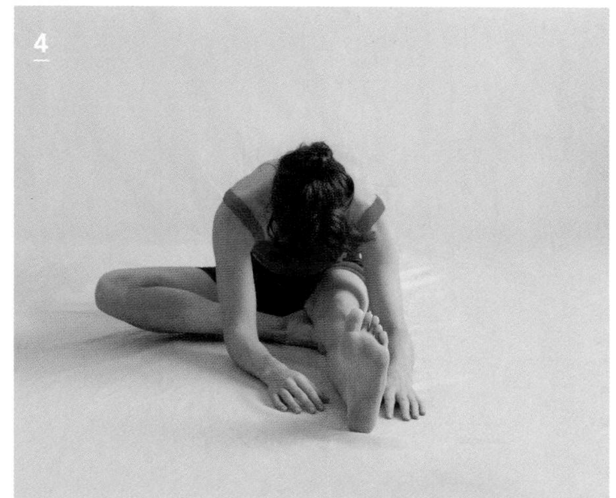

5

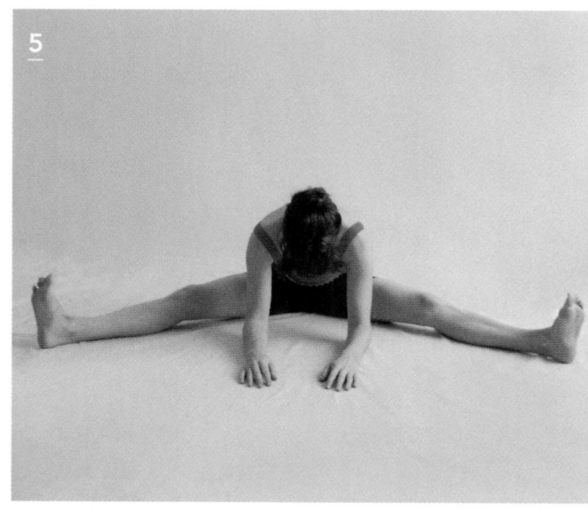

6

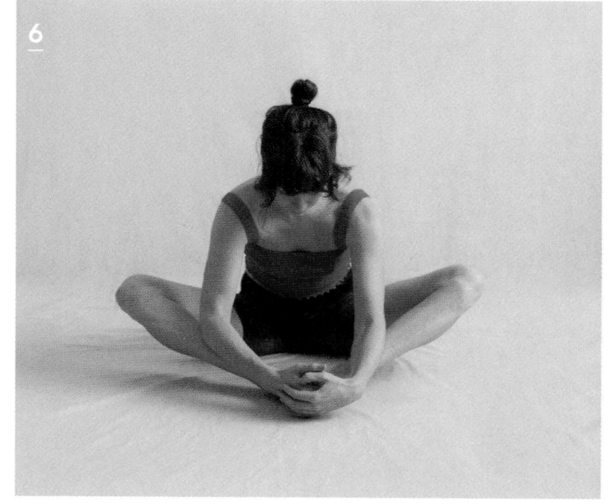

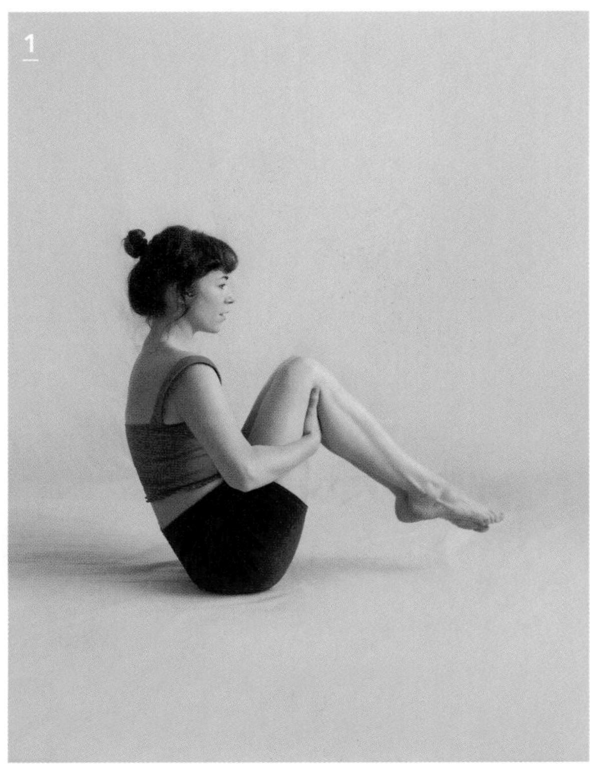
1

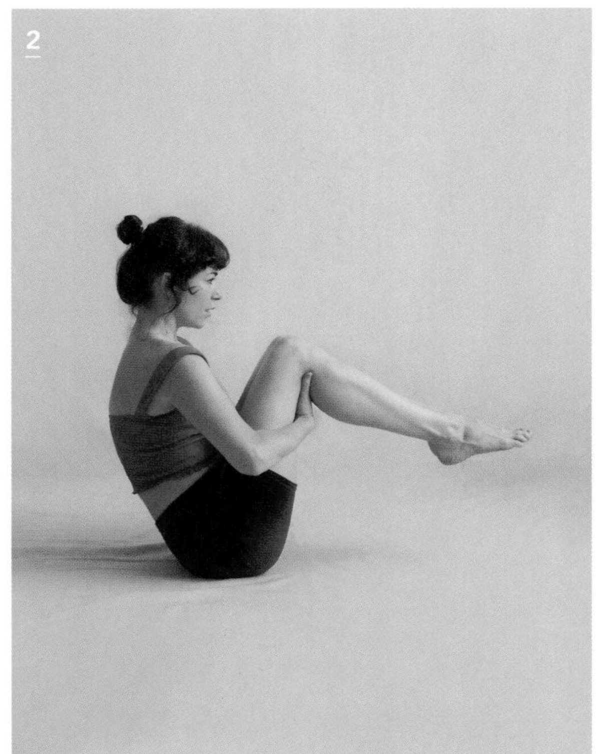
2

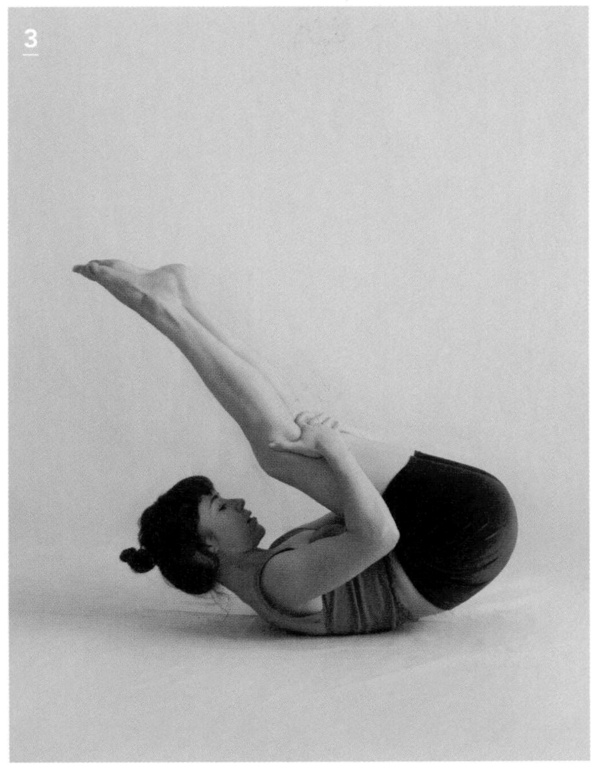
3

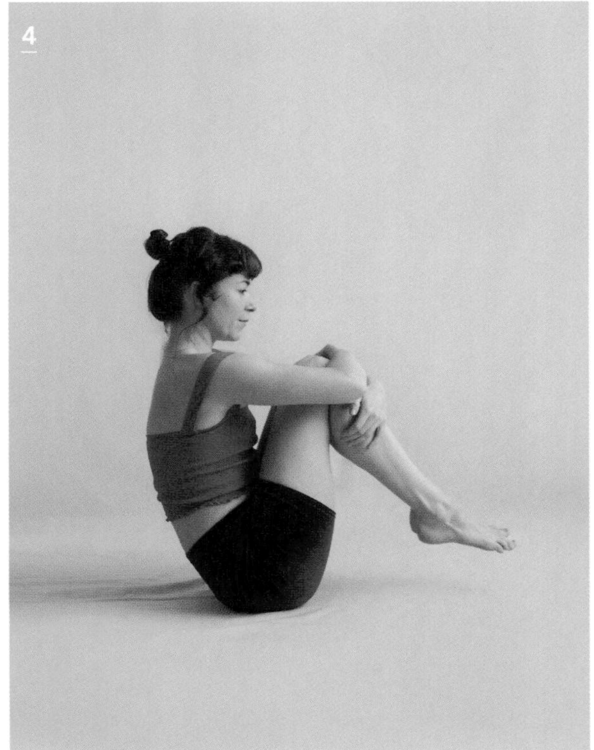
4

## ROCK & ROLL

I can rarely resist sneaking this sequence into a self practice. It's great if the long muscles that frame the spine to keep you upright, called the erector spinae, become a little tense or ropey. I also moderate it to include my glutes, so they receive a little love as well.

**1**

Bend your knees and bring your legs together, tucking the fingers at the back crease of the knees. Lift the feet and begin to squeeze the legs in towards the body. If you're afraid of rolling back too fast, stretching your legs out a little will slow you down.

**2**

Round your spine, hovering back on your sit bones and scooping the navel inwards.

**3**

Allow gravity to tip you backwards, then use the feet to keep the momentum going and pull you forwards and backwards. Your legs will naturally straighten behind you and rebend as you surface.

Notice the parts where you have the most tension or least flexibility – the rocking and rolling will become a little bit jagged, and you'll have to work really hard, or build up to your spine making full contact with the mat.

You can get your glutes involved by rolling up and tipping and twisting slightly to the left, and as your roll back your body will aim to the right.

**4**

End by balancing on the sit bones, then stretch the legs out in front of you.

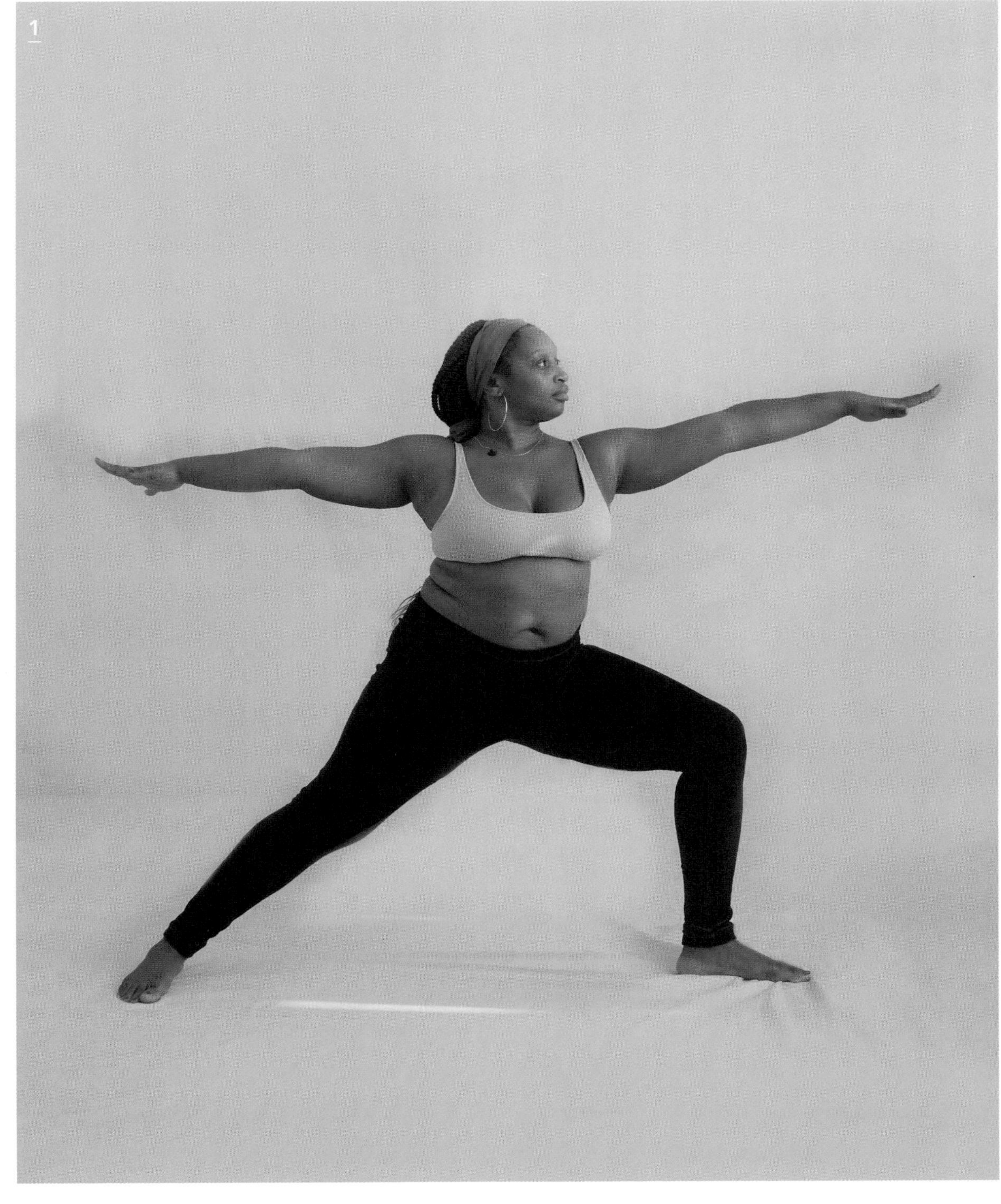
1

## SUN IN MY HEART

This is a flow I return to in my personal practice, adapting and evolving it to include different variations, generally working the upper body and the arms in more fluid or circular flotations.

Standing postures like these feel confrontational, grounding and empowering. I find they tame my disobedient mind and make me feel strong.

**Foundation**

As with all standing poses, consciously setting up the architecture of your foundation through the feet, legs and pelvis gives you more support to liberate your upper body and move freely.

For the first three poses in this flow, the position of the feet is the same:

Stand facing to the right, with your feet parallel.

Raise your arms to shoulder height, parallel to the floor.

Step your feet apart so they are directly underneath the wrists.

Pivot on the heel of the left foot so your toes point forwards, which externally rotates the left thigh.

Turn on the heel of your right foot to point the toes forwards as much as you can, which will internally rotate the right thigh. This is more challenging.

Notice the feet. The back foot tends to collapse inwards, or the toes can sneak backwards. Anchor into the outer right foot while actively lifting the arch and spreading the toes.

Press into the ball of the front foot, across to the mound of the little toe. Focus on smoothing the skin inside the ankle by lifting the arch of the foot.

By awakening the feet, you will subtly tune the alignment of the legs and pelvis while activating the leg muscles.

1

**Vīrabhadrāsana II**

Facing to the right, find alignment with the feet and legs, as described opposite.

Ground through the outer edge of the back foot, and reach through the fingertips of the right hand as you bend the left knee. If the knee goes past the ankle, step the front foot further forwards. Ensure the knee isn't rolling inwards by externally rotating the left thigh, so the knee is directly above the foot. Root through the back leg for strength and support.

The alignment of the pelvis varies from person to person. How far forward your right hipbone is will depend on how open the muscles in your groin are. Once you have the correct alignment of the feet, the rest should follow more naturally. If possible, go to a class and ask a yoga teacher to learn what works for you.

Drop your weight through the sacrum, to lower more deeply into the pose. The front leg stays bent at 90 degrees. Allow the natural curve of the lower spine to flow. If the lower ribs are popping out, soften them into the belly.

Slide the shoulder blades down the back and reach the fingertips actively away from each other, with a bright lift of the heart.

Grow the stem of the neck, broaden the back of the skull and keep the gaze (*dristi*) softly forwards, in one spot.

I usually stay in each pose of this sequence for at least eight breaths. Sometimes I feel the fire and commit for longer, meeting sensation as the challenge and feeling the textures shift in temperature and colour.

*continues >*

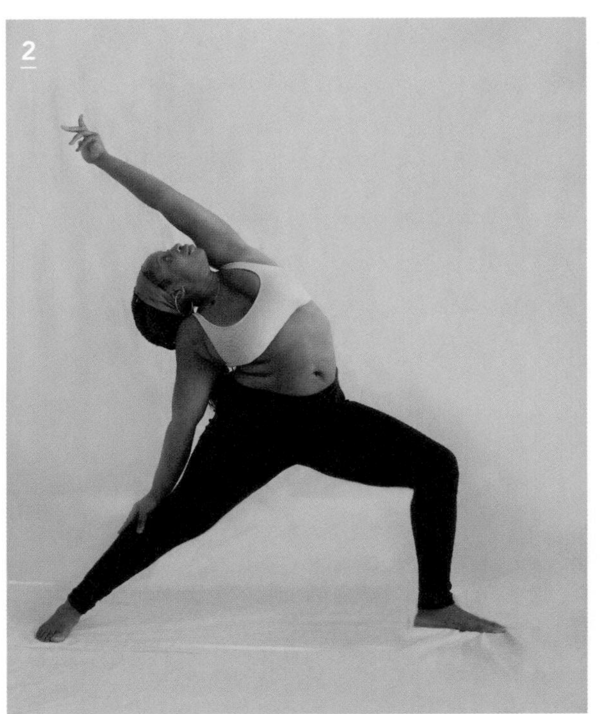
2

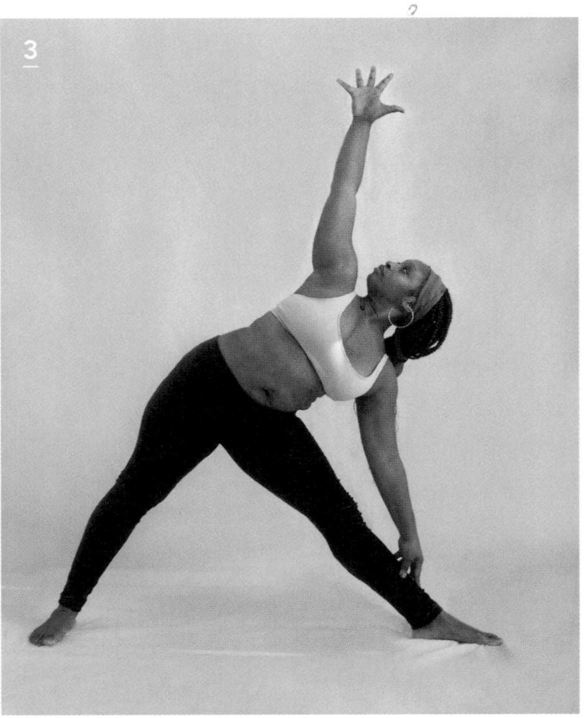
3

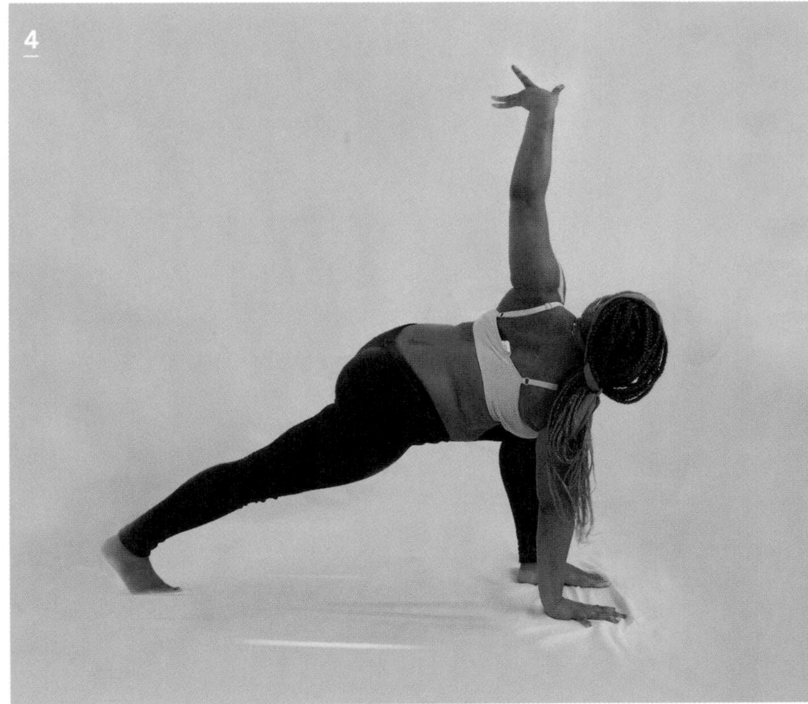
4

## SUN IN MY HEART *continued*

**2**

### Viparita Vīrabhadrāsana

Starting in *Vīrabhadrāsana II*, turn the palm of the left hand to the sky.

As you inhale, circle the left arm skywards as you slide the right hand down the back of the right leg.

Keep the shoulder soft, rotate the chest forwards and lift up from the back of the heart to create a gentle backbend.

**3**

### Trikoṇāsana

Coming out of *Viparita Vīrabhadrāsana*, inhale and straighten the front leg, otherwise maintaining that beautiful alignment.

**Exhale** and lift out of the backbend, raising the torso and reaching the left hand forwards towards your shin, lifting up and out of the left hip socket.

Place the left hand lightly on the left shin. Resist dropping the body weight into the hand. Keeping the legs active, draw the left thighbone into the left hip socket and root through the back foot.

Rotate the right side of the torso skywards, ensuring the right shoulder isn't rolling forwards.

Lift the heart and radiate outwards from the sternum to the fingertips.

Slowly turn to gaze at your right fingers.

**4**

### Parivṛtta Aṅjaneyāsana

Coming out of *Trikonāsana*, circle your right hand forwards, placing it on the ground directly under the shoulder. Allow the back heel to lift, and the toes to face the front of the mat.

Keep the back leg fully energized, as in Plank pose. Activate the thigh muscles and check that the knee doesn't bend. Have both the feeling of drawing the muscles of the legs inwards, while the bones reach out of the pelvis.

Reach the left arm skywards and rotate the chest to twist. Keep the neck long and the shoulders moving down the back to lift the heart.

### Transitioning

I like to add these standing poses into a sequence, like a *Sūrya Namaskār* (see pages 80). I transition from Downward-Facing Dog by floating one leg high on an inhale, then as I exhale, I lunge it forwards between my hands. As I inhale, I press the front foot down into the ground and circle the opposite arm forward then overhead as I make my way to stand in *Vīrabhadrāsana* I, raising the other arm to complete the pose.

## ŚAVĀSANA

*Śavāsana* translates as Corpse pose. This is an invitation to notice the profound shift within, and sense the space without. It's particularly nutritious to practise this restful abandon at the end of an *āsana* and movement ritual, or even after breath work. When you're busy, it's tempting to barrel into the day, but please take this time to bathe in the afterglow of your practice. The more you can relax into stillness, the more receptive your body is to all the goodness you've just worked hard to cultivate. The body needs time to witness itself and just be with the sensations as they come, one rich moment followed by another, each one unique.

Your body cools down fast, so make sure you are cosy – put on some warm clothes or cover yourself with a blanket. If you have a tender lower back, you might like to place a bolster under the knees.

Lie down. Take a little time to arrange yourself, working with the architecture of the body so you feel spacious, in a supported sprawl.

Set your feet wider than hip-distance apart and let them roll away from the body. Place your arms alongside the body with the palms open, receptive.

Press lightly into the elbows, forearms and the back of the skull to gently arch the lower back and raise the shoulders away from the floor. Slide the shoulder blades down the back and slowly return the upper back to the earth.You will notice the wrists shift towards the feet.

Press into the heels, bending the knees to lift the hips an inch or so and pull them in the direction of the feet to tease more length through the spine. Return the hips to the earth.

Lift the heels and move the feet away from the hips. See if you need to release the shoulders again.

Once you've tweaked the placement of your limbs, allow the weight of the body to sink.

Bring attention to your forehead. Soften your temples, relax the skin around the eyes. If your eyelids flutter, open them and then lower them slowly and consciously, as if you're closing curtains.

Soften the jaw. Let the tongue rest heavy. Feel the skull sink, surrender to gravity. Focus on softening.

Envision a liquid quality inside the skull and allow it to spread across the floor. Feel the bones of the face float skywards – the forehead, the cheekbones, the nose and the bones around the eyes. Continue the surrender of the skull into the core of the earth.

Let the top of the neck ease out of the skull. Feel the spread of the shoulders relax and release. Find space in the shoulder girdle. Ease relief into the chest. Feel the bones of the arms weigh down. Soften the elbows, wrists and knuckles and feel the palms taste the intimacy of space. Empty the thumbs, release the skin under the fingernails.

Bring attention to your pelvis, allow it to sink and spread. Feel the thighbones ease out of the pelvis, surrender them into the floor. Let the thighs and the calf muscles ungrip. It takes time. Notice the weight of your heels, and soften the toes as they touch space. Release any muscular tension in your legs.

Allow time to do its thing, letting everything sink and settle. You can't force this process. Just let go of you bones, then let go a little more. Count back from twenty and allow the natural resistance to softness to release.

Lie here for as long as it takes. Most of us are easily distracted. The more resistant the mind, the more essential the process. It's a practice of remembering to come back, again and again.

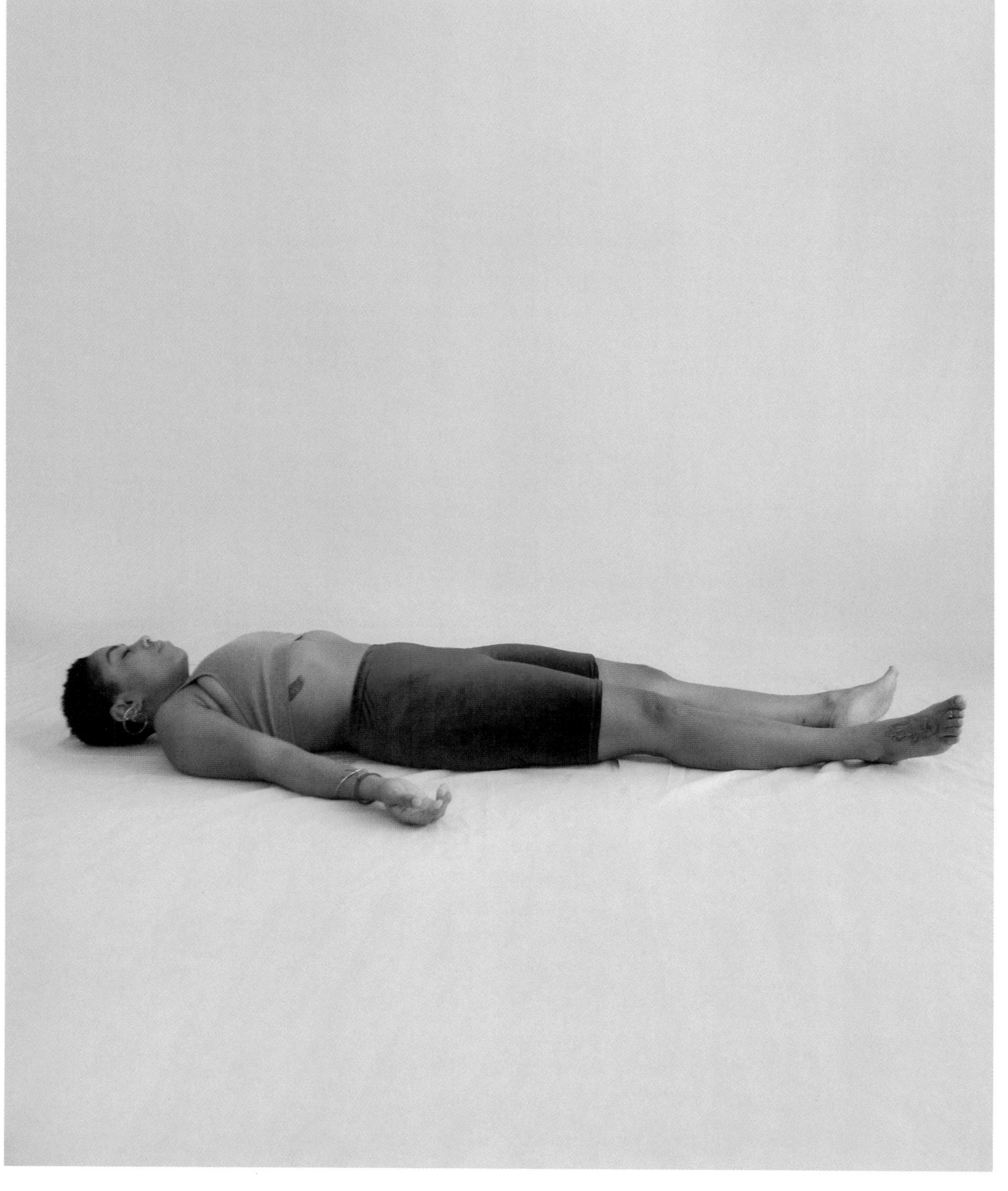

# PRĀṆĀYĀMA

Healthy breathing is a cornerstone to our vitality and creativity. This section looks at how we can rehabilitate healthy breathing habits, explore the breath as a diagnostic tool to understand our physical and mental health, and how to utilize different breathing patterns to create physiological and atmospheric shifts in the body.

*Prāṇāyāma* is much more than this, though. It can transport us into a totally different plane of consciousness, blasting through the banality of the mind into a cosmic state of awareness where our body dissolves into space and time stands still. I use *prāṇāyāma* to help me come home to my body, melt away any stress, light up my brain and soften to receive nourishment and answers.

## WHAT IS PRĀṆĀYĀMA?

*Prāṇā* means life force in Sanskrit, and *yama* is to restrain or control. So in *prāṇāyāma*, we restrain or control the flow of the breath to free and enhance our vital energy, and to expand our mind.

The word inspire comes from the Latin *inspirare*, "to breathe or blow into". It can still be understood to mean inhale, but is most commonly used as "to fill (someone) with the urge or ability to do or feel something, especially to do something creative; to create a feeling, especially a positive one, in a person".

Our vitality, impetus, drive and creativity all come from our capacity to inhale, and *prāṇāyāma* can make us feel better in ten minutes. It's also free – you don't need any space to move and you can do some of the practices without anyone even noticing that you are doing them, at work, in a café or on public transport.

I practice *prāṇāyāma* every single day and have a series of different breathing patterns that I work with to change my atmosphere and bring clarity and focus. I turn to these practices to deal with my emotional health: if I have a shock, a challenging conversation or am just feeling a bit low on power. I also use practices that can induce an altered state of consciousness, where I sometimes have pleasant colourful and psychedelic experiences or a cathartic release (a good cry!)

We breathe all the time, about 20,000 times a day. Ancient yogis believed that our lives are measured not in years, but in breaths. We enter the world with a certain amount of breaths, so the longer it takes for us to spend them, the longer we'll live.

In general, though, we barely notice how we breathe. Yet how deeply and slowly we are breathing is an indicator for our state of mind. The deeper and more fully you breathe naturally, the calmer you will be. The breath is also a wonderful way to anchor the mind in the present and in the body. If you're ever in a panic, focusing on the breath will land you back in your body immediately. A *vinyasa*, or flow, yoga practice with a breath count embodies this knowledge to transform movement into a profound meditation.

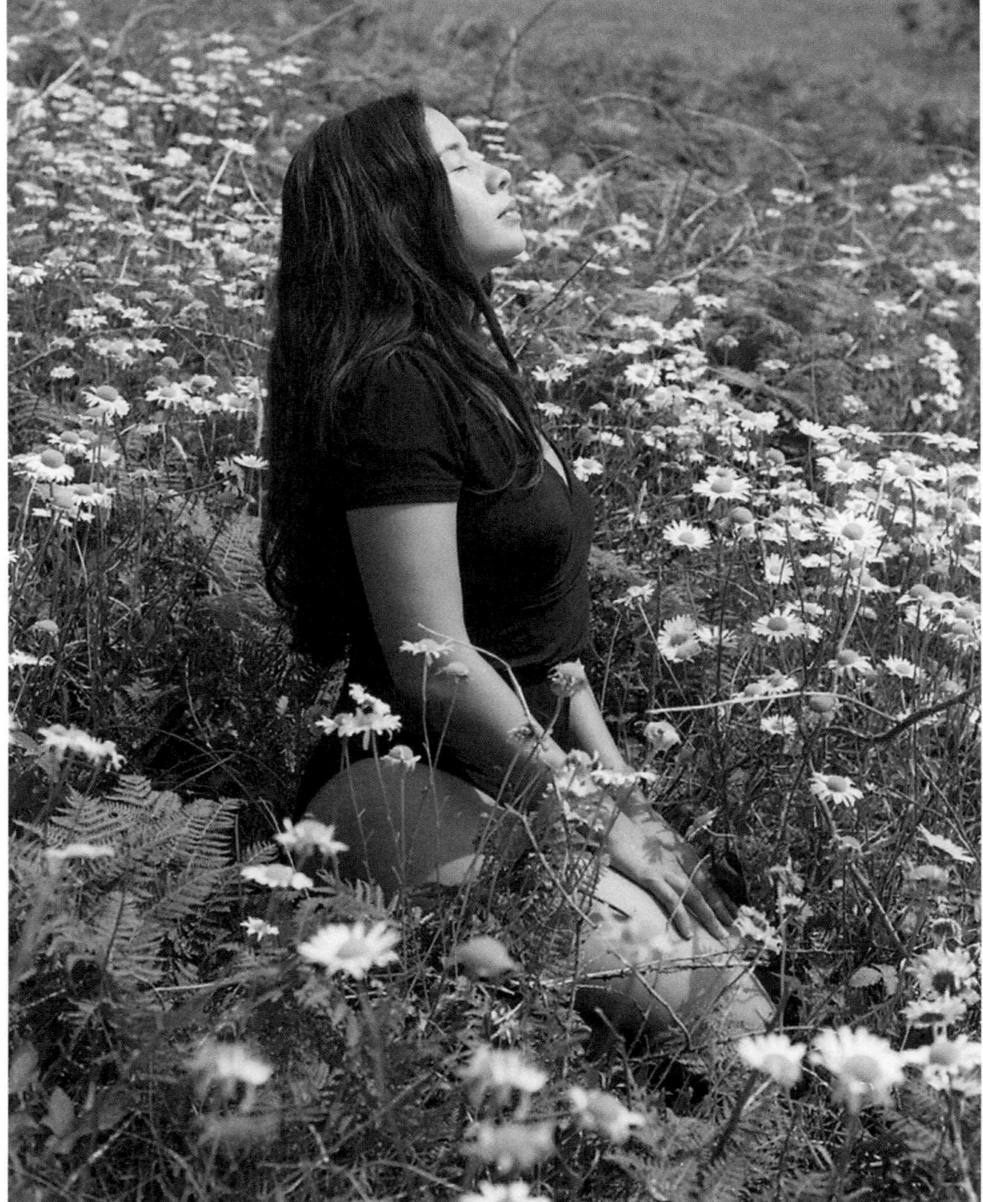

## OPTIMAL BREATHING PATTERNS

Many of us don't have functional breathing patterns. The best way to breathe is deeply – globally (see page 129) or horizontally (see opposite page). The bottom of the lungs is where there is the richest blood supply, and the main function of the lungs is to help oxygen from the air we breathe enter our red blood cells, which will then deliver it to every single cell in our body. The lungs also help us get rid of carbon dioxide as we breathe out. So, deep breathing means more efficient detoxification of our entire body and better nutrition to our cells.

Most of us breathe unhealthily, which is a result of a desk-bound, modern life. When we were babies, we all had a nutritious way of breathing with huge expansive breaths. But from the age of about five, most of our breathing habits changed, and our breaths became more shallow, probably as a result of sitting down at desks at school. When our breathing is shallow, we're only sipping in air and have to work harder by breathing faster. We also recruit muscles around the neck and shoulders to help us, which creates tension.

When we breathe, our ribcage expands, our diaphragm (the dome-shaped muscular shelf at the bottom of the lungs that divides our internal organs from our thoracic cavity) contracts and flattens. This causes the lung capacity to increase and pull air in. The internal organs, including the kidneys, descend a centimetre or two (a bit under an inch), which creates an internal massage that moves the fluid around and keeps us healthy.

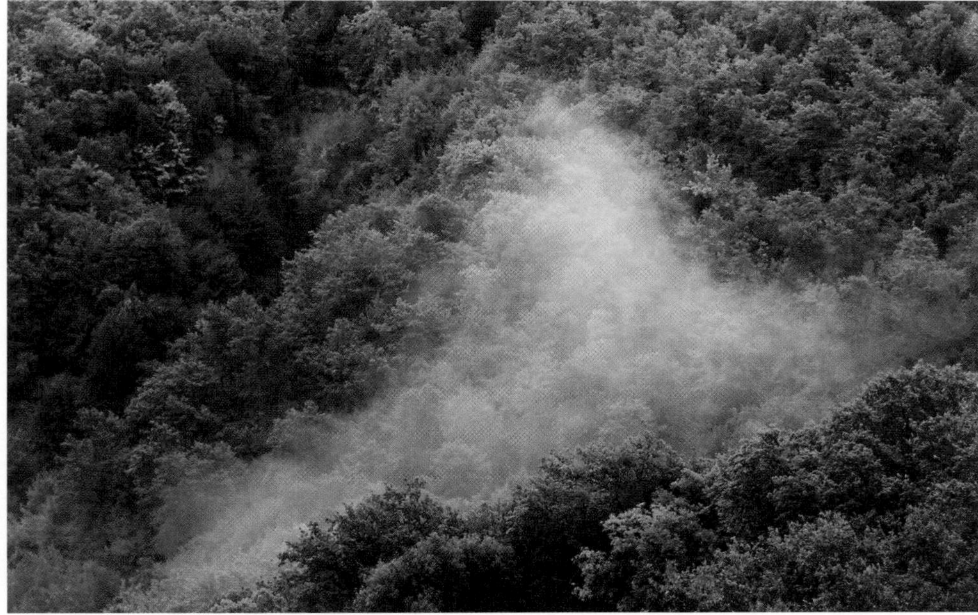

When our breath is malfunctioning, it affects our whole body and life. It influences sleep, memory, anxiety levels, adrenal glands, heart rate and acidity levels, not to mention contributing to back pain.

### HOW DO YOU BREATHE?

Breathing expert Belisa Vranich has devised a method to check on whether you are breathing healthily, with an easy practice to begin to explore better ways of breathing. Take a deep breath in – do you sit taller? As you exhale, do you sit a little lower? If you do, then your breathing is malfunctioning. The best way to breathe is slowly, into the bottom lobes of the lungs, horizontally into the side ribs. As you exhale, you sit taller.

#### PRACTICE

In a seated position, breathe in and round the spine as you curve forward. As you breathe out, sit taller and feel the spine's natural inclination to lengthen. The practices below will help you discover the depth of your lungs and breathe more mindfully.

### THE BENEFITS OF DEEP BREATHING

A breath with a longer and slower exhalation invites the parasympathetic into dominance. The parasympathetic, as described earlier, is our body's relaxation response. It puts on the brakes, tells us we are OK and safe to rest. When this happens, our heart rate slows and we release endorphins, the body's natural painkillers. We also release the chemical called dopamine into our brain, which makes us feel happy.

Deeper breathing improves our blood flow, as we saw above. When we breathe deeply, we have more oxygen in our blood, causing our blood vessels to dilate, which means the flow is easier and we put less pressure on our cardiovascular system.

Deep breathing is also a natural way to relieve anxiety. According to a fascinating study in 2017 by Mark Krasnow, a professor of biochemistry at the Stanford University School of Medicine, a small group of neurons in the brain, dubbed the "pacemaker for breathing" and technically called the pre-Bötzinger complex, communicates respiratory information to another structure in the brain (the locus coeruleus) that is responsible for generating different states of arousal.

These nerve cells spy on how you are breathing – what is going on in your respiratory control centre, whether you are breathing slowly or sipping in air in short bursts. According to this information, the locus coeruleus then sends projections through the brain, which sets in motion a chain of responses that ultimately lead an emotional state of rest, alert, arousal or sleep. So, if we slow the breath, we signal directly to the brain that we are relaxed. The brain will then start a chain of biochemical and psychophysical responses that work with the parasympathetic to calm the whole body.

## BANDHAS

*Bandhas* are energetic "locks" or "valves" within our body that we can engage in order to contain and harness our life force, our *prāṇā*, and direct it into our *sushumna nadi*, the energetic highway threaded through our spine. I use them a lot in *prāṇāyāma*, particularly at the end of a round of breath work. By closing these valves, you can effectively consolidate the *prāṇā* within your body. When I disengage the locks after holding my breath, I often feel this intensely blissful wave of release tingle throughout my body.

I use *bandhas* throughout my *yogāsana* practice to harness my internal power but I also regularly practice consciously releasing them in full. It is important to be able to fully soften and release, for everyone, but particularly for women who are considering having children one day. If you can't fully relax your pelvic floor, you might find the surrender necessary in giving birth even more challenging.

### MŪLA BANDHA

Also known as the root lock, this prevents the most primal, creative energy from escaping downwards, carrying it up to your navel instead. The best way to describe how to engage *mūla bandha* is to imagine you are desperate to pee, but you have to hold it in – it's those muscles. They're at the bottom of the pelvic floor, behind the cervix (for men, it's the muscles between the anus and the testes). Initially, you may find it hard to isolate them and will probably find that the anus sphincter also activates.

Many practitioners engage *mūla bandha* throughout their full *yogāsana* practice, because it elevates the energy, helps cultivate awareness and also fortifies the pelvic musculature, but I move in and out of it depending on the vibe of my practice. Sometimes I am not trying to fly, I merely want to nestle into myself and experience total softness. It's useful to cultivate this discipline when you begin, however, so you become intimate with the physical and energetic sensation and can go on to choose for yourself where to go with it.

**Inhale** deeply.

**Exhale**, letting your navel pull back and allowing the canopy of your pelvic floor to lift. See if you can see a dart of energy brighten through your spine.

**Inhale**, maintaining the sensation of lifting, and observe the containment.

Experiment with this through your practices.

## UḌḌĪYANA BANDHA

The second of the three main *bandhas* is also known as "upward flying lock". When you engage this lock, you feel all of your internal organs lift up, as if your belly has been vacuum-packed and everything is condensed and shrunken together. Energetically, you will also feel a huge lift.

*Uḍḍīyana Bandha* is gets your digestive fire going, gives your internal organs a good little massage and also works on the internal muscles of the lower back. It's also very potent for *yogāsana*, particularly for inversions or when jumping up or through your hands.

To try engaging *Uḍḍīyana Bandha*, bring your feet hip-distance apart on the floor. Soften your knees and rest your palms on the top of your thighs, just above your knees.

**Inhale** deeply, lift your gaze and feel the belly swell, the back stretch and the lower ribs open and flare like wings.

**Exhale**, fold in half over your legs as you empty the breath from the belly.

Suspend your breath – without inhaling, close your mouth, stretch your arms out straight as you lengthen the spine, tucking your chin to your chest, and allow that action to suction the navel to the spine, the belly back and up towards the bottom of the ribs. Stay here for as long as is comfortable.

**Inhale**, lifting up your chin first and letting the body breathe you.

Repeat five to ten times.

## JĀLANDHARA BANDHA

Commonly known as "chin lock", *jālandhara bandha* intensifies the energy in the top of the chest. As you lock at the throat, the energy is directed downwards towards the navel. I generally practise chin lock in conjunction with other *bandhas*.

You can practise this lock either on the end of the inhalation and the exhalation.

Lift the sternum high, drop the shoulders and drawer the chin back into the throat.

To release, lift the chin.

## PRĀṆĀYĀMA PRACTICES

Here is a spectrum of practices that will evoke different emotional and physiological responses. Explore them all, so you know which one to call on when the time arises.

**Pauses as Portals**

Pauses between breaths are elastic, magnetic moments of cosmic stillness. Stopping the breath has an instant effect on the mind. The longer you pause, the more colourful and potentially psychedelic your experience will be. Both the practices below are also incorporated into the *prāṇāyāmas* described later in this section.

**Kumbhaka: Breath Retention**

*Kumbhaka* is the natural pause between inhalation and exhalation. If we begin to exaggerate this stilling of the breath, we notice the mind will also pause. You can do this within your *āsana* practice, when you are holding shapes for a number of breaths. Many *prāṇāyāmas* work with extending *Kumbhaka* to create magical portals of expansion that lead to a profound shift in the mind and the body. The effect of *Kumbhaka* is enhanced by engaging the *bandhas* (see page 124).

**Viloma: Interrupted Breathing Patterns**

*Viloma* means against the grain: *loma* is the direction that hair grows on skin and *vi* means against. Introduce deliberate pauses to segment or suspend the breath. These pauses in the breath are echoed through the mind and are deep places of stillness and knowing.

## DROP INTO PEACE

When you breathe in this deeply poised, mindful pattern, the mind quietens and awareness slowly opens for you. This is an exercise for all occasions, to be practised absolutely anywhere. Here are two simple patterns, both involving breathing through the nose. I was taught the first one by breath expert Max Strom.

**1**

**Inhale**: 4 counts.

**Hold the breath in**: 7 counts.

**Exhale**: 7 counts.

**2**

**Inhale**: 4 counts.

**Hold the breath in**: 4 counts.

**Exhale**: 6 counts.

**Hold the breath out**: 2 counts.

## UJJAYI

This is a rich breath with an oceanic quality. Use it to carry you through an *āsana* practice. It will heat the body and create a gentle sound for you to focus on to engage your mind. Do not force it to sound like Darth Vader.

Breathe globally (see page 129), in and out through the mouth. On each exhale, imagine fogging up a window in front of you. Do this a few times, and then try closing your mouth and breathing through your nose. Re-create the sense of a vibration as the breath whispers around the glottis at the back of the throat. Smooth out your breath. Breathe very softly, so only you can hear.

### Visualization with Ujjayi

To refine your awareness, imagine that as you inhale, you are drawing the breath down from the chest to the pelvic bowl.

Exhale the pelvic bowl up to the heart. Stay with this image. Feel the breath thread up and down the torso. Harness your attention to this visualization.

Begin to notice the effortless wave of *prāṇā* that carries on the breath. Feel it descend as you inhale, and ascend as you exhale.

Allow your mind to catch on to the hypnotic roll of the breath, as it drifts up and down the body. Find that it becomes effortless, light and joyful.

### Kumbhaka with Ujjayi

As you exhale, introduce a light pause at the end of the breath. With this pause, notice the body and mind coming to stillness. During this gap, the awareness rests in the chest and in a pool of light.

Witness how long you want this pause to last: maybe it is just for an instant, before you inhale.

Continue for five minutes, each time pausing, feeling a luminous swell in the heart.

Stay with the wave of *prāṇā* as it moves from the chest to the pelvic bowl. Observe a natural inclination to draw the pelvic floor up as you exhale and pause. Keep the attention on the posture, keep it tall and still.

The breath is easy, no forcing or straining.

To add another layer, as you hold the breath, engage the pelvic floor, begin to draw the belly in and up. Feel the sensation of light in the heart become more pronounced.

Let your mind be totally absorbed in this sensation. You are learning to train the mind and slow it through suspension of the breath.

Allow your breath to relax and neutralize.

If you have time, this is the perfect moment to segue into a cosmic meditation, where you just witness the mind and allow your thoughts to unfold and evaporate, consciously harbouring the quiet and resisting the temptation to engage with your stories.

Stay, kindling the candle of delicate stillness, and see if you transcend the into a timeless place of colourful lakes and pulsing expansion. The trippy stuff takes time to reveal itself – something to look forward to when you've been practising a while.

### KAPĀLABHĀTI: SKULL-SHINING BREATH

This is what is known as a *kriyā* or cleansing technique. It creates heat, wakes up the core, improves circulation and is generally detoxifying. It's an energetic, "lopsided" *prāṇāyāma*, in which you breathe in and out through the nose.

The after-effects of this breath are lovely and are enhanced if you repeat a few rounds. You may feel colourful, light-headed or even dizzy. This is generally very pleasant and subsides naturally, leaving the mind clear and light. The body, especially the hands (which could be tingly) and the face, may have the sensation of a physical permeability, blending with the space around you. You also have a new appreciation of the length of your spine and the space within your body.

**Exhale**, pulling the navel back to the spine.

**Inhale** by relaxing the belly, allowing it to balloon as the air is drawn effortlessly back into the body.

If this is unfamiliar to you, begin by breathing in and out through the mouth. You can place one palm on your belly to encourage the abdomen back, then feel the belly swell as you inhale.

When you are comfortable with your own pattern of breathing, you can close your mouth and breathe through your nostrils.

Practise for about 30 seconds and increase incrementally up to 60 or whatever feels comfortable for you.

Feel the body becoming brighter and clearer.

## SIṀHĀSANA: LION'S BREATH

A deeply attractive breath that relieves tension in the neck and face, releases the throat, energizes and empowers. Good for getting out the frustrations of the day, when you're feeling angry or claustrophobic.

Sit in *sukhāsana* (see page 74), with your palms clasping your knees, and your fingers open like little paws.

**Inhale** deeply through your nose, rounding your back slightly.

**Exhale** with a hissing "ha" sound, opening your eyes and mouth wide and sticking out your tongue. Gaze to the tip of your nose.

You can also do this with Cat and Cow (see page 84), inhaling as you arch into Cat pose, and exhaling through the mouth as you round into Cow pose.

## GLOBAL BREATHING FOR BEGINNERS

A lovely, gentle, three-part breath to help you remember the full capacity of your lungs and set the shape for the rest of your practice.

Lie on your back with your legs bent, feet hip-distance apart, knees pointing to the ceiling.

Soften your shoulders, reach your neck long, tuck your chin in slightly, keep your jaw slack and your face relaxed.

Breathe slowly in and out of your nose, with your palms resting on your belly.

**Inhale** deeply into your belly: feel your palms rise with your breath.

**Exhale** slowly as your belly releases and descends.

Repeat five times.

Place your hands on either side of the ribs, with your fingers pointing towards each other.

**Inhale** into the side ribs. As your lungs swell, feel your ribcage expand in all directions.

**Exhale** slowly: the ribcage closes, the fingertips knit toward each other.

Repeat five times.

Place your palms below your collarbones, with your fingers woven loosely together.

**Inhale** deeply into the chest and the top of the lungs.

**Exhale** slowly and fully.

Repeat five times.

Release your arms by your sides.

**Inhale** into your belly, side ribs, then chest.

**Exhale** slowly from your chest, side ribs and belly.

Repeat this five times, or as long as you would like.

* You can experiment with pausing at either end of the breath, as mentioned in the section on *Kumbhaka* on page 126.

* You can add some movement, to explore how the breath informs how the body arranges itself. Place your arms by your sides, palms down. As you inhale, slowly float your hips up to the sky and lift your arms over your head in synch with the breath. As you exhale, release your arms alongside your body.

## NĀḌĪ ŚODHANA: ALTERNATE NOSTRIL BREATH

*Nāḍī* means channel, and *Śodhana* is purification, so this is a practice that lets stress descend and clarity, space and colour light up the mind.

Bend your right elbow, tuck your index finger and your middle finger into your palm. Use the thumb of your right hand to close your right nostril, and your ring finger to close your left nostril. You will be alternating breathing through your left and right nostrils.

Close the right nostril with your thumb.

**Inhale** through the left nostril.

Close the left nostril with your finger.

**Exhale** through the right nostril.

**Inhale** through the right nostril.

Close the left nostril with your finger.

**Exhale** through the left nostril.

Close the right nostril with your thumb.

Continue for a few minutes, at whatever pace is comfortable to you.

When you are finished, resume your natural breathing, observe and enjoy. Feel a sense of spaciousness and clarity at the front of the skull.

## SITALI: BREATH TO COOL AND RELAX THE BODY

Perfect if it's a really hot day, or you've had a sweaty practice.

Curl your tongue and stick it just out of your mouth, with your lips wrapped around it.

**Inhale** deeply through your rolled tongue.

**Exhale** slowly through your nose.

Repeat for about three minutes and notice the after-effects.

## BHRAMARI: BEE BREATH TO SOOTHE ANXIETY

I love this breath. It's a wonderful way to quieten the mind and create a soothing vibration throughout the whole body. It also focuses on lengthening the exhalation, which reduces the "fight and flight" stress response.

Press your index fingers gently into your ears.

**Inhale** deeply through nose.

**Exhale**, closing lips and making the sound *mmm*, as if you were humming like a bee.

Continue for five minutes, or as long as it feels good for you. When you stop, relax your breathing, sit tall. Observe and bathe in the thick silence.

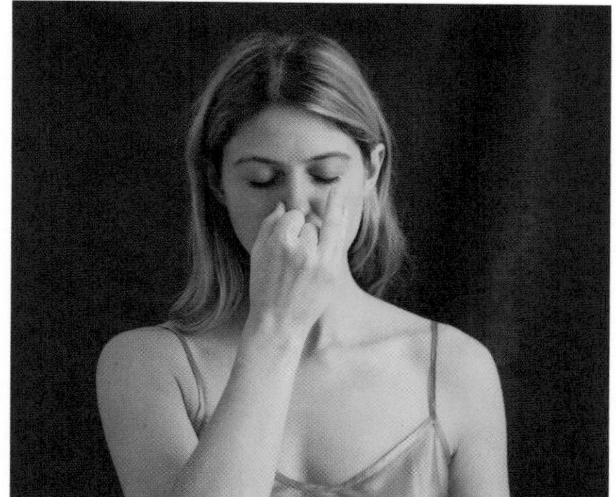

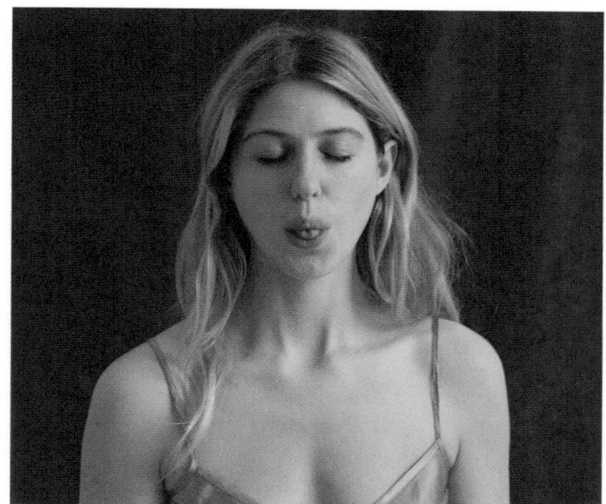

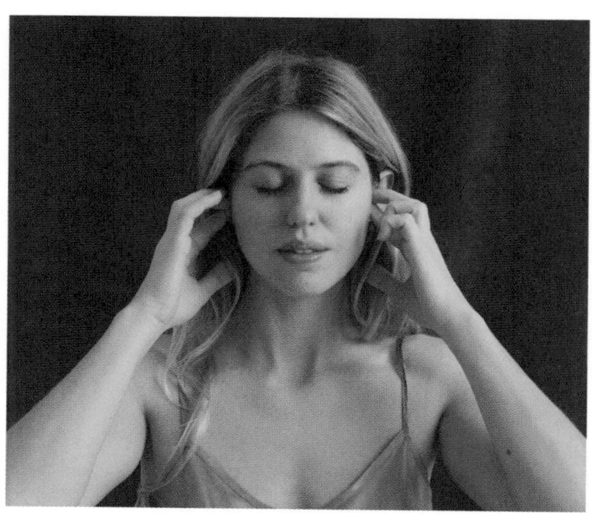

## CAROLYN COWAN'S VAGUS NERVE STRETCH

This is the most immediately soothing *prāṇāyāma* for anxiety or stress. It will deepen the breathing and placate a restless mind. Working with the vagus nerve is a fast-track route to dropping you into your parasympathetic and initiating a potent shift in the emotional and visceral atmosphere of your body. I can't recommend this profound and incredibly effective practice highly enough.

With your fingers linked, make as if you are trying to break your hands free, pulling the elbows away from each other. Resist this force by keeping the fingers tightly interconnected. Feel the arm, neck and shoulder muscles engage.

Now, imagine you are holding a heavy weight with your hands.

**Inhale**, breathing into your belly first, and slowly pull up this imaginary weight, bit by bit on your breath, grounding through the sit bones.

As you reach your hands highest over your head, allow the arm bones to lift the shoulders, pull the upper back higher and stretch the waist. Hold the inhale for a few moments at the top. Tuck your chin in, lift the chest and allow the ribs to flare.

**Exhale**, lifting your chin, lean your head back, stick your tongue out far and stretch your jaw, opening your mouth as wide as you can, and make a hissing sound, as in lion's breath (see page 129).

**Inhale** back to the centre, lift highest with the arms and slowly pivot your head to the right, stretching your neck.

**Exhale** again, audibly, sticking the tongue out, stretching the jaw.

**Inhale** back to the centre again.

**Exhale** to the left, repeating the same actions on this side.

**Inhale** back to the centre, lifting everything high, high, high as you hold the breath at the top.

**Exhale** in the centre, then towards the end of the exhale, slowly release the hands and float them down, finding the arms light and the chest permeable, as a sense of deep peace and tingly softness flows through the body and dust settles in the mind.

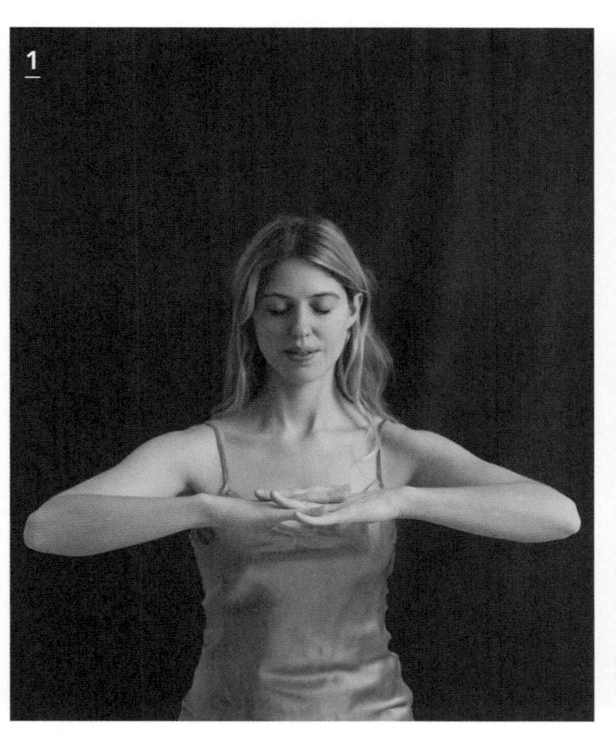
1

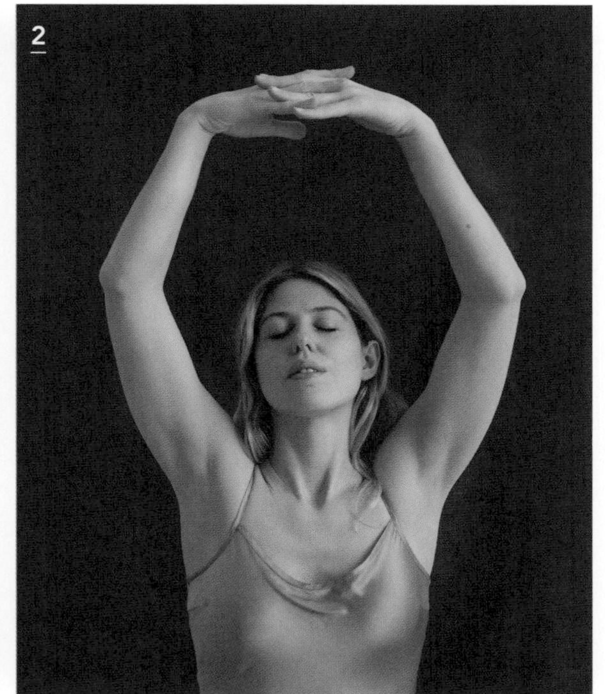
2

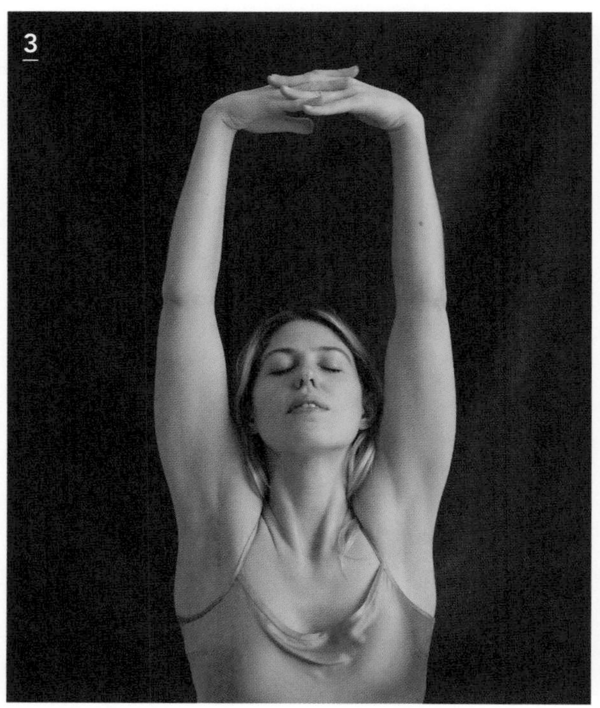
3

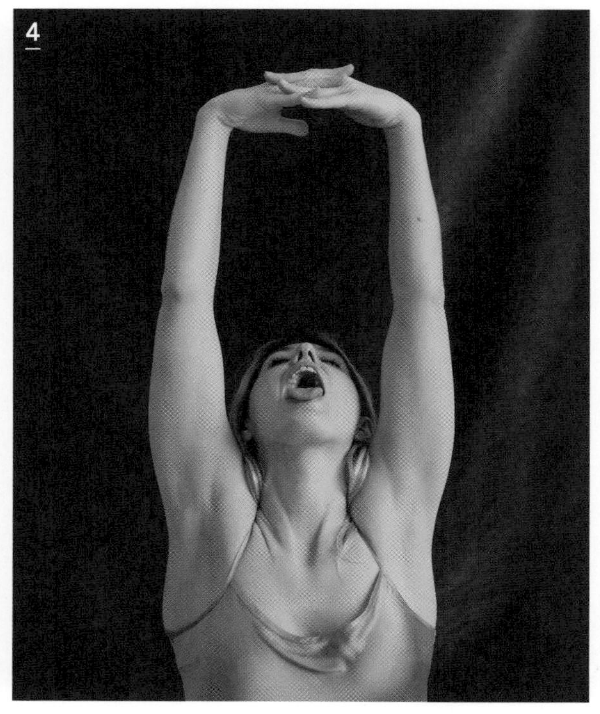
4

## VILOMA INHALATION: ALERT

This is a sweet and short practice to still and brighten the mind, leaving you feeling vivid, grounded and expansive. Great for a little mid-afternoon fix instead of some caffeine.

Sit in a comfortable position. Let yourself arrive and wait for quiet to descend, without working the breath. Observe your inner realm and your personal pulse. The breath is often a barometer of how you are feeling, so observe its texture and length.

Begin *ujjayi* breath, subtly closing the glottis (the space between the vocal cords), so breath can whisper audibly in the throat. Fall into your own cadence of breath.

**Inhale**, feeling the ribs and chest expand.

**Exhale**, maintaining that expansion and lift, emptying the lungs.

Keep doing this for ten slow rounds.

On the next inhale, breathe in to halfway, then pause.

Breathe in to the top of the breath.

**Exhale** slowly, gently, smoothly, until the last drop of air is released.

**Inhale** steadily to halfway.

Expand the ribs in the pause.

**Inhale** full breath.

Continue this for ten rounds.

As you hold the breath at the top, allow the body's natural intelligence to softy engage your pelvic floor, the *mūla bandha*.

After a few rounds of observing this, engage the *jālandhara bandha* or chin lock: lift your chest up to meet your chin, drawing the chin back.

Continue for ten rounds.

In each pause, you softly engage the *mūla* and *jālandhara bandha*. Hold the breath for as long as it feels effortless and natural. If you go beyond this point, you will harden and the practice will be counter-intuitive. Work with the body's natural capacity.

Each time you empty the breath, drink in the spaciousness you have cultivated. Witness how expansive, how broad and open you can become. To borrow a lovely metaphor, think of a jug: each time you breathe, you fill it in all directions: the bottom, sides, back and right up to the brim.

Adjust the length of the rounds to suit your capacity.

Once you have completed the *viloma* practice, allow the breath to relax.

Sink into the stillness and witness.

Feel the global nature and depth of the breath.

Notice the atmosphere of the body, feeling peaceful, grounded and present.

### EXHALATION: SOOTHE INTO SLEEP

This is the perfect breath if you wrestle with yourself when sleep eludes you. You can practise all tucked up in bed or curled up with love. It's also fantastic for any episodes of anxiety or stress – it drops you into a calm place.

Begin by making yourself comfortable, wherever you are.

Scan the body (as always).

Tune into the natural pattern of your breath, notice how it develops and deepens with the simple act of observation.

Cultivate *ujjayi* (see page 127, but do so mindfully, tying your attention to the fine thread of breath as you imagine it entering in a pool through the throat.

Do a few rounds of steady breathing, pausing at top of inhalation and  exhalation.

As you pour air out, feel the emptiness at the bottom. Allow belly to pull into *mūla bhanda*, chest to lift and chin draw back to the throat in *jālandhara bandha*.

After a few rounds, begin to segment the exhale into two parts.

If you are gasping for air, you are breathing too slowly. It needs to be gentle and effortless.

The inhale draws the breath deeply and smoothly into the belly.

The pause in the exhalation slows time and melts the mind.

Do this for ten rounds.

Now divide the exhalation into three parts.

At the end of each part, engage the pelvic floor and retain the expansion of the ribs from the inhalation, through the exhalation.

Continue for ten rounds.

Once you have completed *viloma*, take the deepest, smoothest, long inhale. Hold at the top and soften the body and mind.

Slowly exhale and feel the skin melt.

Bathe in the stillness, looping consciousness through your breath.

# MUDRAS

I love the history and symbolism of *mudras*, and experience a magnetic charge of energy when I work certain ones. In her wonderful book on the subject, Gertrud Hirschi describes *mudras* as "finger power points" and explains that these gestures are understood to be "a mystic position of the hands, a seal or symbol". The idea is that by using certain hand gestures, we can channel and intensify the charge of our *prāṇā*, our life force.

Here is a small selection of my favourite *mudras*. Try incorporating them into your practice, and see if they influence your inner world.

**1. Anjali Mudra**

The universal gesture of prayer. Hands press lightly together in front of the heart, symbolizing the meeting of the masculine and feminine, the universal and the individual, a gesture of you meeting yourself.

*Anjali mudra* is said to balance the left and right hemispheres of the brain. It's used to open and close a practice, with closed eyes and often an *om*.

**2. Jnana/Chin Mudra**

*Chin* means "consciousness", *jnana* means "wisdom" or "knowledge". When your fingers point up toward the sky, it is called *jnana mudra*. When they are directed to the earth, it's *chin mudra*.

This *mudra* symbolizes the union of the cosmic divine (the thumb) and the individual consciousness (index finger). Remembrance of this union is the goal of a yoga practice, and *jnana mudra* is often used to invite a calm, receptive state for meditation. According to Hirschi, "The index finger represents inspiration (energy from the outside) and the thumb stands for intuition (inner energy)."

This is the perfect gesture for seated meditation.

**3. Pran mudra**

Said to work on the root chakra, making you feel safe and grounded, this *mudra* is invigorating and reduces fatigue and nervousness. Pran mudra is also good if you want to cultivate more confidence and motivation.

Touch tips of thumb, ring and little fingers together, while keeping index and middle fingers extended and together.

1

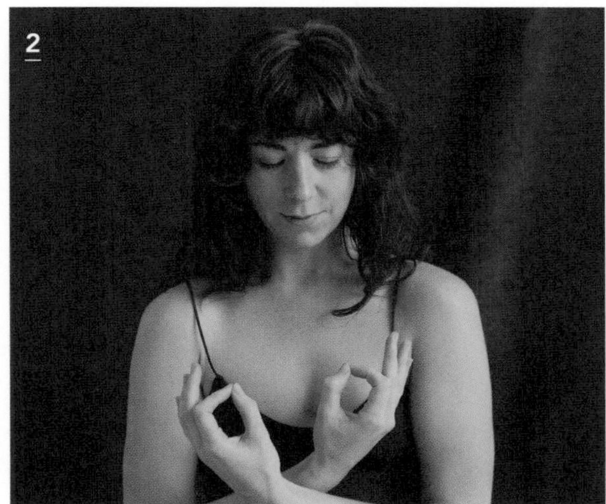


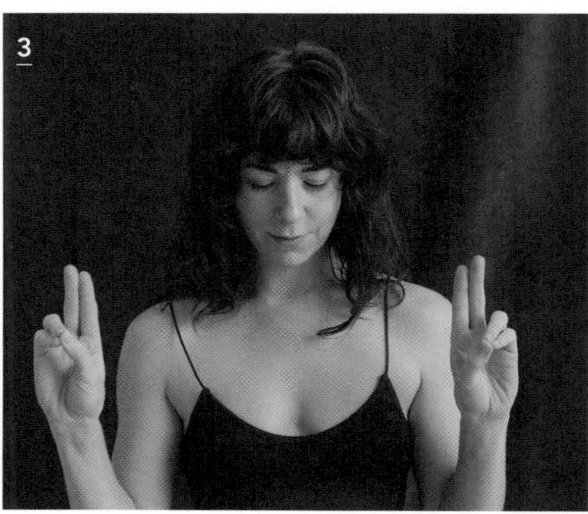

### 1. Ganesha mudra

Ganesha is the Hindu god with the elephant's head, traditionally the bringer of wisdom and remover of all obstacles.

Hold hands at level of heart, left palm facing outward with fingers bent. Right hand faces inward and its fingers clasp fingers of left hand.

Inhale and, on the exhale, energetically pull the hands away from each other without releasing the clasp. Inhale deeply and release.

### 2. Lotus mudra

This *mudra* has a beautiful symbolism. It represents opening to love, just as flowers blossom and open to bees and insects, that in turn allow it to be pollinated and perpetuate. It is pure abundance, and a magical symbol of creation and the divine force. For lonely times of tiredness or misunderstanding – a gesture to the cosmic divine.

Bring hands in front of chest, with only edges of hands and fingers touching on both sides. Blossom hands, keeping both outer edges of palms together but opening fingers as wide as possible. Breathe deeply. Close the bloom by bending fingers and bringing nails to touch.

### 3. Ksepana mudra

The gesture of pouring out and letting go.

Touch palms together, keeping index fingers extended, and interlink the rest of your fingers so that the tips of your fingers press back of hands. Cross hands. There should be a little cave between the palms.

This powerful *mudra* is said to release negative energy and attract fresh, positive energy. Hold it for up to 15 breaths.

1

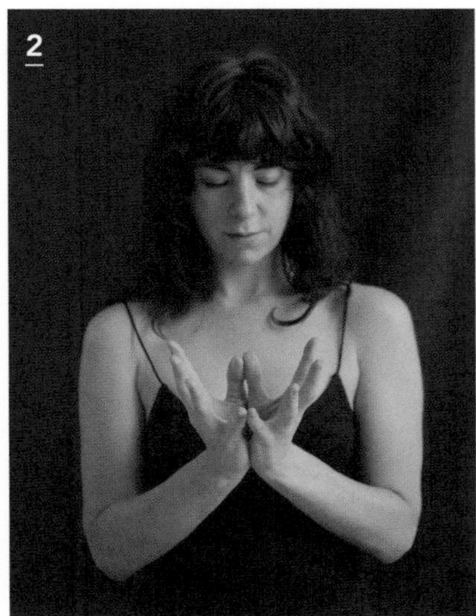


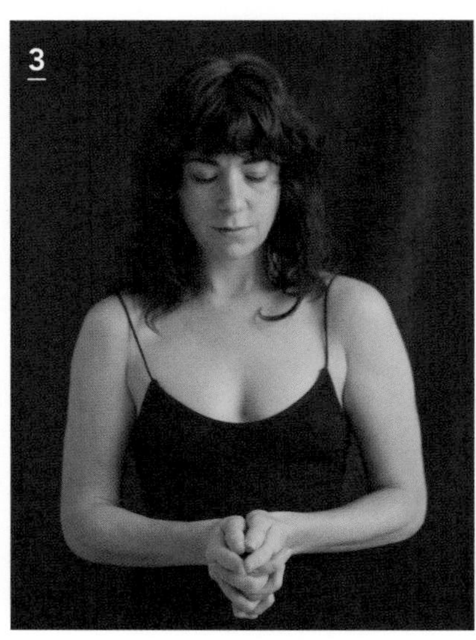

# MANTRA

In Sanskrit, *man* means mind and *tra* means vehicle or instrument. You use mantra to cross the labyrinth of the mind and cut through mind chatter, by focusing on a specific sound or sentence and repeating it until you hypnotize yourself or shift your own perspective. Mantra is a practical tool that can be used in a few different ways:

- throughout a yoga practice, to imbue meaning and poetry into movement;
- in meditation, to anchor the mind;
- when you are moving about your day with a head full of negative babble; and
- to call in something beautiful.

Whether you believe in the law of attraction or not, our thoughts and intentions create emotions within our body that will percolate into the world around us. The language we use to express them has the power to crystallize them as truths. We create self-fulfilling prophecies on a daily basis, and mantra is a wonderful tool help us select what we would like to manifest and attract. We use mantra to take control of our mind, shift our perspective of ourselves and the world around us, communicate positively and to call in what our heart desires.

## OM – "THE HYMN OF THE UNIVERSE"

*Om* is said to be a primordial sound, a matrix of sounds that contains all vibrations. If you're reading this book, you've probably chanted "om" at some point. You may have tuned into its magnetism and connected to its vibratory qualities. If it made you feel awkward, that's OK. Perhaps choosing your own personal mantra will be more useful for you.

*Om* is sometimes spelt *AUM*, which is a more accurate translation of how this word is written in Sanskrit. If you sound out *AUM* as you chant, notice that the A vibrates in the throat, the U vibrates at the top of the mouth and M is a powerful vibration from the lips, through to the top of the skull.

*AUM* is also said to represent the layers of consciousness.

**A** – is the waking state

**U** – is the dream state

**M** – is the state of deep sleep

At the end of *AUM* is a pause, a silence like negative space. It is experienced poignantly after chanting. This silence symbolizes the state known as *Turiya*, or Infinite Consciousness, that transcends all other state of consciousness.

### SO HUM

A simple mantra from the Vedas to remind you of your eternal connection to the universe and its deep mystery, *So Hum* translates as "I am that", with hum or "that" representing all of creation and the universal infinity that is breathing through us all.

Try repeating this during seated meditation.

Inhale: *So*

Exhale: *Hum*

You can set an alarm and build up to anywhere from 5–15 minutes.

### CHOOSE YOUR OWN MANTRA

If some of the Sanskrit chants seem too abstract to you, then feel free to create your own little collection of personal mantras. Here are a few ideas to get you going:

I am loved.

I am in control of my actions and emotions.

I can do this.

I am power.

I am beautiful.

I am enough.

I have everything I need.

Love is all there is.

I am a voice for peace.

I am strong and fearless.

# MORNING RITUALS

No matter how busy I am, I always do something in the morning to welcome the day. I tailor my morning rituals depending on how much time I have, how busy my day is, how I slept and how my body-mind is feeling. I use one or more of the practices below, depending on how spacious my life is on that day and what I am working with or seeking.

### PRĀṆĀYĀMA OR MEDITATION:

I meditate and practice *prāṇāyāma* for up to half an hour every morning. The more disobedient my mind is, the more active it is when I wake up. I cherish this time in the morning to anchor myself within my body, to witness who I am and to usher in some space so I can move into the day refreshed and grounded.

### YOGĀSANA, RUNNING OR SWIMMING

I practice *yogāsana* or run five days a week. I was never a runner when I was younger, so pushing through the wall and coming out the other side has been very empowering for me. It makes me feel strong and alive. When I am busy, I have to be careful not to choose a run over practising yoga. It's easier to run in stressful times, as sitting still and moving slowly through the chaos is much more uncomfortable and challenging.

I would recommend mixing it up, but be careful not to hide from yourself. The more challenging it is for you to be with yourself, the more necessary it is for you to bring yourself home.

### DREAM YOURSELF AWAKE

I keep a notepad by my bed to jot down my dreams before my mind becomes too cognitive. I find dreams are a way for me to access a deeper part of my consciousness, to see the primal parts of myself that I hide during my waking life. My dreams reveal things about my relationships, work and deep longings and fears. You too might find recurring symbols or scenarios. The more you journal, the more easily you will remember and track your dreamscape.

### SACRED SPACE

I have an altar at home with objects that are precious to me. It's a space to honour the divine, to celebrate people I find inspiring, sacred symbols or depictions of goddesses that represent an archetype I am drawn to. When I wake up, I light a candle, burn some sage or palo santo and watch the smoke dance as the invisible becomes visible. If I'm feeling negative I work with the gratitude practice on page 144 to consciously orientate myself into a positive bias.

Sometimes I chant or set an intention for the day. Not only does it remind me of the beauty of life, it's poetic and feels intimate and magical.

### NO SOCIAL MEDIA, TECHNOLOGY OR EMAIL

This is a matter of mental hygiene: protect the sanctity of your morning space before you have performed your rituals. Don't let people or work intrude before you have set yourself up for the day. If you let it in, it might distract you from nourishing habits.

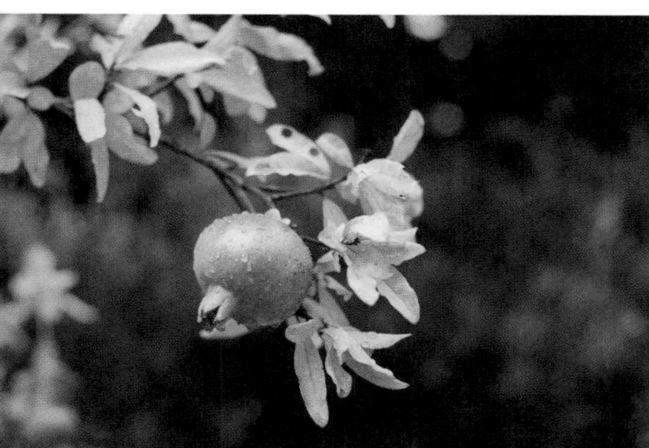

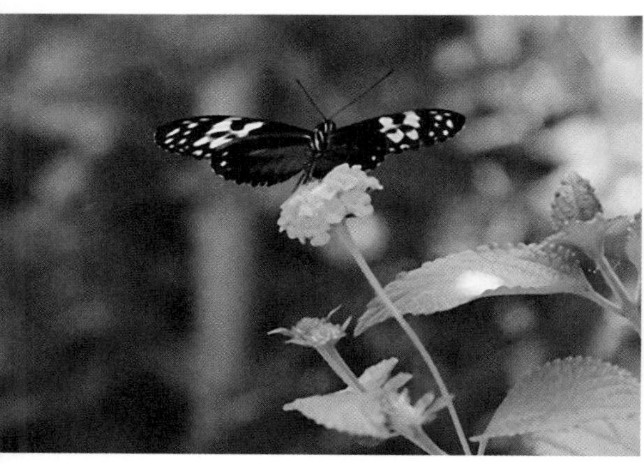

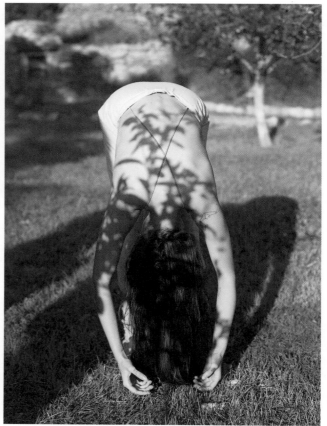

## SUN IN WINTER

Sometimes we get stuck in a rut of negativity and lose perspective. This practice is a beautiful one to reorientate ourselves, dropping us into the present, halting a loop of unhelpful thoughts and dwelling in the grounding, comforting practice of gratitude.

Softly close your eyes and take a moment to arrange and arrive in your bones.

Feel the the weight of the pelvis blossom on to the floor.

Grow the spine out of the hips and lengthen the back of the neck.

Soften the shoulders down the back and elevate the heart.

Stillness descends. Allow for silence. Let the breath breathe the body from the inside out.

From a space of safety and softness, silently say to yourself:

"I have gratitude for my breath. However rich, shallow, coarse or smooth. I am grateful for this breath that sustains me.

I am grateful for my body. However graceful, strong, easeful and comfortable it is. I am grateful. I have a body that can hold me here, for these few minutes.

I am grateful for my mind. I am grateful that I am the witness. I can observe my thoughts, whether they are dreamy and colourful, or dark and angry. Whether they're peaceful or restless, grounded and deliberate. I am grateful, for I can be the witness."

Sit and invite the feeling of gratitude to permeate through the whole being.

Think of one or two things that you are grateful for. Stay with these gratitudes, and say to yourself silently:

"I am grateful for ..."

See that once you find one thing to be grateful for, other things will begin to bubble up and come to you.

Some may surprise you.

But even noticing one or two can lead to a wide web of gratitude.

Bring your palms to touch.

Give thanks to all the people who have made it possible for you to sit here today.

Rub your palms together until they heat up.

Raise your palms up to your eyes and feel the warmth that you've just kindled.

Give thanks.

Slowly blink your eyes awake. Open the webs of your fingers. Release your palms on your lap.

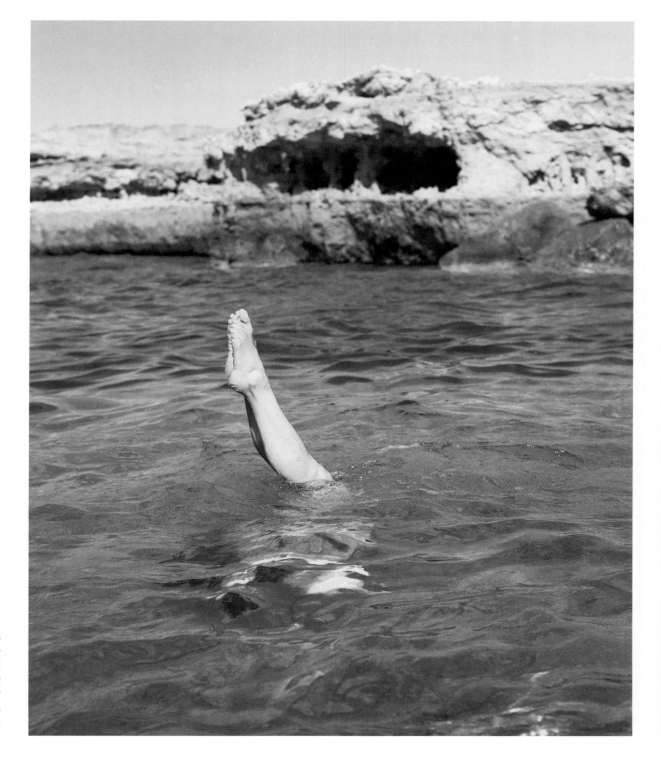

# CHANGE YOUR LIFE

There are times when you're in a rut and need to explore the reasons why you found yourself in this space, so you can map a way out and create a nourishing environment for yourself in all areas of your life.

Here you will find some ideas to help you choose the questions, in order for the paths to reveal themselves to you. The ideas here will prompt a process of self-enquiry, or *svādhyāya*. You can begin to add to them, break them down and answer them yourself.

If you're going through a really rough patch, I'd recommend getting a good therapist. Sometimes you need a professional help you get back on your feet again.

You can do a lot of work yourself, but it's so beautiful to have the support. Seeking a sister circle is a powerful way to feel held. Sitting with sisters will reveal to you the universality of your challenges, which is very reassuring. Someone may have also experienced the same thing and come through the other side, which will be inspiring and empowering for you.

The essence of all the ancient teachings is one of awareness - the art of noticing. When you are stressed, anxious, restless or depressed, your mind is occupied with its own stories, stuck in a negative feedback loop. You miss a lot of what is going on around you until it's too late; you've already been hijacked. This makes it more challenging to extract yourself from unhealthy situations or deploy the safety measures that help you catch yourself in time.

I used to go through a full kaleidoscope of feelings, just in one day. I still do sometimes, but after many years of practising, I have begun to notice better what it is that is that nourishes me. Now I am better equipped to take careful steps to do more of the things that find inspiring, and swerve, or better manage my energy around people and situations I find deplete me.

Once you begin to look after yourself, you will still experience some of the same situations, but you'll be able to keep your centre and respond to them in a way that honours your boundaries. When you are nourishing your mind with space and quiet, your mind will open, your memory will improve, you might see more connections and your intuition will be amplified.

All of this means that you are better placed to make better decisions and communicate more clearly. You will be embodied. You'll be able to witness your emotions as they arise, and start to see patterns and triggers. Once you notice these, then you're able to do a little detective work and try and figure out why it is these situations are triggering.

Have you ever wondered:

- ○ Why you never perform as well as you think you can in a particular work situation?
- ○ Why you don't feel good enough around a certain person?
- ○ Why do you always get drunk or high around certain people?
- ○ Why do you always do what your partner wants instead of asking for what you like?
- ○ Why do you always have a downward spiral after summer?
- ○ Why do you think you can't receive pleasure?

Sometimes, you'll be able to figure out a solution on your own. It might be as simple as: because you're too tired, unprepared, you are very capable but you have a block, because you are not expressing yourself creatively, or giving yourself the time to do the things you enjoy, learn and grow. Other times, the answer will mean much deeper work.

I've placed a few more general questions here to get you started. The answers to these might be surprising, and should be a strong indication of where you can make positive changes in your work, home and social life. For example, there are things that we might think are trivial, but they are actually the key to making us feel more empowered or fulfilled.

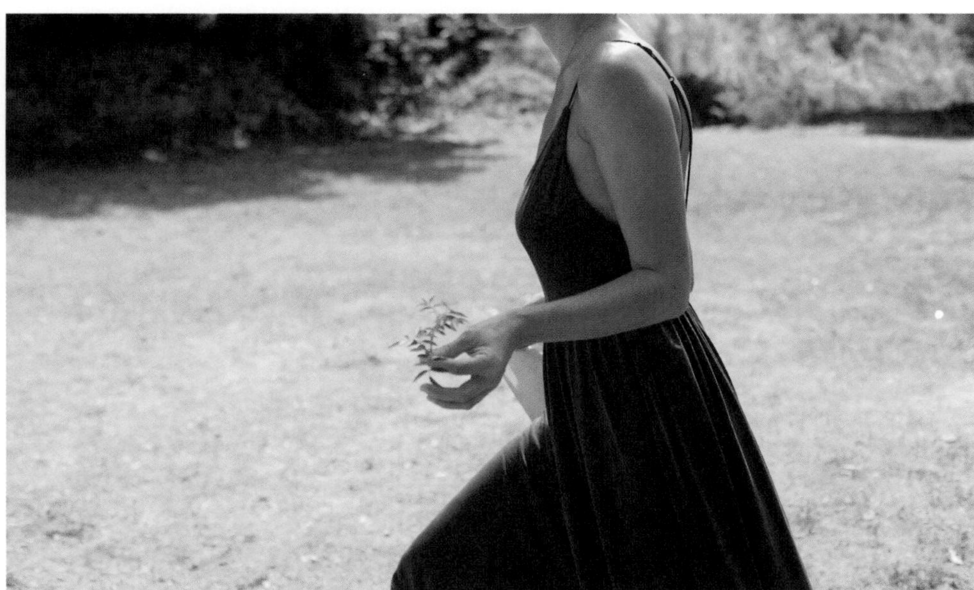

Take a notepad with some pencils; make it beautiful to you. It's a way for you to author a life of pleasure, fulfillment and peace. Write down the following:

- What are you naturally good at?
- Can you orientate your work around these skills? Are you doing this enough? Are you giving yourself credit for the times when you shine?
- What would you like to learn? Do you have a list of areas in which you'd like to grow?
- How can you begin to bring learning into your life? Are there books, courses, podcasts that you can weave into your life to start your journey of learning? Can you put some time aside weekly to allow yourself to explore?
- What situations do you find stressful? There are often simple things we can do to manage our stress. Prepare yourself well, rest beforehand, take breaks, use the tools you have to get you through it, have a reward for afterwards.
- When do you feel most confident? Write a list of the situations in which you feel good, light and natural. Orientate your life around doing more of these.
- Whose company do you enjoy the most?
- Who lights you up? Who do you feel brings out the best in you? Where do you feel safe and cherished? Seek out these people and places more.
- When and where are you most happy? It may be the same answer as some of the questions above, but is there a particular place, activity or person that always inspires happiness? It could be a walk on the heath, cooking at home, or dancing. Noticing can help you appreciate it and weave it more frequently into your life.
- What gives your live meaning? Do this more and savour it when you're enjoying it.

QUESTIONS FOR DEEPER WORK

Some of these questions may be more uncomfortable or triggering, so choose to explore them at a time that is right for you, when you have support and the tools in place to do the work.

- What triggers come up in work, friendships or romantic relationships?
- Is there a pattern of behaviour? Do you always melt into your partner? Do you give too much, or too easily? If so, why? Do you feel you are not enough, or not as good as your partner?
- Are you attracted to partners who are violent? Do you play the role of rescuer to make you feel powerful, or do you hide from responsibility and play the child or victim? Do you go on the defensive?
- Are you living your truth?
- Are there times when you tell yourself or others mistruths to make the situation easier for you? Do you deliberately mislead people to make yourself look better? Are you living a life that honours your truth?

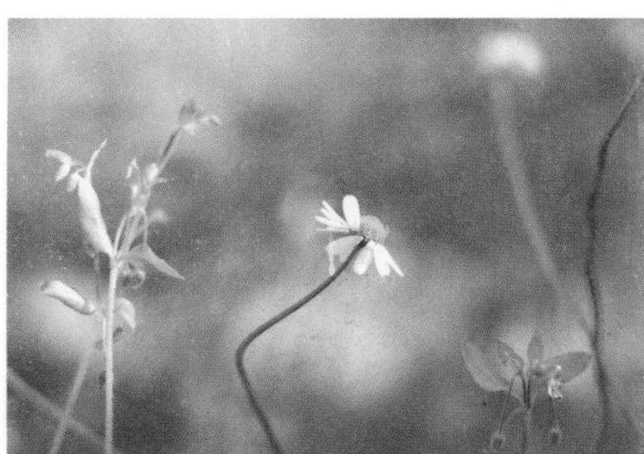

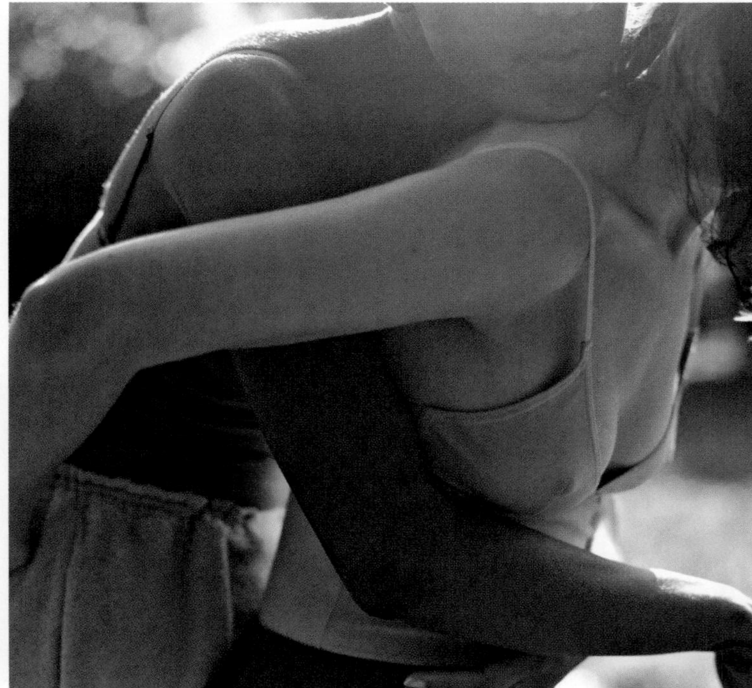

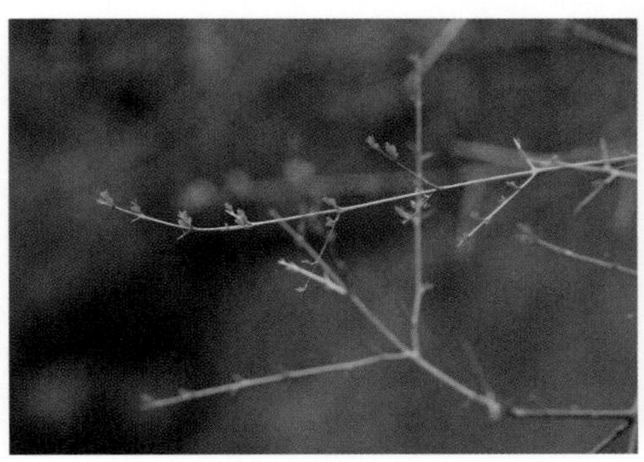

○ Are you able to communicate clearly? Do you know what you want and do you feel comfortable asking for it? Do you find it difficult to even speak sometimes? If so, how can you start to open up, find your voice and speak your truth?

○ Do you have healthy boundaries?

○ Do you make rules for yourself to honour parts of you, and your life, that you'd like to keep private or protect? Where have you felt your personal space has been invaded? Do you always get swept away with the tide? Do you let yourself do what is easiest instead of saying "no"? Where have you lost yourself to someone else? What can you do to make sure you honour what is precious, what is pleasurable and nourishing to you, even if it means saying no to someone else?

○ Do you have some habits that are never nourishing or productive, for example, unhealthy eating or sleep habits? What can you do to prepare yourself and make it easier to take the actions that will make you feel good? Do you feel lazy? Are you disorganized, which may make your life chaotic? How are you with money? All these unhealthy habits have solutions; you just need to acknowledge they are there and carve out the time to create a structure that allows you to work on them.

○ Are you attracted to people who treat you kindly?

○ If you are around people who are not kind, why? Do you only value people you think are powerful or cool? Are you blocking relationships that could be more inspiring or nurturing? Are you wasting time with people who don't care as much for you as you do for them? Who could you reach out to who is good for you? Treat them kindly too.

○ Who do you often feel uncomfortable around?

○ Why do you think you are uncomfortable around this person? Is it because they are not aligned with you, or is it something else? If you feel that they're not right for you at this point in your journey, give yourself permission to spend less time with them.

○ Who do your give your power away to? Are there some people in your life who you feel take your power? Or who you you feel dimmed by them? Can you create healthy boundaries to honour yourself? What can you do to empower yourself? If you feel lacking, how can you top yourself up?

The answer is always in you. You are your greatest teacher, and you are enough. You just have to find the practices that help you discover yourself.

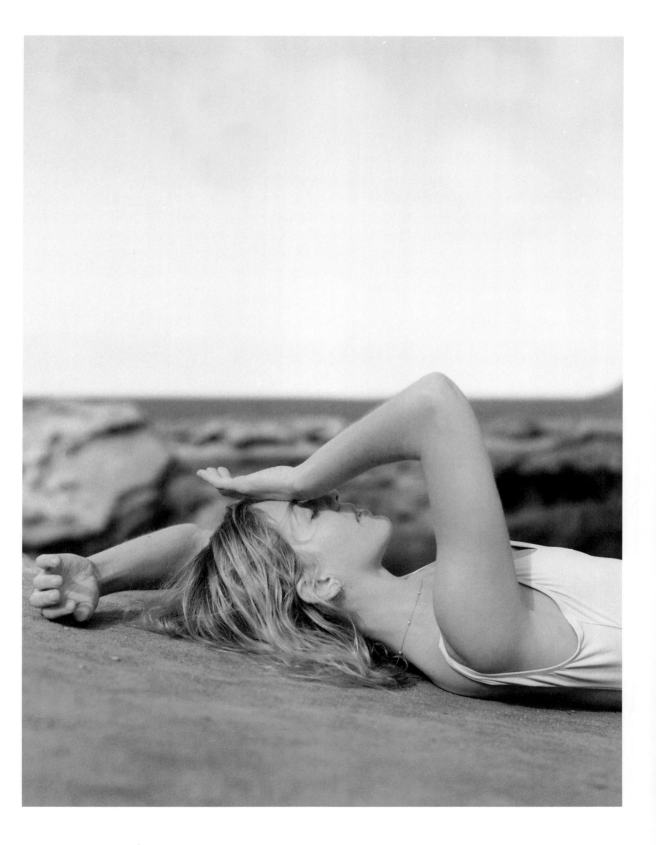

# 4

# SIGHING INTO STILLNESS

*"Pain is important: how we evade it, how we succumb to it, how we deal with it, how we transcend it."*

AUDRE LORDE

# MORTAL COIL: MENTAL HEALTH

I'm super-sensitive, and always have been. I was bullied by the girls at school and developed painful psoriasis all over my body and sometimes my face. This is a skin condition that's like eczema, but almost impossible to cure with medication because it's partly psychological – a visceral lesson in how the flesh echoes the mind. At school, to avoid the girls who bullied me, I sometimes hung out with the boys, climbing trees and building dams. Other times, I withdrew into my own world. I immersed myself in the magical realms of books, spent hours daydreaming or loved to hide away, watching and listening to adults.

*Experiencing the most dramatic spectrum of emotions and regularly confronting my shadows have given me direct experience of change and transformation.*

I observed people. They fascinated and sometimes scared me. I also *felt* them. I sensed their anger, their sadness and their insecurities. I saw the energetic dynamics in a room. This used to be confusing and overwhelming. I felt everything too much, and at boarding school there is little opportunity to process information quietly. But now I know it's a gift that I am learning to trust and work with.

I feel fortunate to have found a career in which I am surrounded by beautiful souls and practices that continue to facilitate my healing and growth. If anyone is testament to how yoga and meditation can create lasting and sustained healing, I am it incarnate. I've changed so much in the last couple of years, and it's all down to these practices and being in a nourishing community. That's not to say I don't hit lows, but I'm much better than I used to be at managing and tempering them when they arrive. Instead of seeing my depression as a weakness, I've realized how much it has taught me. Experiencing the most dramatic spectrum of emotions and regularly confronting my shadows have given me direct experience of change and transformation. That truth lives and breathes in me as a human and as a teacher.

Depression demanded that I make decisions to help me find a nurturing and supportive way of living. It forced me to cut out things and people in a way I wouldn't have had the courage to do if it hadn't been essential. I would never have discovered our magical community and practices without it – I'd be a completely different person. My life is richer because of it.

### BREAKING THE PATTERN

I have fairly typical characteristics of depression. It's not just a low, or even the deep sadness you experience after heartbreak or grief, though it can be triggered by these. It's as if your being has been hijacked: you lose all sense of yourself and your purpose in life. When talking to someone who might be suffering, it's important to understand

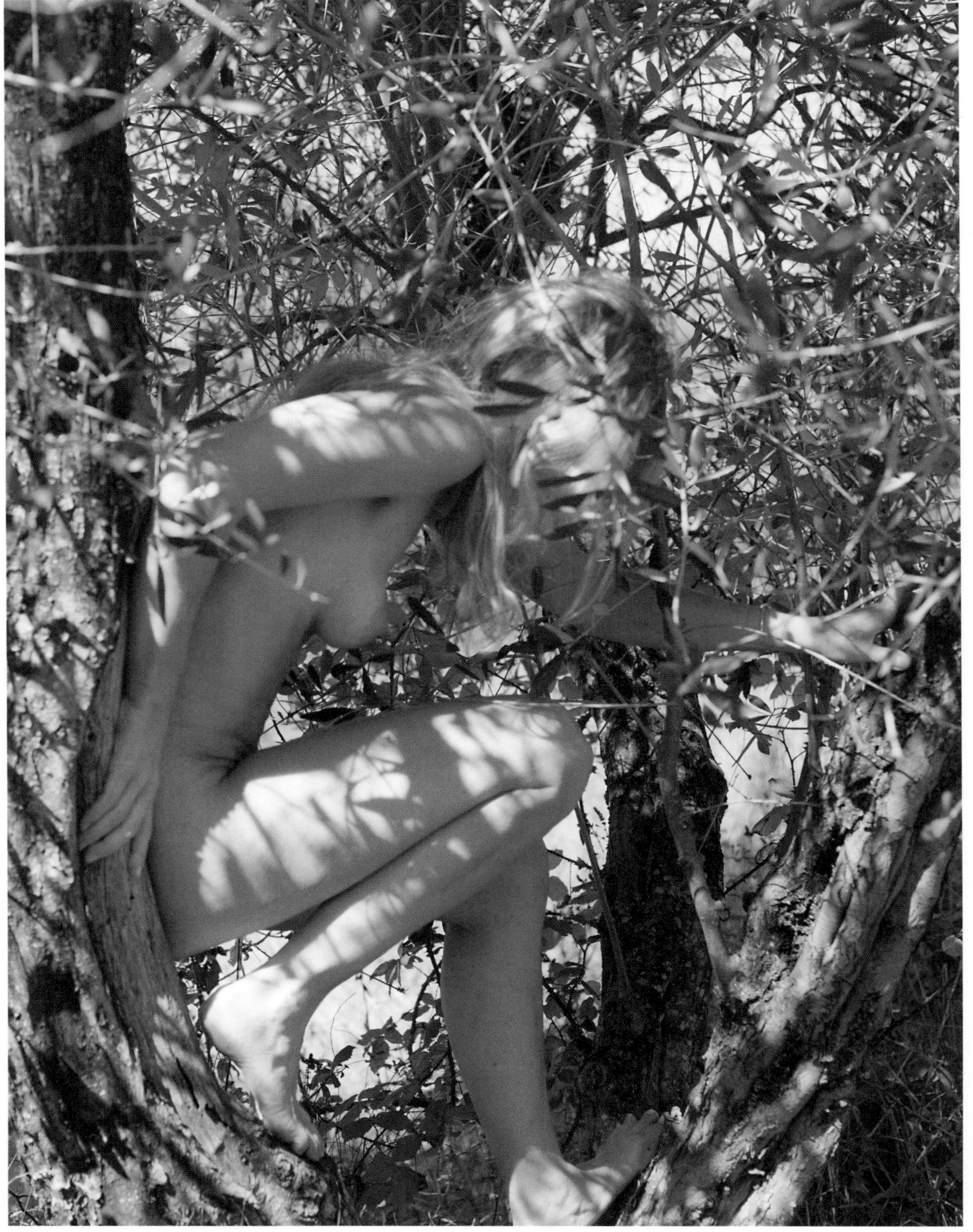

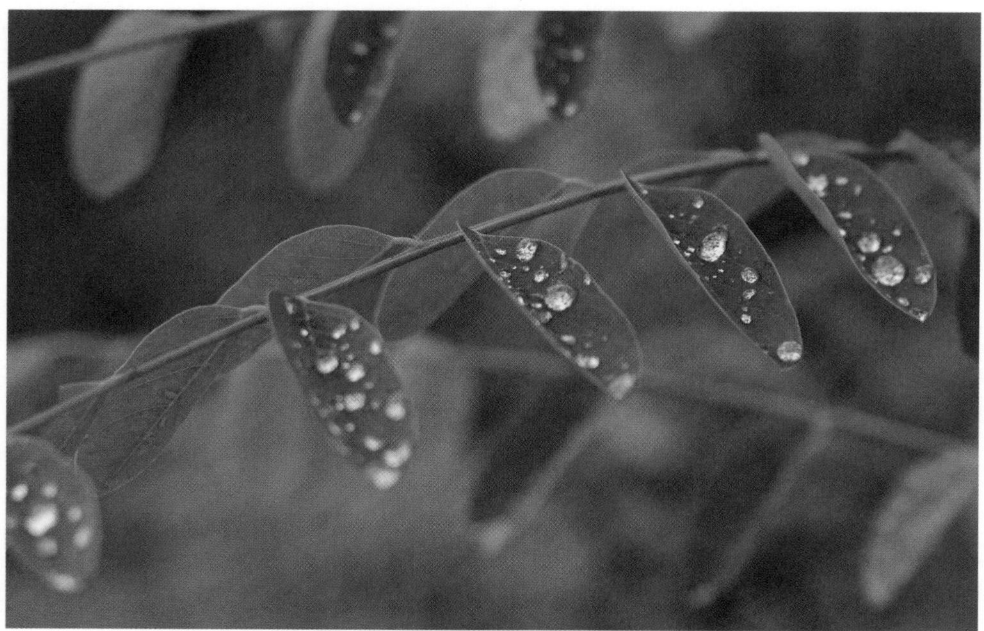

that all they need is to be loved, seen and heard. They don't expect or want you to do anything to heal them. Feeling your constant love and presence at a point of deep vulnerability is powerful enough.

For me, when I am in one of these depths, I feel as if someone has chopped me up into separate parts, and that these segments are operated from a mind that is hovering in a marshmallow a foot or so above my head. Sometimes the signals from this external control booth are fractured, which leaves me paralysed and numb. There is also an operating delay. In tandem with slow signals, the body has to make extra effort to gather itself together to move through space, which is thick and tangible.

Everything feels artificial and full of effort. Thinking becomes almost impossible. Planning for the future appears futile because the present is so long and low. Food tastes of nothing. When I talk, my voice is alien – I hear it as an echo from a far away land. Day-to-day becomes an exercise in fake life and every night I hope that in the morning I will wake up and feel natural again.

Then, totally out of the blue, I do. The miracle of vitality and delight returns to everything. It's so instant that it feels as if the darkness never happened at all. Each time I surfaced, I told myself that it was the last time, that I was cured. Which, of course, meant that I never made any progress. In denying that it was part of me, I

*... the brain is always evolving and adapting, meaning that we have great potential to rewire our circuitry and develop powerful new habits...*

would feel even more helpless and scared when it caught me unawares and hijacked my body. It didn't help, of course, that until very recently there was little dialogue about depression and it was considered somehow shameful and abnormal.

A big step to getting better and empowering yourself is knowing as much about the illness as possible, so you can make informed decisions about how to recover and then to stay well. One of the sources that I found most useful was Sharon Begley's *The Plastic Mind*, a great account of the long journey some tenacious scientists embarked on to uncover the inner workings of the mind; how this related to ancient Buddhist wisdom surrounding the mind; and a number of "mindful" practices that are born out of the tradition.

## MAKING NEW CONNECTIONS

The work documented in *The Plastic Mind* led to the groundbreaking discovery of neuroplasticity – the ability of the brain to form new neural connections throughout life that allow it to reorganize and renew itself, and adjust its functions in accordance with its environment. Changes in the environment influence how the brain functions, so we can consciously create a particular environment to kindle the changes that we would like to make. But what the studies included in the book also demonstrated was that training the mind to alter the way you think and engage with your thoughts can act back on the brain. This is important, because it confirms that we can heal after traumatic experiences, and have the power to change how we think, which can make a difference to our emotional landscape.

The revolution of neuroplasticity contradicted the prevailing dogma that we are stuck with the brain we inherit or develop in childhood. Instead, it demonstrated that the brain is always evolving and adapting, meaning that we have great potential to rewire our circuitry and develop powerful new habits or learn endless skills, all the way through adulthood. This is really inspiring – we can all pick up a new language, an instrument and learn how to surf. Most importantly, we can consciously cultivate more positive thought patterns, which change our perception of the world and mean we can rewrite our story. It's actually our lack of belief in ourselves, often caused by misinformation, that is the biggest handicap.

If we undertake the journey of getting to know ourselves and our oceanic inner world, we can better understand the thoughts and processes underpinning our emotions, and the impulses and behavioural patterns that shape our personalities and determine our futures. We can reform and redirect them to become positive and joy-affirming, which will, in turn, shape who we are and lead us to continue to unfold. This too is yoga – consciously exploring and reinforcing the connection between the mind and the body.

## THE BRAIN-GUT CONNECTION

Ninety percent of serotonin is found in the digestive tract. That whole area is soaked in a variety of neurotransmitters, brain proteins and other psychoactive chemicals. The gut is home to the enteric nervous system, also known as our "second brain", which sends and receives impulses, records experiences and responds to emotions. It functions independently of the central nervous system and peripheral (autonomic) nervous system, but communicates with the central nervous system through the vagus nerve, which is the main highway in the autonomic nervous system, and has long been understood to be the repository for good and bad feelings (see page 132 for an excercise that works with the vagus nerve). This understanding is embedded in our language: think of that sinking feeling you get in the pit of your stomach when you realize you've forgotten to do something important, or the way you consult your gut feelings when making a difficult decision. We experience butterflies of excitement and, even more viscerally, the upset stomach caused by stress hormones.

*The gut is also called "the second brain" and is home to what is known as the enteric nervous system.*

The gut has its own ecosystem of trillions of microorganisms (mostly bacteria, but also fungi, viruses and primitive single-celled organisms), called the microbiome, and exploring whether this is a key regulator of brain function – that is, whether these microorganisms send messages to the brain that influence its function and your behaviour – is one of the most exciting areas in medicine.

In the gut, the microbiome breaks down food, fights off infections and boosts our immune system: it affects every single system in our body. The gut also has a huge influence on our moods: scientists are slowly revealing more links between the gut and the brain, showing that gut bacteria can alter the biochemistry of the brain and affect our mental state as a result. So the microbiome is also important for brain development and social behaviour.

## THE MIND IS MORE THAN THE BRAIN

There is another way to look at working with mental illness. Traditionally, it has been considered that "brain states" – that is, the patterns of neurons firing in one place and neurotransmitters docking in another – give rise to mental states. This is the theory underpinning taking medication for mental health problems. However, as many yogis and Buddhists have known for centuries, there is a part of the mind that is separate from the chemistry of the brain.

According to this philosophy, consciousness is independent of the circuitry of the brain. You see this immediately when you meditate. You cultivate a state of mindful awareness and become a witness beyond your own stories. You observe thoughts and feelings as they simmer to the surface, fracturing the continuum of stillness and space. The more you train the mind, the more it stretches into the quiet, so you

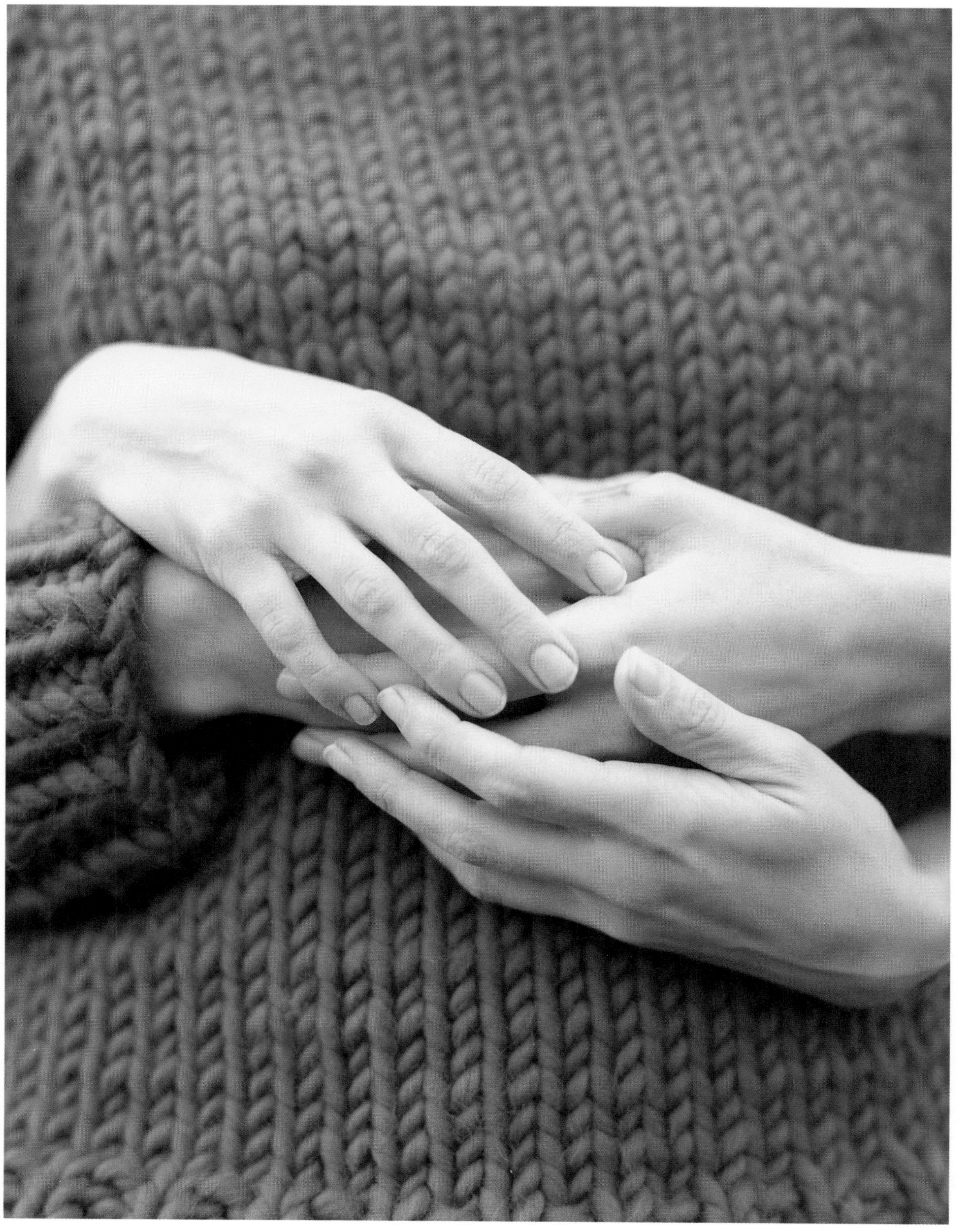

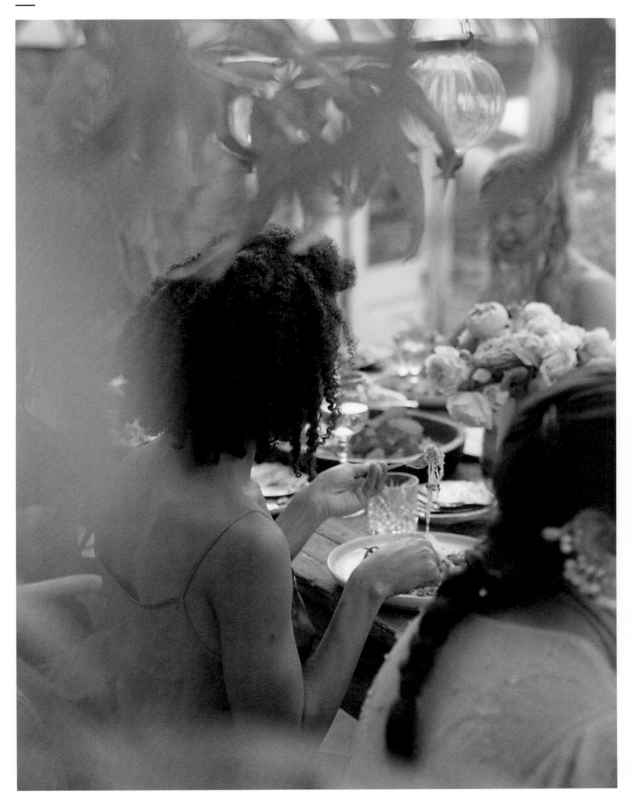

can soak up the peaceful expanse and become mindfully aware of your inner world. This cultivation of distance enables you to manage your emotional response to your thought patterns (and also events as they happen in your daily life). Instead of considering brain activity as controlling mental activity, you discipline the mind to change the brain state.

In this way, you are not focusing on the cause of depression, but instead finding a way to deal with the resulting emotions, thoughts and behavioural patterns. The distance that mindfulness allows enables you to strengthen the gap in which you can understand that depressive thoughts will transport you back to that place of darkness. This in turn can lead to imprinting a system of belief that may make you vulnerable to depression. In *The Plastic Mind*, the cognitive psychologist Zindel V Segal is quoted as saying:

> *The experience of depression can establish strong links in the mind between sad moods and ideas of hopelessness and inadequacy. Through repeated use, this becomes the default option for the mind: it's like mental kindling...The experience of depression imprints a tendency to fall back on certain patterns of thinking to activate certain networks in thinking memory.*

So, a sad mood could activate this whole depression network; if we allow ourselves to fuel it with a sad environment and negative thoughts, we will further entrench our brains by strengthening the circuitry and adding to the memory bank.

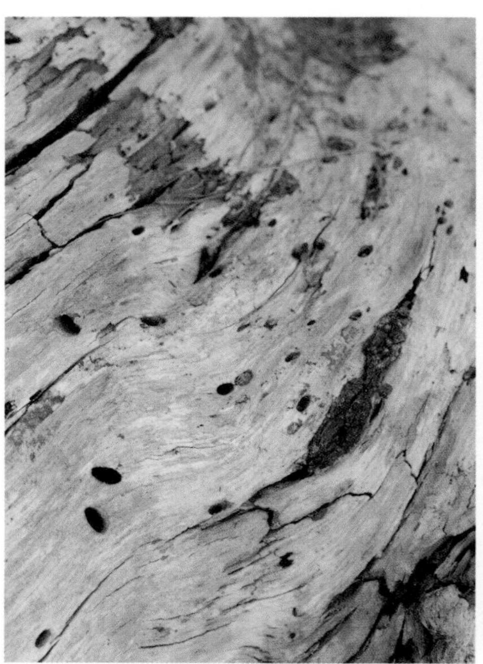

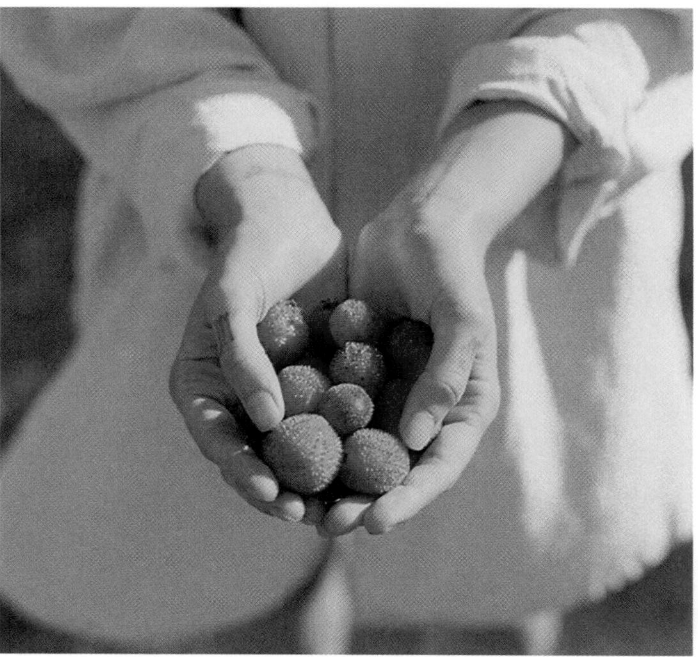

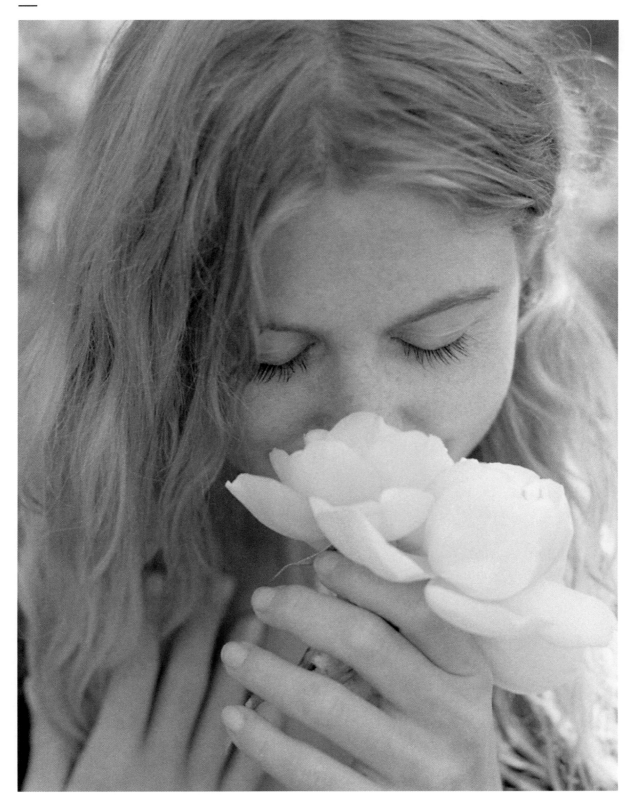

Actually, Patanjali, the compiler of the *Yoga-sutras*, was on to this around 400 BCE, when he wrote:

*When disturbed by disturbing thoughts, think the opposite.*

This is where cognitive behavioural therapy can be useful. It teaches you how to retrain your thoughts, so they don't lead into a negative spiral down the abyss. Once you can identify the triggering experiences and dysfunctional thoughts, you can have control over them and change them. So, whenever you catch yourself thinking something negative, you can turn it around. Think how many thoughts you have in a day. Thousands and thousands. Sometimes your head is like a radio on repeat, and if the script is endlessly negative, you're going to start believing what it says and who you tell yourself you are. You'll then be trapped in a churning cycle.

But if you repeat life-affirming mantras, you can create more positive thinking circuits in the brain. This will modulate the negative analytical circles of thinking and your reactions to negative thoughts and feelings. It's a helpful way of remembering that thoughts are not facts; mindfulness expert Jon Kabat-Zinn says they are more link

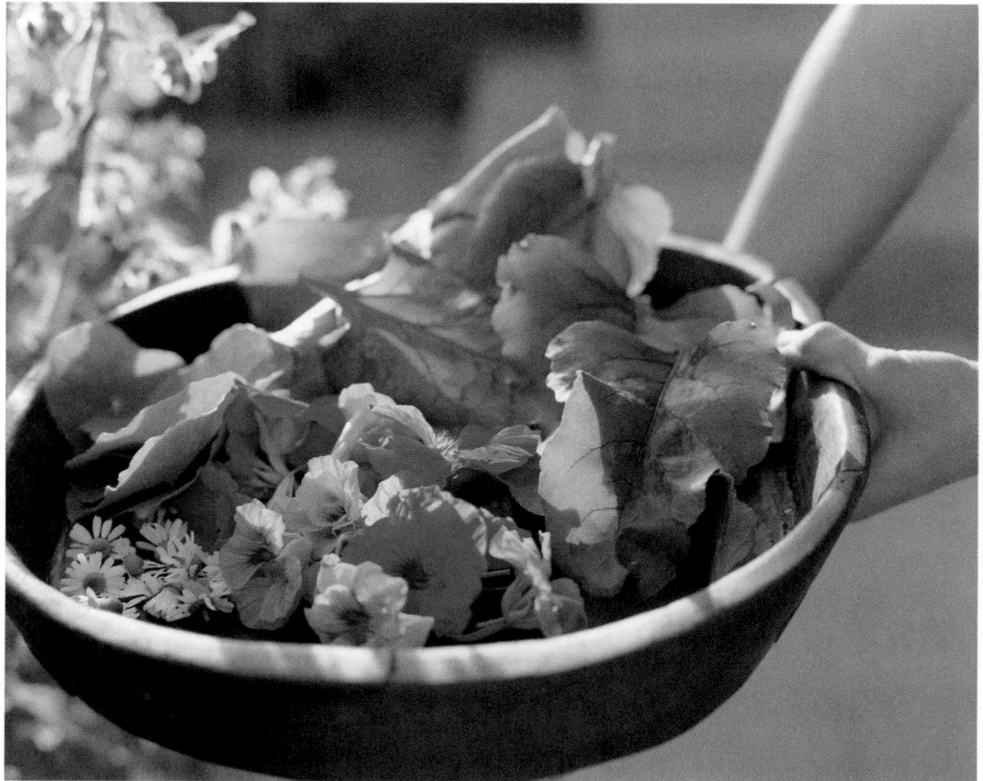

"events" and need to be regarded as such, although it's also important not to blame yourself and then load your "negative thoughts" with more "negative" connotations. This is where ancient Buddhist and yoga techniques sing. Instead of labelling thoughts as "bad", you accept that they just are. You don't need to judge them – they come and they go like clouds in the sky.

If you also make the effort to sweet talk, instead of criticizing yourself, then you begin to believe your new narrative and weave a new circuitry of positivity and joy. The mind is able to "act back" on the brain and you just have to trust in that before you discover it yourself. The brain works like a muscle, and if we consciously participate in certain exercises, the part of the brain that is dedicated to managing this function will expand in tandem with the practice.

We are complex creatures who need to be nurtured, stimulated and inspired in many different ways. We need a global approach to loving ourselves. Through managing my own mental health, I have created an infrastructure of practices and rituals that ensure I stay well, and which I am now able to share with you.

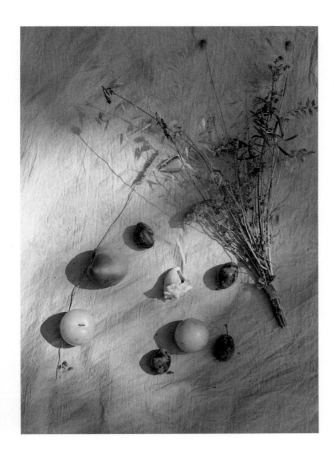

*If you also make the effort to sweet talk, instead of criticizing yourself, then you begin to believe your new narrative and weave a new circuitry of positivity and joy.*

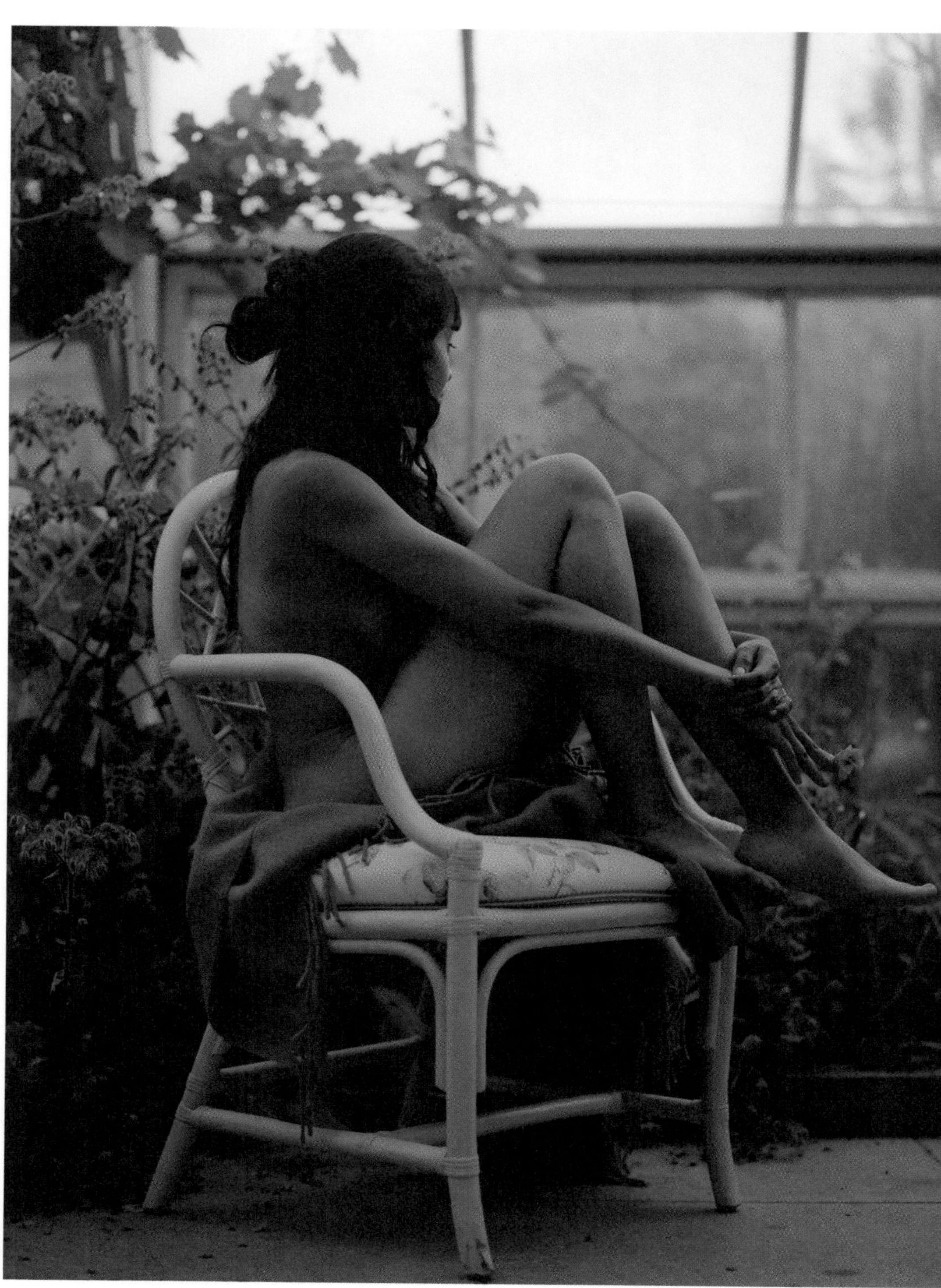

# SHADOW WORK

It took time before I was willing to acknowledge my depression fully, and this is often the case for our "shadows". It can be dark and uncomfortable when we embark on this journey. There will be moments of uprooting that cause doubt and deep vulnerability. At times, it seems that the closer we look, the darker it is within. Ugly parts of ourselves that we thought we had expunged years ago will surface again and again until we meet them face on and claim them as part of our human history. If we deny our darkness, its grip on us only tightens in its toxicity. Anything that we try to hide from ourselves, or the outside world, reverberates louder internally. I have the wonderful Carolyn Cowan (my Guardian Kali) to thank for an introduction to much of the material here. Carolyn and I have hosted events together, and she has also worked with me personally, as a therapist.

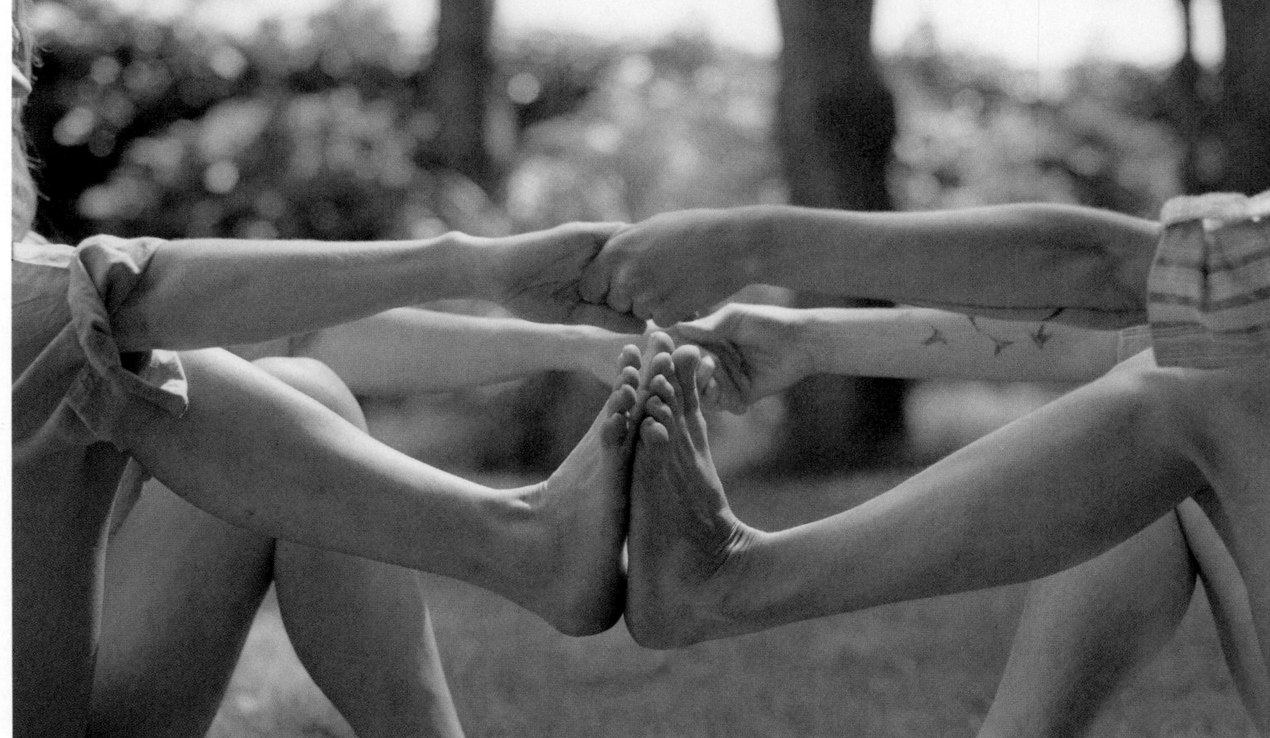

Our shadows are the little gremlins inside us that feel greed, jealousy, desire or the need for power. We ignore them because they elicit uncomfortable feelings of shame or guilt. To summarize these crudely, guilt is "I have done something wrong". Shame is "I am something wrong". These old friends, guilt and shame, cut deep. Absolutely no one wants jealousy to sear through them when they look at their friends' achievements, or feel the hot flare of unsolicited desire. These emotions are all-consuming and distracting. In our shame, we are secretive about them and this unwittingly endows them with power over us. They dominate through denial.

Shadow work is when we open our eyes to these parts of ourselves that we'd rather forget. We recognize them and take ownership of them. Slowly we begin to free ourselves from feelings of shame. This is liberating and empowering.

For me, the writing process was a massive exercise in shadow work. I spent a huge amount of time on my own. I read endlessly. I spent hours in my thinking mind, turning ideas inside out. At times, I tried to write myself out of the book, rather than speaking the truthful tenderness as it breathed through me.

I eventually surrendered into a vortex of growth, with all the growing pains that accompanied it. I didn't run away. It was as if I processed everything that I had learned over the last few years and saw all my shades. I had a lot of time when I was just with myself, which was gloriously liberating, but also very lonely and challenging. I had dark dreams that dredged up old trauma. I woke up many nights feeling unsettled, exhausted from the gauntlet of ghosts.

Fears moved back up to the surface. Fear of failure, judgment, rejection, abandonment. As I tuned into myself, I also attracted people and situations that triggered me deeply. I mean, there is always more...

## TAKE YOUR TIME

Emotional clarity and hygiene are really, really important. We so often gloss over things, but emotions become magnified when they're repressed. It's not always easy to identify where they come from, so we need to carve the time to sit and really feel into them. For example, if you experience fear in a social situation, and you can recognize that feeling and understand why it is there, you can more comfortably be with it, and work through it, by noticing the sensations in your body and staying present. This will empower you hugely in the moment.

Reflection, sharing circles (see page 184) and therapy help you see how you act when you respond from the shadowland. The more you observe, the more work there is. But that's not because you aren't making progress – it's only that before you didn't notice. Essentially, they all come from our own feelings of fear, loss or lack. For example, if you are feeling jealous of someone, it is because you are experiencing a lack in your own heart or you are catching your own potential, expressed through someone else. So identify where that feeling comes from, and see what you can do to make you feel good in your own body, career, relationship or whatever it may be.

*Emotions become magnified when they're repressed. It's not always easy to identify where they come from, so we need to carve the time to sit and really feel into them.*

What I now realize is that, yes, I am really sensitive, so I need to manage this if I'm in intense spaces with thousands of people. But also, I was on edge because of being bullied as a child and, in some deep, forgotten place, my body remembers – even all these years later. So, if I am not in the right mood, or in a group of people who I feel very safe with, then I get really triggered. When this happens, I want to get the fuck out of there. So I just honour it. It's cool. I also don't take a load of drugs, because that's obviously not very helpful. You need your wits about you to negotiate with your shadow.

We often experience our shadows in relationships, of course. In fact, this is one of the key ways in which we experience shadows, because they are mainly triggered by other people. If something keeps coming up, if you feel angry toward someone and you're not sure why, you need to think where that emotion is coming from. Either it's your own business you need to deal with on your own, or your anger is justified and you need to speak your feelings truthfully.

This is for the sake of your own wellbeing and integrity, not for anything to do with the other person. Most negative feelings lose their power once they are spoken aloud or written on the page (see page 147). You have also to be prepared for the other person not to meet you in that place of honesty – which is very hard. To speak your vulnerability openly and not have that honesty met is challenging. But everyone's on their own trip. I used to find it hard to speak about triggers, feelings and emotional needs. I'm much more comfortable about it now. It's empowering and cathartic.

Another gift that writing this book gave me was the excuse, as if I ever needed one, to practise quietly and deeply. I felt much closer to myself, to my heart, to the expansive beyond. Everything was magnified, which meant some emotions were distorted. I was very raw. So be aware, if you're doing deep work, that you need time and space to be gentle with yourself and to integrate. Feeling so deeply will sometimes surprise and unsettle you. It did me, and I should be well used to it. The world may be too much. So take care. Be tender with you.

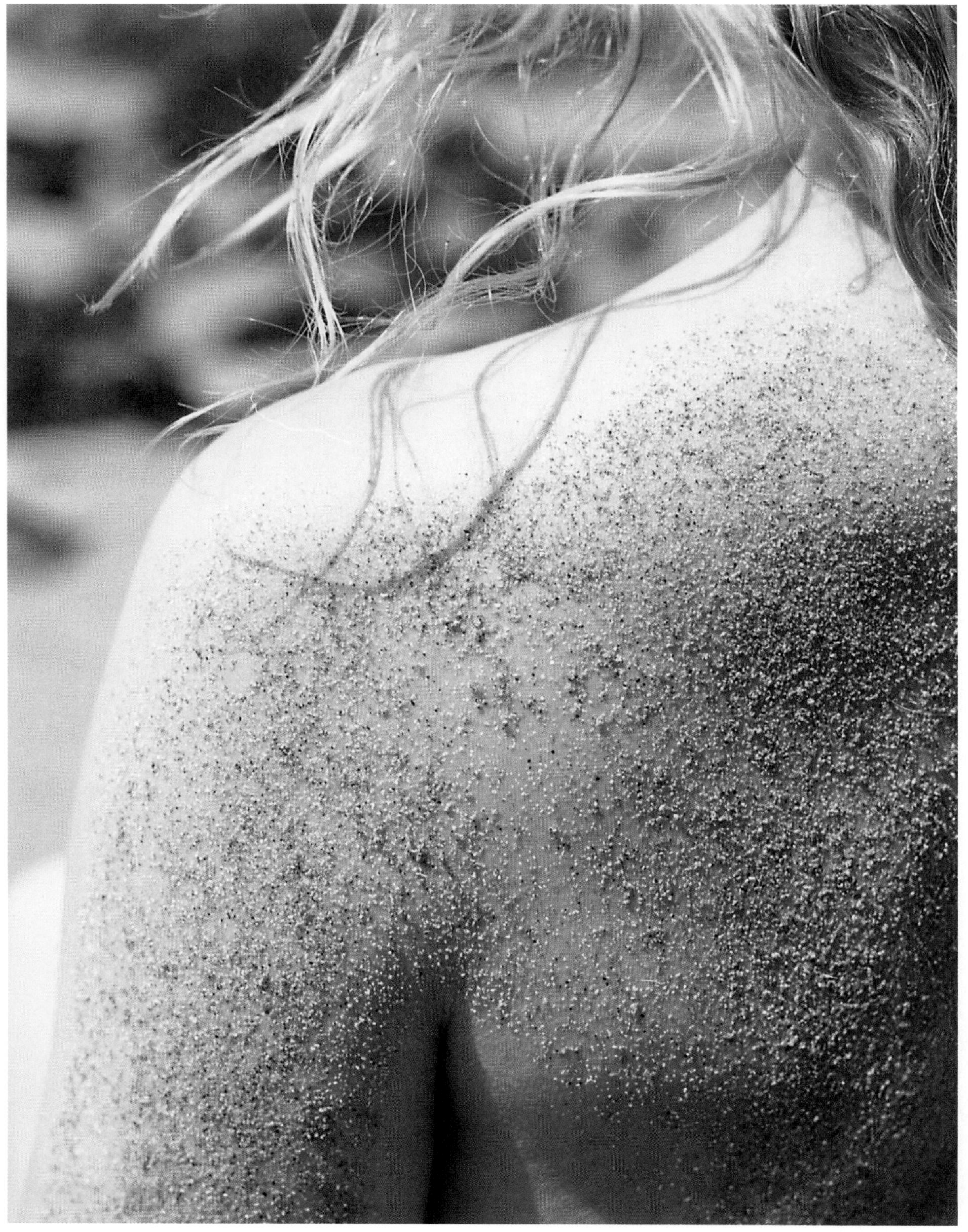

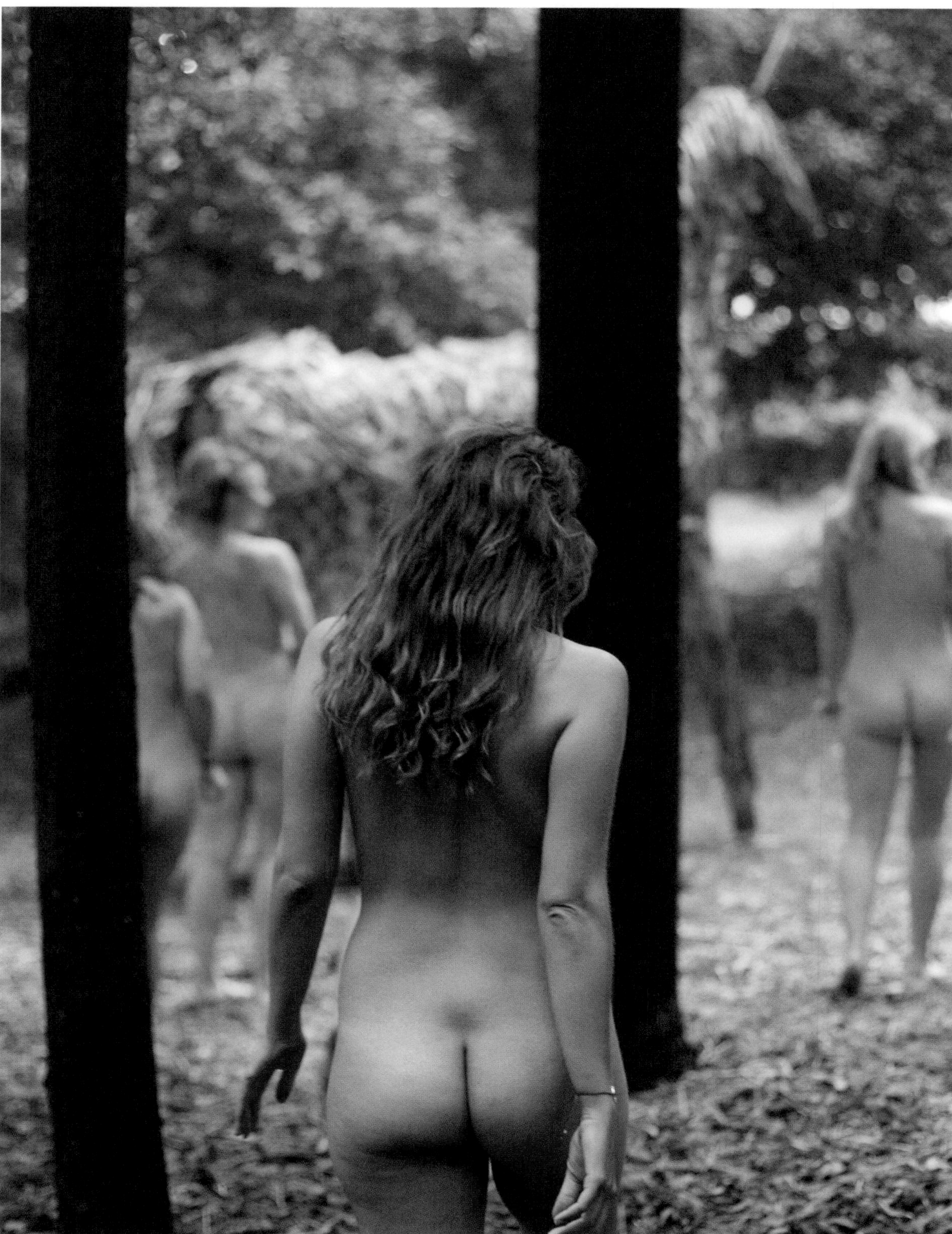

5

# IN THE COMPANY OF WOMEN

*"The earth is at the same time mother, she is mother of all that is natural, mother of all that is human. She is the mother of all, for contained in her are the seeds of all."*

HILDEGARD OF BINGEN

# COMING TOGETHER

I love all of our Secret Yoga Club offerings, but women's work inspires and transforms me the most. I've found that a group of women in a safe space is the best environment for me to continue to interrogate who I am and who I want to become. When I sit with my sisters, I feel a sense of homecoming, a sweet feeling of community and openness that is always refreshing.

Most women I know have, at some point, experienced something that has temporarily dimmed their sense of power and potential. Perhaps they never befriended their bones or smiled at their reflection. Maybe they couldn't find where their talents slept and have lost the will to wake them. It could be a steady eroding of confidence in an unsupportive relationship or environment. Or perhaps there are more obviously traumatic experiences of domestic or sexual abuse in a woman's past. We may have no idea, and I'm often shocked by what's beneath the surface. We all are tender. And brilliant actors.

We all need to belong, to be welcomed just the way we are. We want to be cherished, encouraged to share our talents and teach our craft. We want our emotions to be received and honoured. We want security in the knowledge that we will be held beyond this evening, month or year. Whether this is by a lover, our kin or our chosen family of like-minded humans.

There are endless ways we can gather as women. At SYC, sometimes we work in celebration, through worshipping our bodies and finding nutritious ways of sharing and singing. Other days, the deep calls, and we use the safe space to delve into our dark and shadowed swampland, to do the work that is essential for explosive blossoming.

We can sit together, in a peaceful hum of creation, exploring the ancient crafts that were woven into the seam of our grandmothers' lives. Or we can just gather, enjoying a glass of wine, letting the conversation carry its natural course through the intimacy of uniquely universal stories, sometimes sharing fascinating skills and channelling Baubo – the bawdy old woman of Greek mythology – in eruptions of filth and deep belly howls that shake through our body and bring tears to our eyes.

This work watered me when I was dry. It helped me release deep trauma and shame that I inherited from the women in my family and have carried through my whole life. It opened up language for me and guided me to use my voice, to find the right words to carve an equal and supportive relationship with my partner and heal a broken relationship with my mother.

The wisdom here helped me learn about and love my body. Awoken by breath and movement, I expanded my awareness of my menstrual cycle and finally unlocked my own orgasm. I discovered how to take the time to find what turns me on, how to use words to communicate the ways in which I like to receive pleasure. This was more liberating than I had ever imagined, and the feeling of self-sufficiency and satisfaction translated into other areas of my life.

The explorations here are only a starting point. There is much more to discover and unlock. But I hope this will mark the beginning of your own treasure hunt.

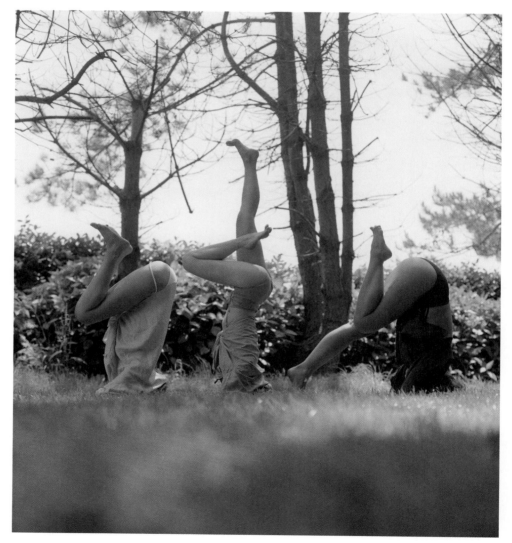

# RHYTHMS & CYCLES

It's really useful to connect with our hormones and, if we are in the menstruating phase of our life, to our monthly cycle and map out our emotions and energetics so we can plan our life schedule in harmony with our internal rhythm. If we begin to understand our seasons, we can learn whether we are experiencing hormonal influences as feelings, or if our emotions need to be investigated and honoured as a real and valid reaction to a situation. Once we learn the language of the complicated inner realm, we trust ourselves more and have better control over how we move through the world.

Being a menstruating woman is a wild and mystical experience. In ancient societies, the time of bleeding was sacred and the connection to the lunar phases and natural cycles was ritualized and celebrated. Yet the majority of us move through this part of life without even awakening to the latent creative, psychological and spiritual dimensions of our monthly cycle. I've found that practising menstrual-cycle awareness is an invaluable tool for life and stress-management. By charting my own seasons through my cycle, I began to understand my own nature, through the ebb and flow of my personal energy, *prāṇā* or chi. It wouldn't be too much to say that it was another form of awakening.

Much of the knowledge I will explore in this chapter is channelling the wisdom of two luminaries, Uma Dinsmore-Tuli and Alexandra Pope. I'm very grateful to have found their teachings and rediscovered my menstrual cycle anew, through using their practices as a way to deepen my connection to this personal lair of power.

Long gone are the days when women retired to the red tent for celebration, ritual and a nurturing five days of singing and stories. It has just become a time of the month that arrives with inconvenience for some, or a feeling of nauseous dread for others, sometimes without warning, other times with far too much warning (tears, anger, tiredness). It's easy to pass through each cycle without ever exploring what happens when we aren't bleeding, always experiencing it solely as menstruation, a time of permeable vulnerability when our clarity is overwhelmed by a surge of potent emotions.

I'd never really been too bothered about my period. There was nothing of particular drama or note. When I was in my twenties a mistrust of the pill led me onto a hormonal coil, which cancels out your periods all together. So I bypassed the monthly release and disassociated completely from my cycle.

A few years ago, I started to pine for my monthly bleed and disliked having a foreign object in my precious uterus. It felt unnatural for my womb not to have this time to cleanse and let go. I disliked the idea of alien hormones being artificially placed in my blood. I wanted to feel them truthfully, and to chart my developmental process.

So I had my hormonal coil removed. I've since welcomed each shedding with a feeling of fresh gratitude for the potential held in my womb. I've been amazed to see the patterns appear, and feel more settled in the comfort of knowing what to expect of my seasons and my energy. It has also been really interesting to see how it affects, and is affected by, my stress. I once went away for a month and had a huge amount of anxiety due to work and personal circumstances. I felt energetically imprisoned in my own tension and missed my bleed for ten days. Finally, I returned to my partner and my home. The next morning I awoke to feel the relief of a full bleed. It was as if my body had been holding out for harbour.

It had been so long since I had periods that I was unprepared for the sheer force of the mood swings. Once I was immersed in them, I couldn't understand them as a chemical shift of the seasons, and therefore couldn't temper (*ahem*) my behaviour accordingly. They just engulfed me. I've since become better acquainted with my cycle, and now think of it as a powerful tool for self-care, and I hope you will too.

As always, please consider the information here as the beginning of your journey. Do take the time to further explore anything else that calls you. If you are currently having periods, then keeping a diary for recording your emotions and energy levels may reveal interesting patterns.

## FOLLOW YOUR SEASONS

The menstrual cycle is a fascinating process. Most females who have reached this stage in their development will experience the bleeding more formally known as menstruation on average once every 28 days. But the cycle is actually divided into four stages that map the process as the body prepares for pregnancy by secreting hormones to prompt changes in the ovaries and uterus that allow the cycle to occur.

These four stages can be equated to the four seasons of the year, and tuning into them is one of the most powerful tools for what Alexandra Pope calls "body literacy" – a form of self-knowledge and empowerment. Instead of experiencing menstruation as a problem or "curse", it becomes a gift and shapes a template for how you experience your flow of power through each month. Once you understand this, you can map your creative, work and social engagements in accordance with the natural rise and fall of your moods and vibrancy. So the current carries you.

If you are not already mindful of the atmosphere of your body and the waxing and waning of energies as you move through the month, this new self-awareness can be radical. The invitation to open up and unfold into the natural expression of your energy will bring about a total shift in consciousness and the way you live your life. Taking notes each day, as you move through the cycle, is a really profound way to check in with yourself and make an inventory of your emotional landscape.

If you find that you periodically become exhausted, then this can help embolden you to make the changes that you need in order to live a more nourishing life. Saying "no" around your autumn and winter (see "The Sesaons", opposite) is a great place to start. You'll find that resting during those seasons enhances your health and ultimately makes you more productive. Carve out space in your cycle to be quiet and reflective, no matter if it's only ten minutes of meditation, or a bath during menstruation. Even if you have children and a busy work life, there are little pockets to be cherished as yours.

If you have just given birth, I've been told the return of menstruation can feel like menarche – that's the technical term for the first time you ever had a period. Some women find that their cramps have disappeared and they are able to enjoy their bleed for the first time. Or they begin to live more fully, really relishing the surge of vitality in the first stages of the cycle and noticing a real blossoming of creativity on certain days. Before I started on this journey, I'd never paid particular attention to my ovulation. Now I find it exciting to feel this twinge in my ovaries and to catch awareness of what I imagine to be the release of the egg. It has given me a sense of renewed awe and wonder, and anything that bestows your body with a sense of sublime appreciation is definitely worth the effort.

It's important to remember that although there are archetypal seasons, absolutely everyone will experience their cycle differently. There is no right or wrong. Be open to yourself and willing to accept the patterns that arise for you.

# THE SEASONS

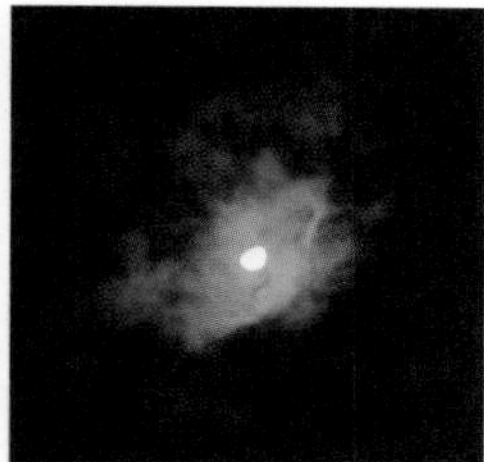

**Winter**

Bleeding phase (moontime)

Archetype: wise woman, crone, visionary

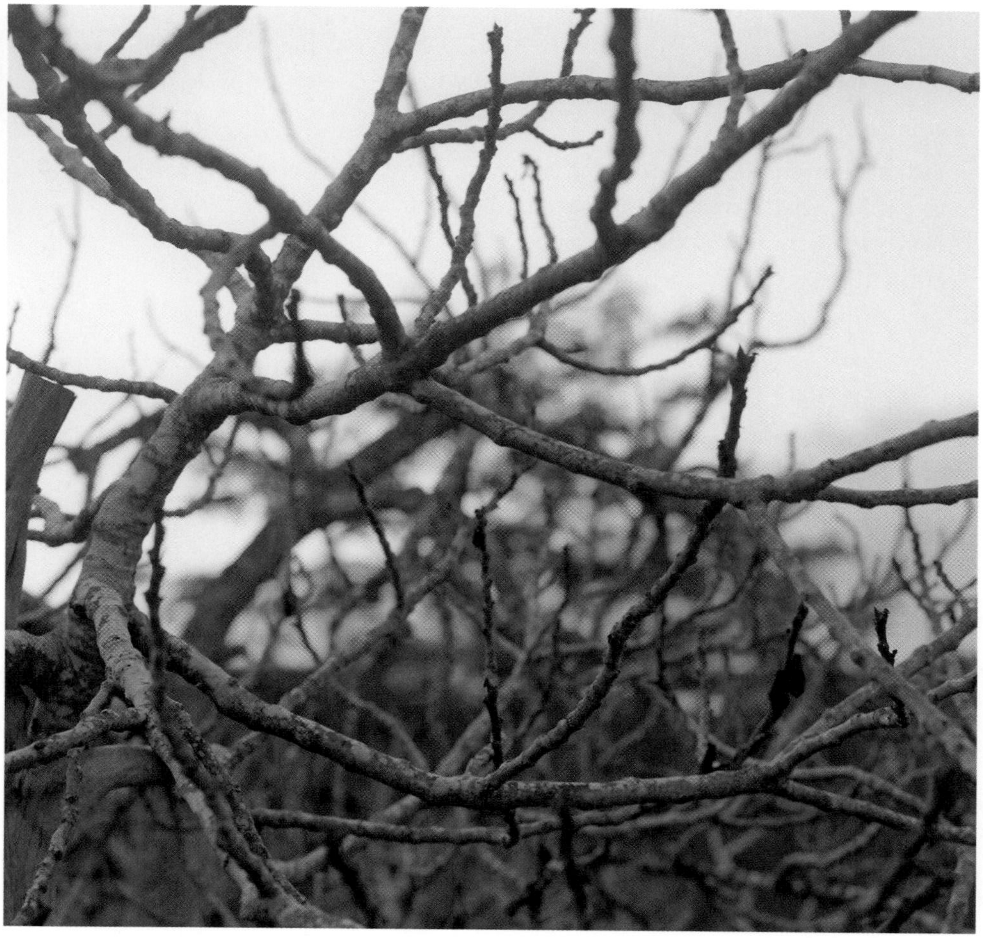

This is the period of menstruation, but it is also both the beginning and the end of your cycle (in a regular 28-day cycle, this would be would be days 27 to 5, for example – the last days of one cycle and the first days of the next). As you are bleeding, you are preparing to ovulate again.

The energies for this season are surrender and psychic expansion. You'll feel sensitive and permeable. It can be challenging to be still and hibernate, when you are used to pushing and pursuing. There are times when I've been shocked at how difficult it is to force myself to rest, when the urge to be active has been almost overwhelming. I've had to push through feelings of guilt and woo myself into a more restful state.

Typically, your winter is a time of softer energy, reflective, creative and permeable. It's a time of introversion, a space where you can surrender and turn within. This is the perfect opportunity to take a little break (where possible), schedule in some time alone.

Allow for a pause. Practise gently, explore yoga *nidras* (also known as yogic sleep), womb meditations, go for walks in nature, check into sister circles, take long baths, cook, garden, read, write, have a massage, allow yourself to receive. Take naps, lie in, step away from emails and social media. Do things that inspire you and notice if creating this space for softness and receptivity results in more creative inspiration and ultimately more productivity.

I've found that grasping for things creatively in life and work is not as productive as I used to expect. If we are constantly pursuing something, it lacks the grace and originality that happens when we create the space to receive. I've often found my winter illuminating in terms of problem solving and creative practices like writing. I meet things that seemed elusive or challenging with authenticity and ease. Ultimately, I've found that taking some time out (which I've been very bad at doing in the past) has led to a surge in productivity and the self-esteem that follows. Taking time out leads to a surge in productivity and the self-esteem that follows.

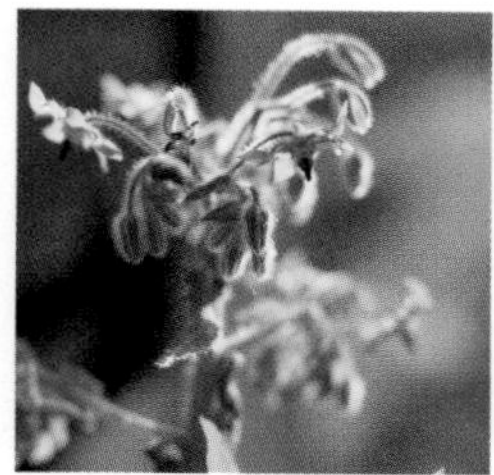

**Spring**

Follicular phase

Archetype: goddess, maiden

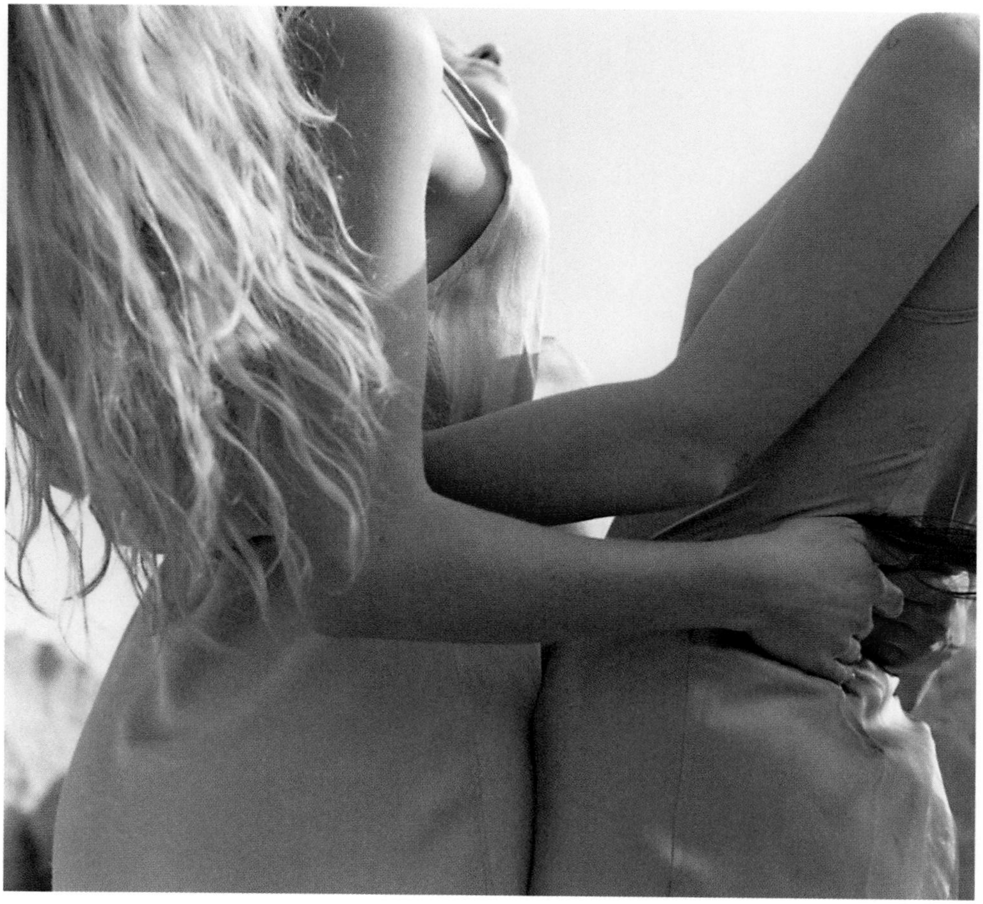

As the follicles in the ovaries mature in preparation for ovulation, this is a really magical time of regeneration and rebirth, with a feeling of being cleansed and renewed. It's a transition from a reflective space of inner quiet to extroversion and becoming. During this phase (days 6 to 11 of a 28 day cycle) your estrogen levels rise and your energy levels flourish. Your spring is absolutely ideal for research and plotting, physical activity, taking on challenges or being a social butterfly. It's a time of heightened productivity and focus.

With ovulation imminent, you feel potential, an element of excitement where possibilities blossom. It's a time of power and motivation, bringing a feeling of inspiration and playfulness. This is a wonderful time to assert yourself, to say "yes". To step into your power, feel confident and excited by life. A great time for fresh starts, feeling energized, independent and supported by the universe.

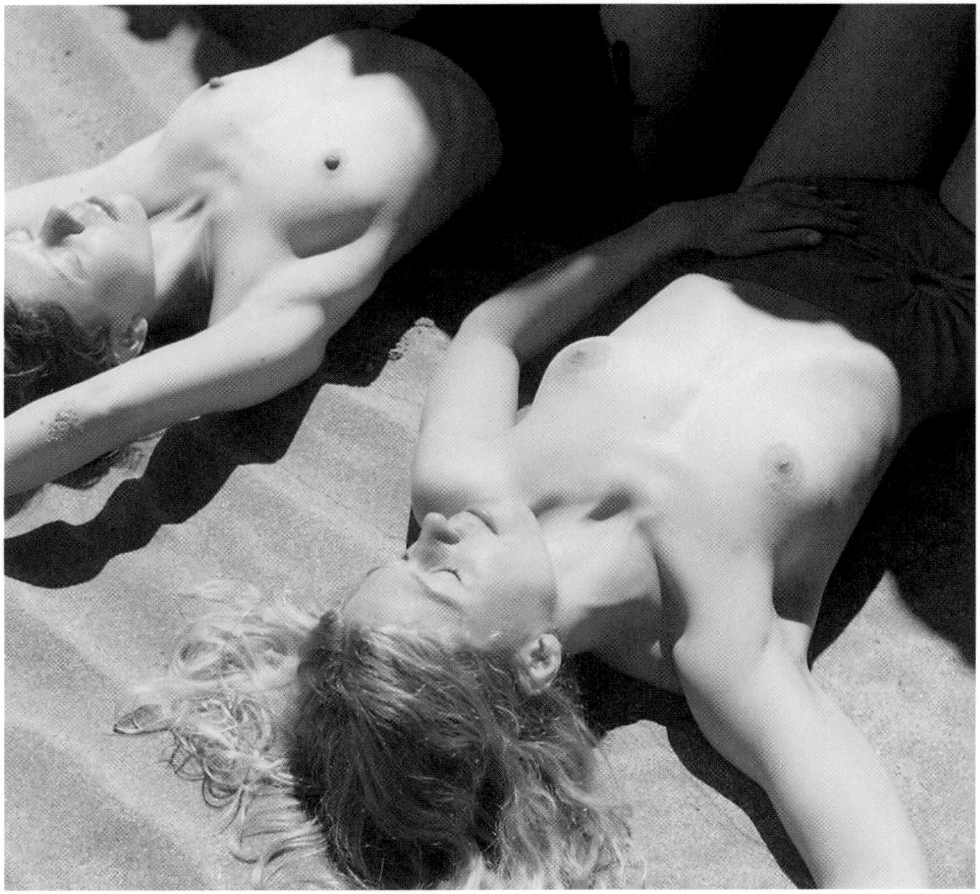

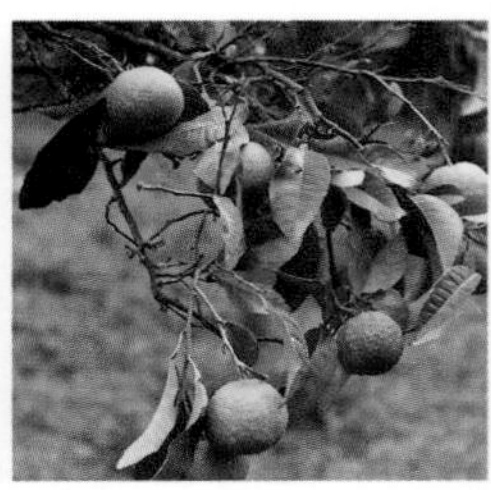

**Summer**

Ovulation phase

Archetype: mother, healer

If your body functions on a regular 28-day cycle, you are likely to ovulate around day 14, so days 12 to 19 are a juicy time of power, expressive extroversion, self-celebration and vitality.

Our busy culture tends to value this season the most, as a time of pursuit and tangible achievement. You may experience your summer through feelings of liberation and exhilaration, vibrancy and self-confidence. It's a time to be a social butterfly (again!), to take part in the community, to invite friends round and cook for them. You can really be strong and hold space for others, as your vitality is effervescent. It's perfect for a time of performance or public speaking.

This is the period of fertility, so you might experience a surge in your sex drive and a heightened experience of pleasure. It's a wonderful time to ask for what you want, both in the bedroom and in life.

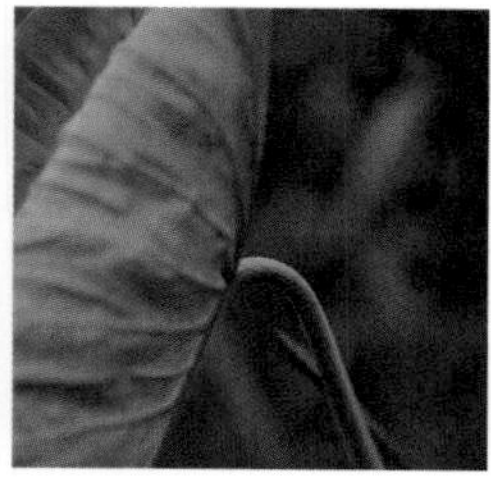

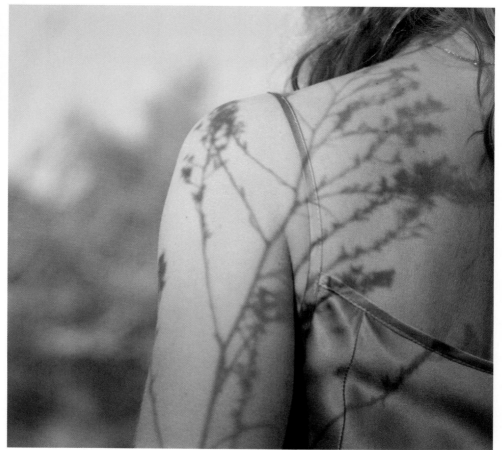

**Autumn**

Luteal phase

Archetype: wild woman, priestess, enchantress

With levels of the hormone progesterone (which prepares the womb for pregnancy) at their highest, this is a time of tension and complexity as we negotiate our way through a dramatic shift in our moods and energies. As we experience the poignant change in our inner atmosphere between days 20 and 26 in a 28-day cycle, we'll be challenged to balance the wrestling energies within us with honesty and integrity

Following on from summer, we might carry some of the sting with us, asking that we use our power with discernment, by selecting which emotions require action and which are best left to settle and evaporate as the winds change. This is when your inner critic comes into the field, to question you and criticize you, chastising you for any perceived fault.

At this point in your cycle, your hormones will dip and leave you with lower energy, feelings of irritation, less coordination and an urge to be still rather than active.

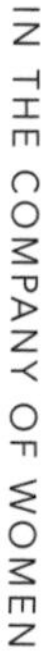

## HONOUR YOUR CYCLE

Your life will really begin to change when you honour your body by consciously inhabiting its seasons and cooperating with its natural dips and surges. The best way to do this is either to create a monthly chart and keep a brief diary each day, mapping out your cycle, or to download an app to help you keep track.

Once you begin to cultivate menstrual awareness, you tune in to your needs and begin to surrender to the natural demands of the body. The body responds and becomes more powerful and creative.

This idea comes from Alexandra Pope, and I absolutely love it. First of all, it's helpful to imagine a dream for your bleed. Choose the most delicious place you can imagine yourself dwelling. It can be anywhere: a sunbed on a golden, beachy paradise, a big beautiful bed in a hotel where you're hand-fed figs and grapes. Once you figure out your absolutely ideal situation, you can reduce it and identify the elements in it that you can incorporate into your daily life.

For example, if I imagine that I want to be far away in a tropical place being pampered and fed, it probably just means I want some time out and a bit of healing touch. So I book myself a massage and commit to being offline in the evenings. Sometimes, I ask my man to do something with his friends so I can have a candlelit bath and watch something dreamy that I've been saving for a rainy day. Or I go to bed super-early and dive into a book.

I used to find it very difficult to say no. This is not uncommon, particularly in yogis, who tend to be people-pleasers. Of course, this meant I used to tire myself out doing things that I'd prefer not to do. So either I had less energy for the stuff that was important to me, or I ended up feeling a little bit frayed.

If this sounds familiar, then the time of the month when you are bleeding is the most precious opportunity for you to learn to say no, even if this is not what people want to hear. Guard this as a sacred time for you to reflect or reconnect. This will mean that you will greet your period with relief and gratitude, which is a sacred shift in itself. Once you set this intention to spend your precious time more mindfully, you experience a change in how you carve out your days in general.

Starting a chart is not only wonderful for helping you establish boundaries, and great for noting moments of introversion or extroversion, but it leads you toward a more sustainable way of living. In tuning into yourself, you will learn to be guided from within, which is essentially what any kind of mindful practice like yoga is all about. It will help you to cultivate self-compassion as you modify your expectations of yourself according to your emotional and energetic landscape.

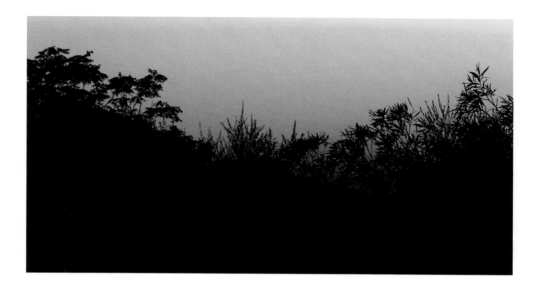

It will also create a feeling of deep self-trust, where you can experience your emotional life and your hormones more reliably. We've all been there, darting off snappy little emails that seem totally reasonable. Or barking with exasperation at partners who can't do anything right, only to feel sheepish once we realize we've been usurped by hormones. There is absolutely nothing more frustrating than being taken by surprise by your period, or someone pointing out that you might be coming on, before you notice it yourself. By committing to mapping your cycle, you ensure that you're in control. You can pre-empt yourself, and perhaps warn your partner, children or colleagues that your bleed is about to start, which will give them the invitation to treat you with more generosity.

Here are a few ideas for things to chart on your cycle:

- ○ Mood
- ○ Energy level
- ○ Sleep
- ○ Dreams
- ○ Motivation
- ○ Sex drive
- ○ Creativity
- ○ General feeling of health and wellbeing

If you are low on time, just note energy and mood. A few words will do. But try to be disciplined about keeping your chart going, so it becomes an integral part of your life. The regularity will enable you to see recurring themes and patterns as they arise, and prepare for them in the future.

# WONDROUS WOMEN

Women's circles are a beautiful way to connect to our sisters and see how our personal story weaves into the big picture. Once you sit with women, you realize how precious this is as an antidote to the busy extroversion of everyday life and the nectar for all the times you give.

Each woman offers up secrets, unfolds, and is rewarded for her bravery when her stories echo and reverberate through the her-story of the other women around the room. It's comforting to hear communal experiences; it's also inspiring and empowering. I always leave sister circles brimming with wonder for all of the mystery and strength of womankind. And I am also seen, heard and held.

It is in circles where the deep work is done. The shadow work. That is to say, we sit and we talk about the things that we are processing, some light, much dark. Here, we expose our stories, bound and tangled through layers of flesh and clay. Here, we free ancient secrets suffocated in the depths of our bones. Here, we unearth the seeds we rejected, fearing lest they take root. Here, we recognize the terrifying and magnetic pull toward excavating our little chambers of longing, the ones slowly burning away in shame and fear.

These experiences, the shadowland ones, can be unsettling and confrontational. We can feel undone as they demand we examine the foundations of our being, whether we have unconsciously inherited them or spent a lifetime carefully building them. We all layer, weave and colour our lives into our bodies, so that it is as if we are viscerally dissecting ourselves, burrowing deep through the sludge to reach light.

Once we give voice to our darkness, it loses its power and we can carefully cleave it from our soul. So when we talk about experiences that leave us feeling guilty or ashamed, we also release that shame and lighten our load. These deeper conversations still bring up fear, of course, in the invitation to step out of familiarity and into the naked unknown. Whether our past has been filled with joy or pain, it still feels like our identity, and it's not easy to let go of experiences and emotions that have cloaked us (to use Carolyn's Cowan's metaphor) our whole lives.

At SYC, most of our woman's events involve a meditation and intention-setting, then a somatic practice – a form of healing and empowerment experienced as movement through the body. Once we have created this physical opening and eased out of our contraction, we perhaps feel able to expand energetically and emotionally.

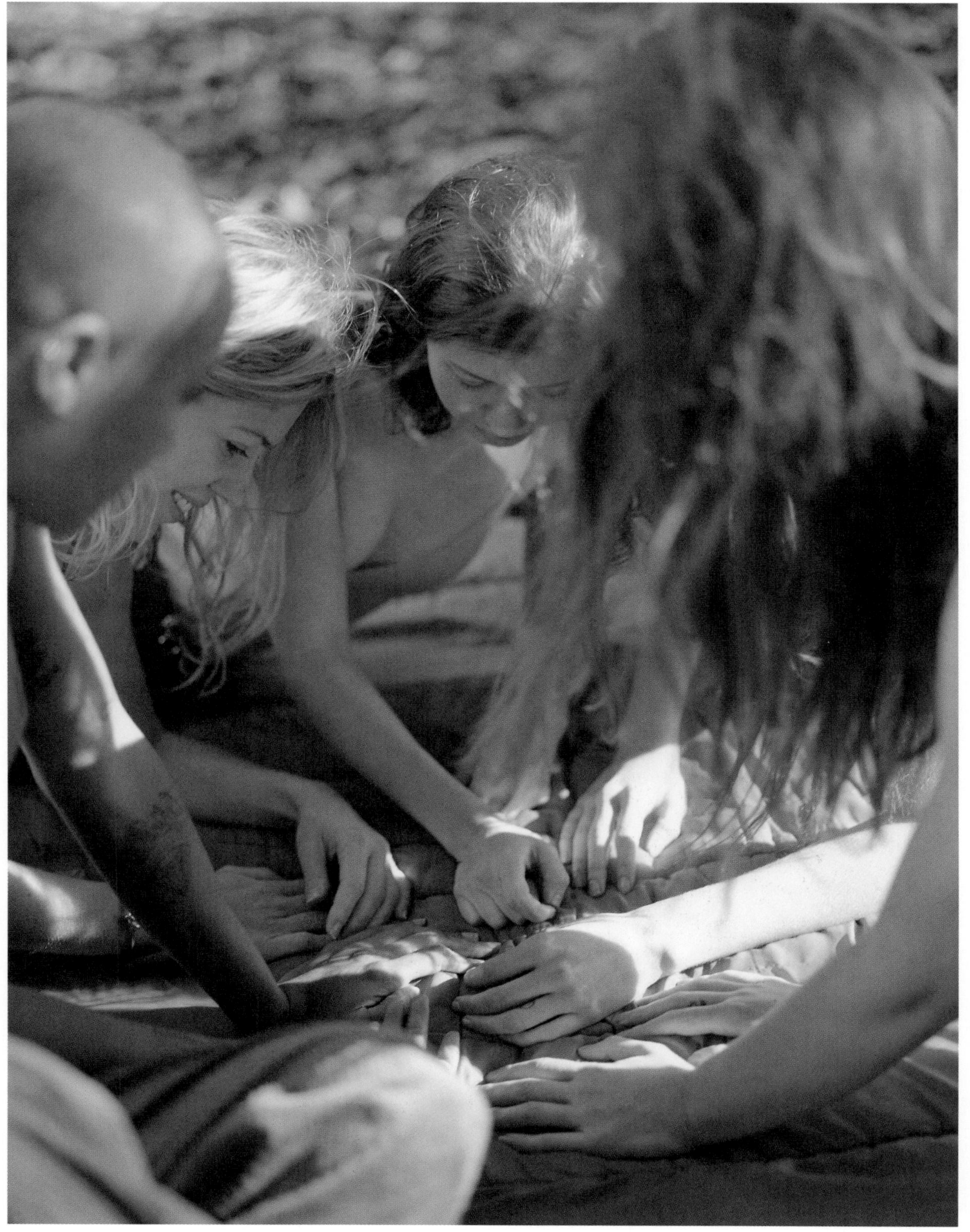

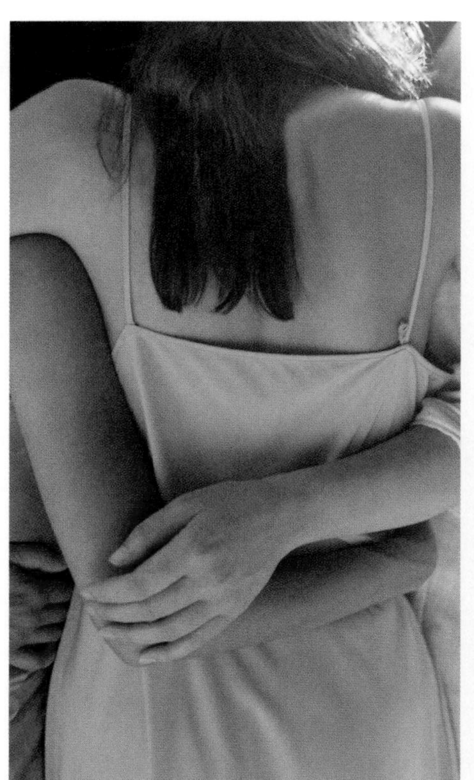

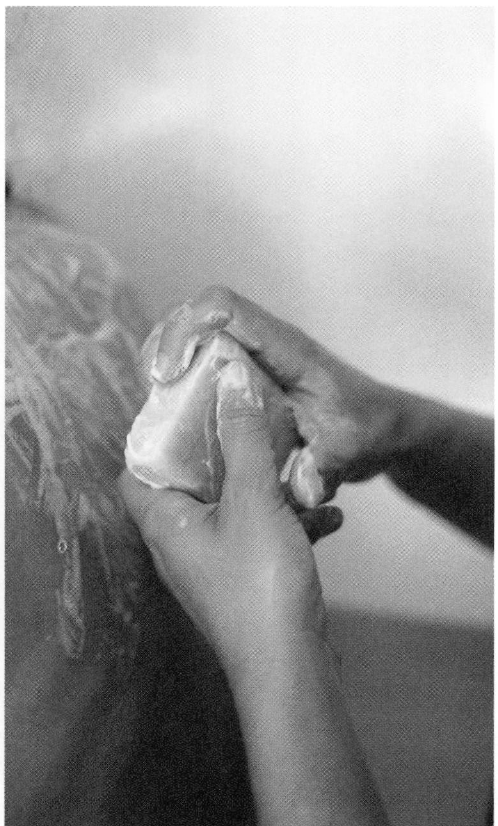

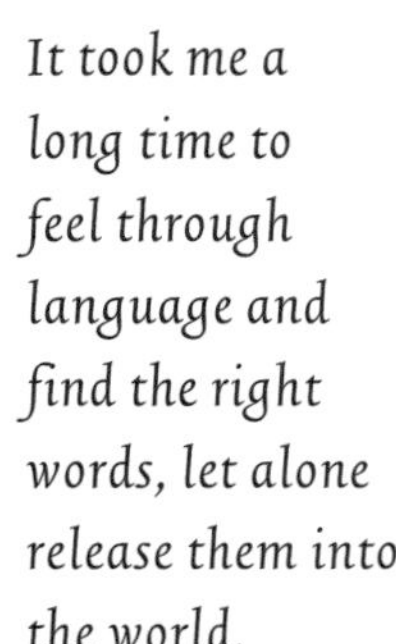

*It took me a long time to feel through language and find the right words, let alone release them into the world.*

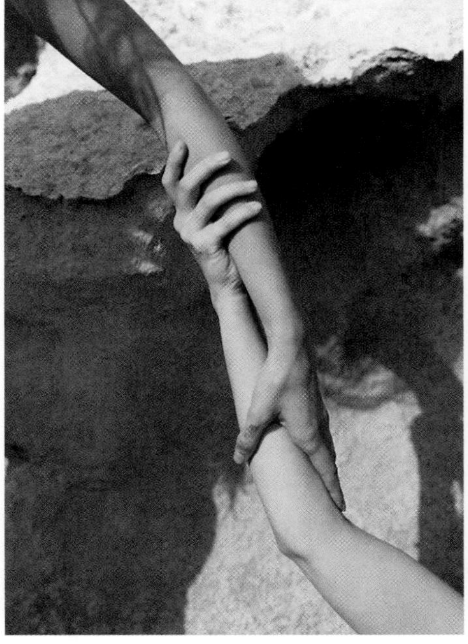

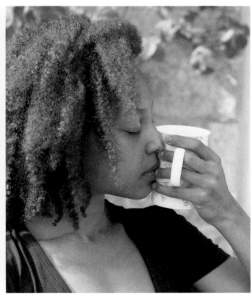

The sessions also always incorporate an element of sharing, sitting in a circle with sisters and putting voice to experience. For some, the chance to express is deeply poignant. If you're not used to speaking out, this is a very powerful practice.

It took me a long time to feel through language and find the right words, let alone release them into the world. I know that being given the gentle time to explore myself verbally made me think and then act differently. As each woman in the circle speaks, it's natural to think about what it is most present for you. I used to become very nervous and eat my words. I'm often surprised at what's beneath the surface, at which little things refuse to be ignored. It's cathartic.

These practices force us through a labyrinth of emotions and thoughts that we would otherwise have circumvented. But "the only way out is through". In these circles, we identify things and people that make us feel diminished, and uncover what it is that we need to welcome into our lives, where we have neglected ourselves and which boundaries we may have dissolved and need to resurrect. Sometimes we are so busy extroverting that we don't see what it is that we actually need. Here, we discover this together. It's like the most wonderful, heartful form of group therapy, at a fraction of the price.

In these circles, the same themes surface again and again: women wanting to be more to everyone, dividing their bodies into two to be mothers and lovers, caring for their baby and feeling guilty about missing freedom, identity and income. Many times, I listened to shimmering and intelligent women talk about feeling eroded by a masculine environment at work. Women struggling with the sadness of caring for an elderly parent, or supporting a partner by managing the domestic duties, feeling overstretched, undervalued and unseen, lonely and longing.

Some of us were redefining what it means to be a woman, what we had inherited from our ancestors and what we were cultivating for our future. The thing that I was most shocked by, which the #MeToo movement revealed, was how many sisters had been sexually abused and were moving through the world, quietly carrying this wound with them, living with fear and dissociating from their bodies or sensuality.

I wanted to create a space for women. I saw how much we could learn from each other, how each story was uniquely universal and how speaking it would help others find their voice. I thought about my mother. She had a violent, alcoholic father and she used to stand as the buffer zone between him and her mother. Her childhood was hijacked by a hypervigilance that has only recently begun to abate.

It has been my great joy to see her bloom over the last few years, to absorb her into our community so we can rediscover each other outside the limiting paradigm of mother and daughter.

I often think that if there had been a sisterhood supporting her, as there is for me, she'd have been held and maybe discovered a way to empower herself. When I think about our future children, and what kind of environment I would want to grow into them, I know that there is so, so much work to be done and I want SYC to be part of the change. Gathering together, we can support each other, help each other heal and evolve, find solutions and plant seeds for the new world. It's all possible.

## CREATING A WOMEN'S CIRCLE

Creating your own women's circle is easy. Once you create a framework, it will unfold for you very naturally. Here are some tips to creating your own circle.

### INTENTION OR THEME

Identify what your intention is in initiating this circle. This gives all the sisters a focal point for conversation and clues to help them explore their emotions. An example of a more practical circle is creating a safe space to explore and discuss starting your own creative project. This could include creative expression, creative practices, fear of exposure, fear of failure. Another example is an exploration of motherhood: questions regarding identity, negotiating motherhood with other roles, guilt or exhaustion.

### GATHER

Invite your circle to your home, set the space with candles and palo santo or incense. It's nice to have some tasty bites or drinks. You could also ask people could to bring food with them to share.

### THEME

It's good to select a theme, so there is a starting point for conversation. This can be anything, from the cycle of the moon or other astrological insights to choosing goddesses from pagan or Hindu mythology or working with the seasons.

### LANDING

It's really important that everyone land together. We have such busy lives that we tend to arrive somewhere on the crest of our emotions, sometimes scattered and a bit uncentered. As the host, you can welcome everyone into the circle and guide people through a brief meditation, read one out or find one online to guide you

Take about 5 to 10 minutes, allowing everyone to gather themselves up and sit in stillness to see what is there, empty out the day and tune into their emotions.

## NAME SHARING

Once you come back, and open your eyes, invite everyone to smile and look at their sisters in the circle. Take it in turns to go round sharing your name and bringing one or two emotions into the space.

For example: I'm Astrid and I'm feeling relaxed and open. Or maybe, distracted and exhausted. Make sure you share first and say something honest and heartfelt, to set the tone for everyone else.

## PRIVACY

Take a moment to acknowledge that you are setting a sacred space, and that what is shared is private and will not be spoken of outside this circle. People may talk about their own experience with others, but not mention that of a sister. This creates a safe vessel for people to open and speak freely.

## NO JUDGMENT

Please make a point of mentioning that this is a space free of judgment. We all have ugly, contracted feelings; this is where they can be shared to begin the catharsis of release, and prevent toxic emotional energy from curdling into shame. In sharing, people are taking ownership of their voices and their personal experiences. One of the beautiful things about this is that we find that each woman has her unique story, but that story is always universal. In listening to our sisters, we will find echoes of our own experiences, and each woman has her own profound wisdom from which we can learn. I always leave circles feeling inspired.

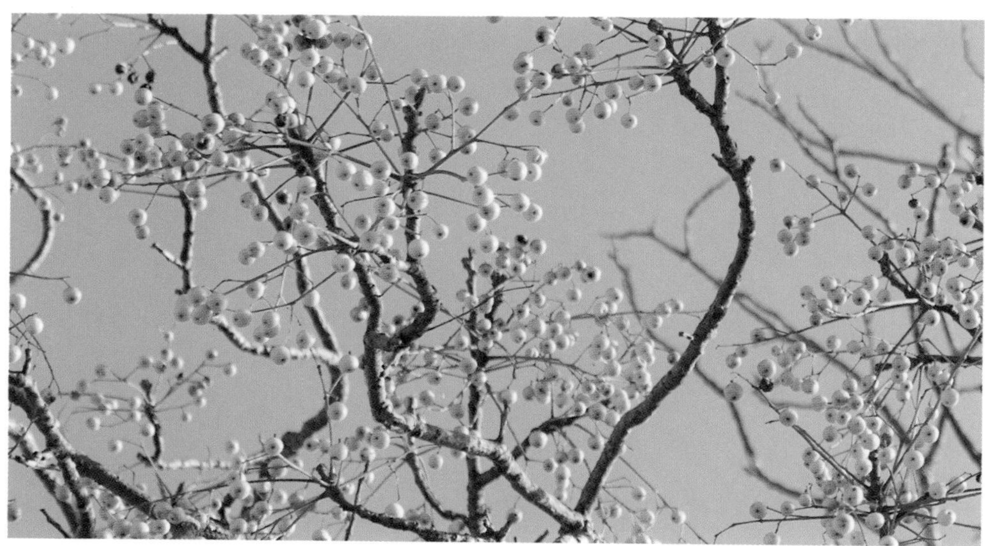

However, the intention is a sharing circle. This is not a space for a woman to be directed, for anyone to think they have the answers to another woman's life. It's not for anyone to tell another woman what she "should" do, unless a sister specifically asks for help.

### SPEAKING

In my experience, people can get nervous if we go round in a circle, clockwise or anticlockwise. Instead of listening fully to sisters, they jump ahead to plan what they would like to share. I can't remember where I heard this, but if you invite people to speak as they feel called, like "popcorn", people will wait and wait and wait, then *pop*! They're ready to voice the thoughts that have been accumulating. This way, some people can decide that they would prefer not to share, either at all, or only speak a few words.

It's totally normal to get nervous and feel awkward. You get used to it, I promise. The more practice you have, the more naturally and succinctly you'll be able to gather your thoughts. Try not to judge yourself on what other people are saying; just speak your truth and that is perfect.

### CLOSING

It's important to thank everyone for coming, to honour all that has been shared, to sit with it for a few moments, let it settle and also create a space where people can release anything that may not be theirs.

You can ask people to go round sharing a word, as you did at the beginning. Perhaps this might feel like the right thing. In which case, close with a meditation and potentially set an intention.

You can also close by chanting *om*, which has a grounding effect. There is the option to hold hands. Do whatever feels right at that moment.

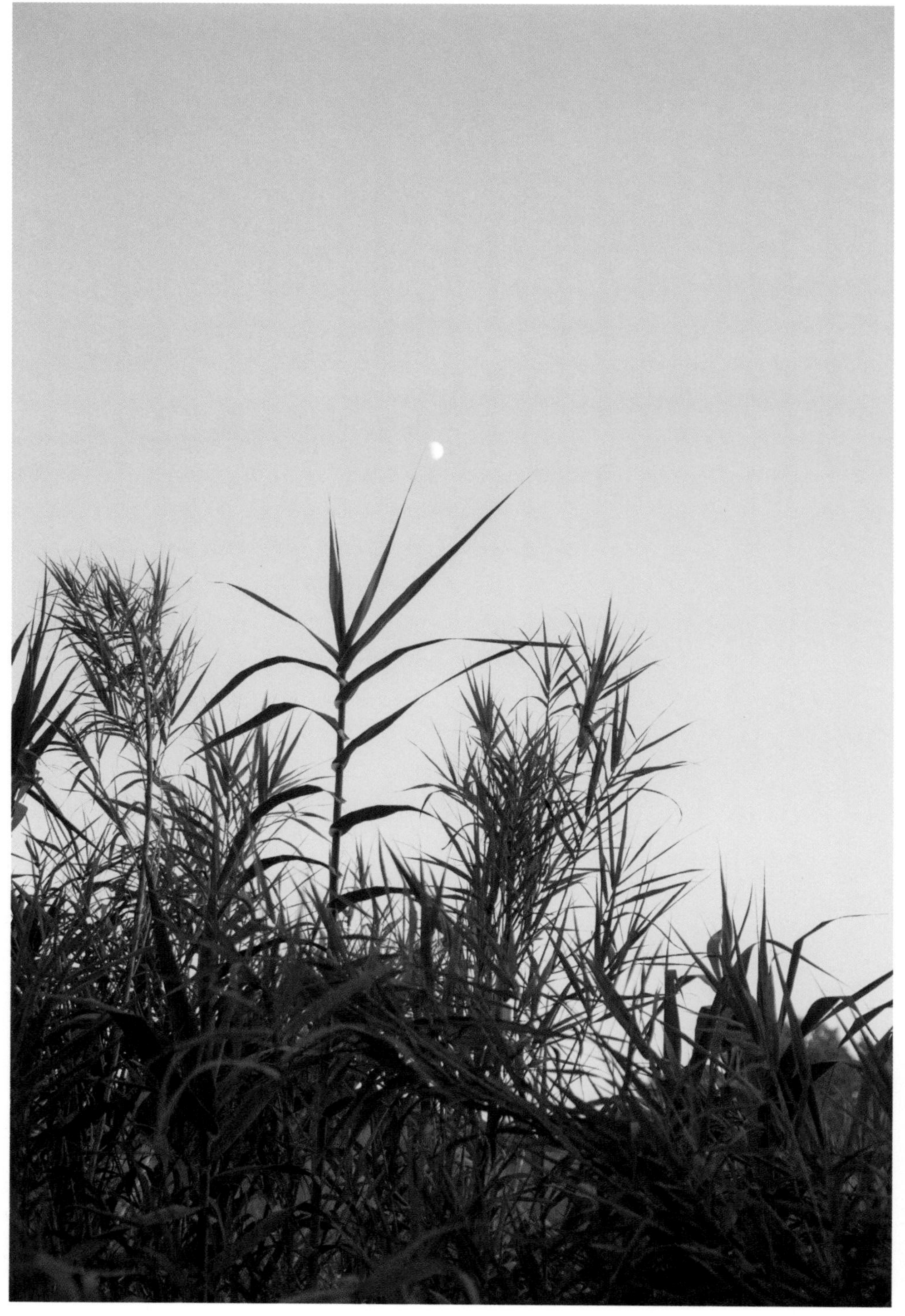

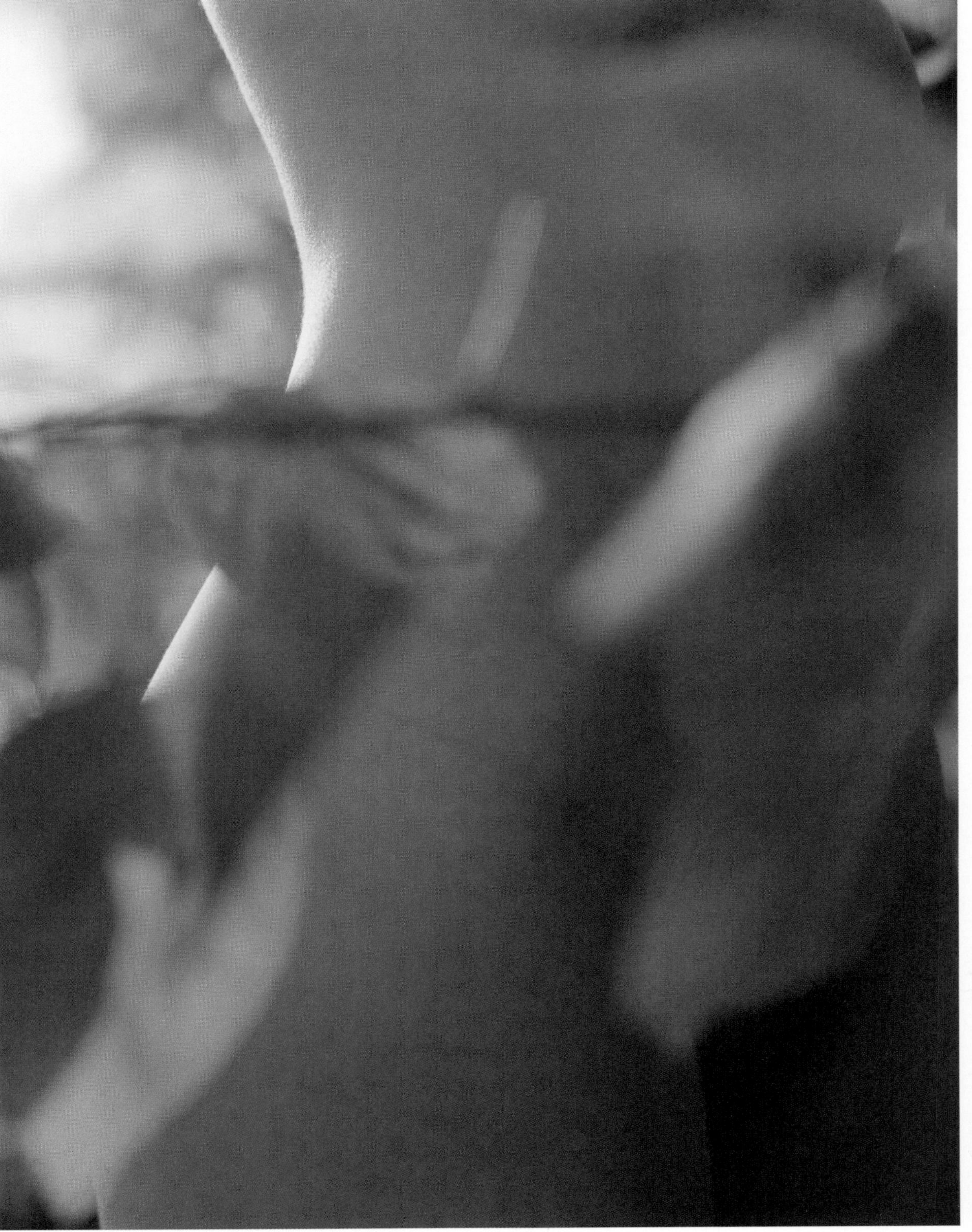

# 6

# EXPANDING WITH PURE SENSATION

*"Sexuality is one of the ways we become enlightened, actually, because it leads us to self-knowledge."*

ALICE WALKER

# THE SIGNIFICANCE OF SKIN

All living creatures need attention. We're thirsty for tenderness. We flourish with attention and care. We yearn to be seen, heard, appreciated and encouraged. We long for intimacy, for a primal, visceral connection with other souls. We want romance, to be met at the shore of our hearts and carried into the deep.

We want to feel the powerful current of connection charge through our bodies. To be electrified by a touch that brightens our bodies and awakens our *prāṇā*. We truly want to be held. There is a deep need for us to experience our bodies skin on skin, the weight of another human on our being. To be stroked, soothed, celebrated and adored.

We need to unlearn our shame and conditioning, particularly in relation to our bodies and their desires. We should celebrate and unlock our latent sexuality and harness our innate sexual power to reach a higher state of consciousness and revitalize our senses. This power is a gift, and it's a wild awakening.

The skin is our body's largest organ and it's the interface between our interior realm and the exterior world. It's the very first sense that we develop – as eight-week-old foetuses in the womb. Through our skin, we experience the texture, temperature and temperament of the physical plane. It's how the world feels. Skin brightens with excitement, stands to attention in fear and carries the tantalizing shimmer of arousal.

You'd expect us to give a lot more attention to the significance of skin. After all, our skin tingles with curiosity, it wants to explore. Think how often we capture our own attention by allowing our hands to roam, tracing our fingers on tempting textures: a wooden table, a grainy plane of paper, the face of a loved one or a patch of grass. Touch is a very pleasurable invitation to escape a chattering mind and dive into the present moment.

Touch is also a very natural part of our humanity and an integrated part of life. I've always craved tactile experiences. I hug strangers in greeting. In my yoga practice, I like to move slowly, until space becomes tangible. I love eating, am happiest with a delicious sip of wine on my tongue (I feel there's a crossover between taste and touch). I walk barefoot in mud and grass, swim naked whenever possible and even plunge my body into cold water to feel the shock of presence in my flesh. I'm always reaching out for my boyfriend for a little touch of his head or face. I love to touch.

Our society is afraid of touch – we've become prudish and sterile. Maybe it reminds us of our proximity to the animal realm, through the primal desire or longing it awakens. Or perhaps it exposes our tender vulnerability and simplicity. But touch is incredibly healing. Our bodies respond to being touched, we respond to touching.

Some of the most obvious benefits are (should you need an excuse):

- Hugging can lower blood pressure, particularly in young women.
- Hugging can lower the heart rate.
- The more hugging, the higher levels of oxytocin in the blood. Along with a number of other benefits, this encourages social bonding. Wounded animals been shown to heal faster when given oxytocin.
- Touch stimulates the brain to release endorphins, which improve our mood and reduce stress levels.

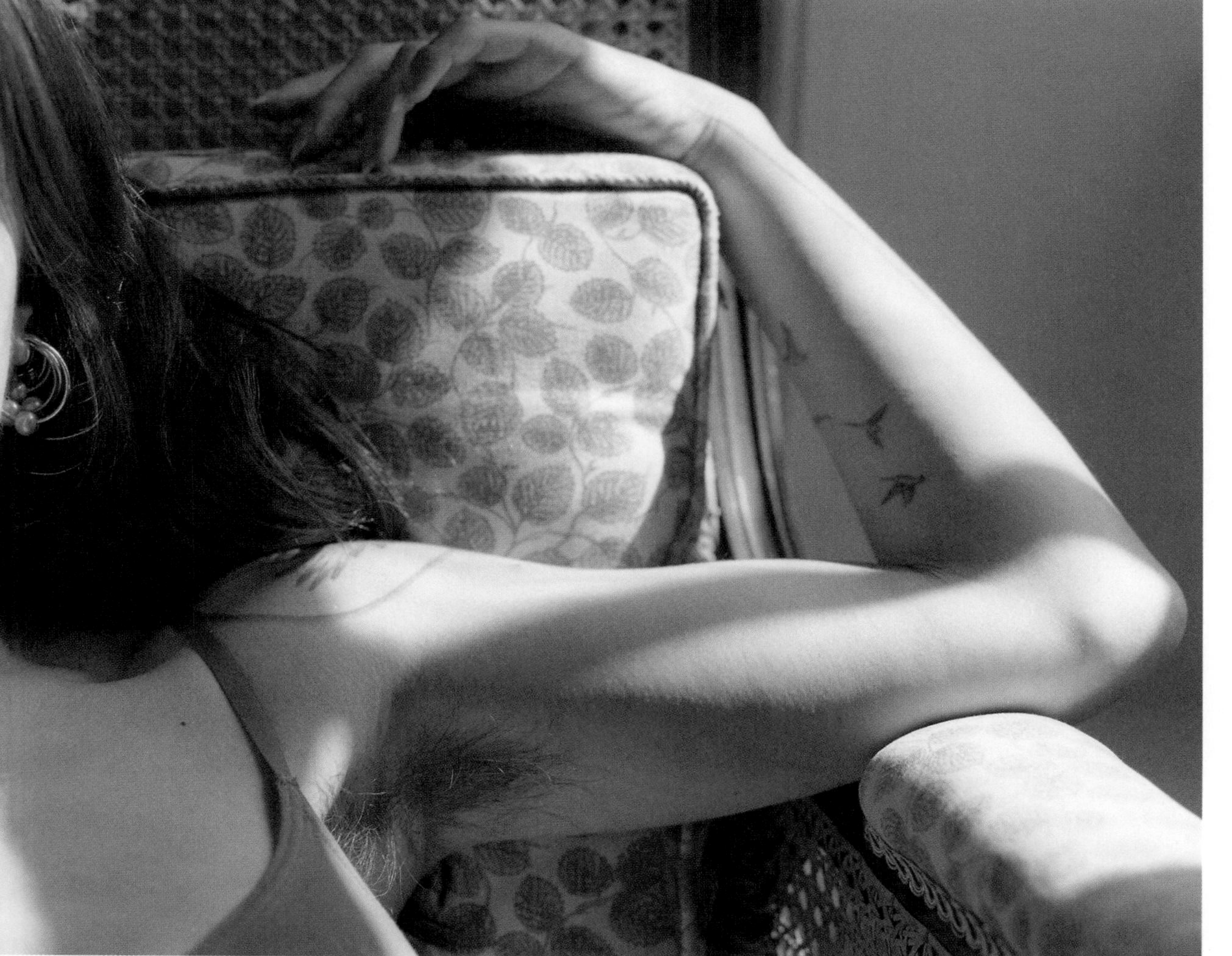

There are ways that you can receive the nourishment of touch, in a safe space, without an agenda. I notice that when I am under pressure, my yoga practice isn't always enough. I still feel tense, I feel the cortisol coursing through my body, particularly when I'm premenstrual. My limbs are heavy, my forehead compressed and my little heart picks up its march in a way that can feel unsettling. So I take myself to healing hands and wait for the fizz of stress to dissipate.

If you need convincing further, a recent study carried out at the Cedars-Sinai Medical Center in Los Angeles revealed that people who undergo massage experience measurable changes in their body's immune and endocrine responses. According to the study:

- People in the Swedish massage group experienced significant increase in the percentages of white blood cells, which play an important role in defending the body against disease.
- Swedish massage also caused a large decrease in arginine vasopressin (AVP), a hormone believed to play a role in aggressive behaviour and linked to increases in the stress hormone cortisol.
- Swedish massage caused a decrease in levels of cortisol.

So get yourself booked in for a little massage of self-love.

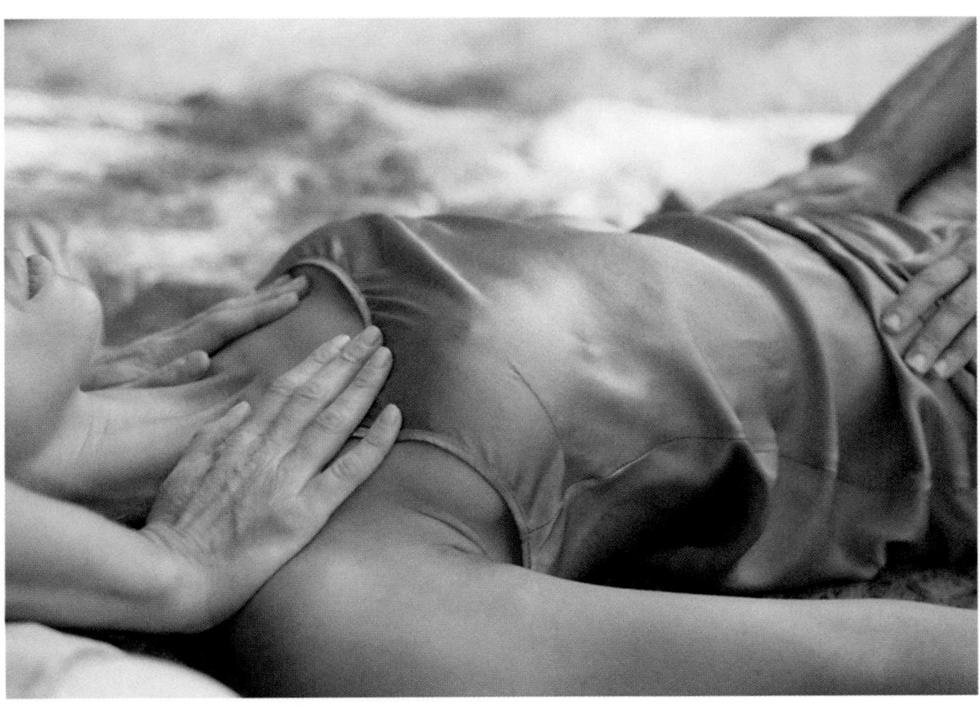

## SELF-MASSAGE

I know: it's not quite the same as someone else attentively washing all the stress out of your limbs, but self-massage can be a beautiful way to reconnect to your physicality. It can also be surprisingly luxurious.

You can adapt this into a little morning ritual, in which case you'll probably need to skip the romance and just focus on the massage. I have a friend who does this ritual every single morning.

If you have the time, take a nice long soak in the bath. Case studies show that we relax more in soft romantic spaces, so make it sweet with cosy low lighting, some candles and sage or palo santo and play dreamy music. Then you want somewhere comfortable to lie down, so a bed is ideal, or a big towel on the floor. Watch out for oil, though.

Start by sitting in an easy position, but feel free to move around and find a way of working your body that feels good for you. Take your time. You might want to weave a few intuitive stretches into the movement. Make it special. Be present and slow. Let your fingers educate you on where they need to go. Linger in the tender spots, experiment with pressure and breath, allow a few sighs to release.

### FEET

Poor things, our little feet. So precious and so neglected. We barely look at them, yet they carry us everywhere. We have 26 bones in our feet (that's about one-quarter of the total number in our bodies), about one hundred muscles, tendons and ligaments, and almost 200,000 nerve endings per sole. Feet are highly sensitive, intricate networks of architecture and they love to be touched.

Notice how open and receptive they feel after you have given them attention. Walk around and see how they feel.

Cup your right foot in one hand and cover it in some nice-smelling oil. Then hold it with both hands, fingers along the front of the foot and thumbs facing the sole. Let your thumbs slide down the foot, slowly fanning outward, massaging down the curve of the arch and across the top of the sole, just below the toes. Repeat as often as feels good to you.

Now cup the inner ankle with your right hand, then wiggle the fingers of your left hand between your toes, like little toe dividers. Place the thumb of your right hand in the arch of the foot, pressing gently, and slowly circle the wrist of the left hand, holding the toes.

Release the toes, then use the fingers to trace down the gap between each toe, massaging as you go. Noticing how much longer each individual toe is, how deep the bones go into your foot. How interconnected everything is.

Use thumb and forefinger to massage the little joints by squeezing them with a little bit of pressure and rolling them in a circle. Continue with the pads of the toes.

When you're done, repeat the process with your left foot.

### LEGS

Rub oil into your legs. Pay particular attention to the calf muscles, fanning up and down, as before. Stretch out your leg and cup the calf muscle, with both thumbs pointing down the front of the shin toward the feet.

Press the pads of the fingers into the belly of the calf, and slide the fingertips away from each other, horizontally across the calf, as if you were closing your hand. Move your fingers up and down the leg.

Use the tips of your fingers to massage a circle around the knee.

Then continue the same action up the legs to the thighs, squeezing the flesh, fanning with the thumbs, experimenting with rubbing and squeezing. See what feels good. Place your thumbs into the crease of your hips, hold them there for a few moments, then slowly move them around toward the crest of the hipbone, grasping and kneading, responding to your body. Notice how small the gap between the top of your hip and the bottom of your ribs is.

When you have finished, repeat with the other leg.

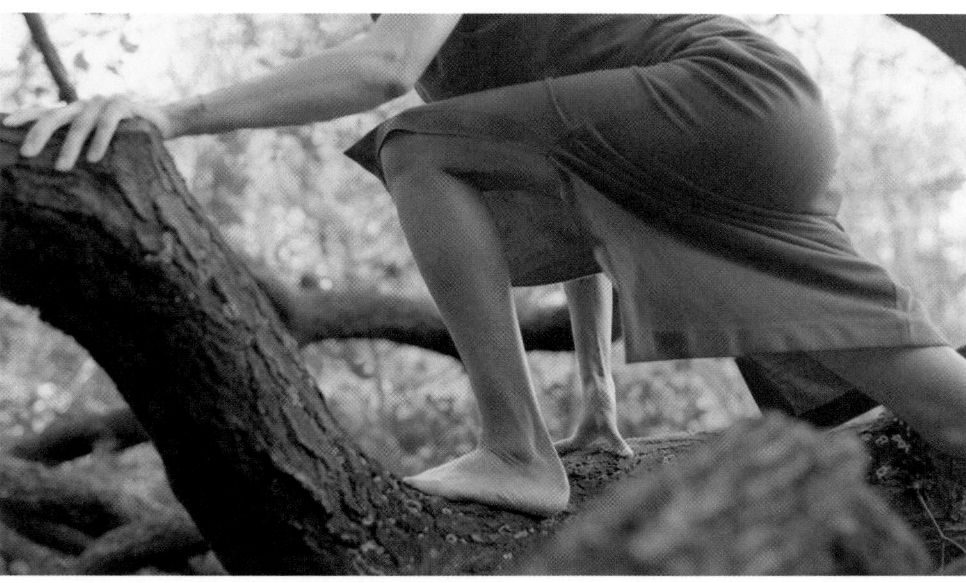

GLUTES

The glutes or gluteus maximus muscles are the large muscles in the buttocks. Plug your fingers into the dimples at the top of these muscles and use circular motions, pinching, sliding and stretching the fingers across the flesh. You can even get in there with a tennis ball and roll around a bit.

In a seated position, slide your hand under one side of your bottom, with the palm cupping the cheek, so you are sitting on your hand. That bony little golf ball you can feel is one of your sit bones. Make little circles with your bum, so you're massaging around the sit bone. Then do the same on the other side.

BACK

Use both hands to cup the back of your hips, with your thumbs pointing toward your spine. Trace along the back crest of the hip, massaging with your thumbs. Walk the thumbs around the lower back, moving upward. Pinch the sides of the waist, sliding the thumbs from the middle of the back toward the waist as you do so. Press thumbs into the two long muscles flanking the length of the spine, called the erector spinae. Trace along the ribs and follow the thumbs forward, plugging and holding them into the armpits as the fingers massage the front of the chest.

CHEST

Gently pinch the flesh at the front of the chest. Slide the fingers down and around the breasts before cupping them, massaging them gently and with care. Circulate the fingertips up and down the breastbone. Tuck and press them gently under the collarbone, continuing the massage. How amazing is it that your lungs fill your chest up to above your collarbones? Can you feel this with your fingertips, as you take a deep breath in?

SHOULDERS

Bend the right arm across the body. Cup the left shoulder girdle. Burrow the right thumb into the girdle, massage and squeeze around it. Navigate the palm up toward the neck, using the four fingers together on the back of your body, with the heel of the palm on the front, to massage the shoulder blades: squeezing, kneading and exploring. You can use the left hand to cup the right elbow, and further encourage it into and down the back.

Repeat on the other side.

ARMS

Start with the right arm and move the palm down the arm, kneading, squeezing, exploring and pressing with the thumbs and fingertips. Circle the elbow. Press the four fingers down the length of the forearm, finding, pressing and easing the tender gaps and spots. Massage around the joints of the wrist.

### HANDS

Holding the right hand in the left, fan and knead into the central well of the palm. Burrow the fingertips into the space between the web of bones in the palm. Rub all the joints in circular motions, then press and knead the fleshy parts of the hands and the pads of the fingertips. Circle the wrists in one direction and then the other.

### NECK

Cup your neck with both hands, bringing the heels of your palms to kiss at your throat. Press and rub the back of your neck, up to the base of the skull, down to the top of the shoulder and in between the wings of the shoulder blades. Press the hands up to the base of the skull, along the bone at the back of the head, following along to the back of the ears, the neck, under the jaw, the front of the throat, burrowing gently behind the jawbone and back up again to behind the ears. Turn your head to the left, tuck your chin into your neck and follow the muscle from the base of the skull behind the ear, down the length of the neck to the clavicle. Repeat on the other side.

### FACE & HEAD

From the neck, massage the fingertips in circular motions up and around the skull with the fingertips meeting at the front of the skull and the thumbs nestled into the temples. Follow the fingers down the forehead. Move around from the top to underneath the eye sockets, pressing into the flesh. Find the gap under the cheekbones, move under the mouth and onto the chin. Touch your index fingers on the bridge of your nose, then slide them down the length of your face, toward the ears. Return to the bridge of the nose and follow up the forehead, fanning as you go.

End by just cupping your beautiful face, closing your eyes and taking a moment to feel. Then lie back and drink in the blissful melt of relaxation.

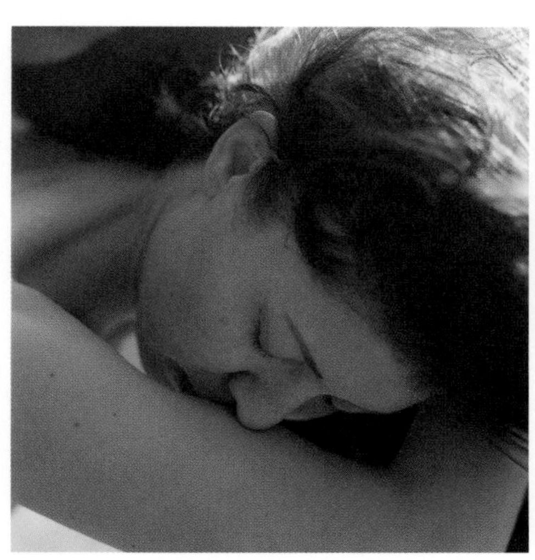

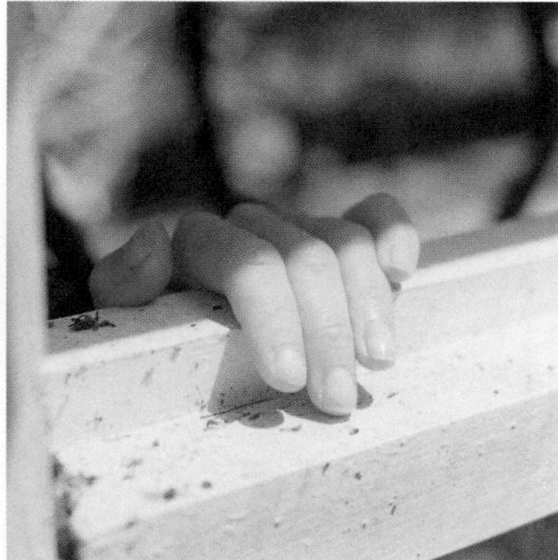

# NEO-TANTRIC RITUAL OF TOUCH

*...when we find a space of quiet through meditation, breath work or movement, we cleave our mind from the churn and witness our stories unfold.*

I'd expressed an interest to a friend in exploring this more sensual, energetic work, so she passed on an invitation to an event she was going to. I decided to go based purely on her recommendation and didn't even investigate. I found myself en route to the event before I'd even sat down and read what it was about.

The description was exotic and mystical. It talked of Tantra and energy work, celebrated Mary Magdalene, and it mentioned Christ Consciousness. It also stated that nudity was optional, which almost made me spit my tea out. But I continued on the journey, interest piqued, spine bright and skin alert.

I arrived at an innocent-looking and Spartan venue in north London. By day it was a yoga school for children with learning difficulties. Today it was moonlighting as an unlikely cocoon for a group of women of all ages, shapes, sizes and sexual orientation, seeking many different things: sisterhood, community, warmth, connection refuge and also excitement or desire.

I could feel the different energies mingling in the room. We sat in a circle, each with her own colour of excitement, anticipation and fear. No one was talking. Everyone was waiting and watching. Guessing and projecting. Looking for clues in clothes and stories in eyes.

The teacher came in, a twinkle, half sprite, half woman. She shared her story of sexual promiscuity, shame and abuse. Sex had been her drug and her body had become burdened with too many, too much. So she'd turned to healing herself in the way her skin responded to most: touch and love to replenish the energy coursing through her that had been so depleted through years of carelessness.

She'd moved in Tantric circles with men, but found that there was a predatory undercurrent and hadn't felt safe. So she began to explore women's work. How to open up the heart through the body, and how to bring warmth into the soul by revitalizing the subtle energy with touch and intention.

The first practice was to dance. But the room was sparse and bright and the music on the speakers was tinny, not nearly loud enough to drown out the inhibitions of a large group of women. The teacher then asked us to close our eyes and, rather unceremoniously, to "sacredly disrobe" and sit down. She turned the music off. The room fell silent and 30 little birds fluttered in 30 chests. I sneaked a peek, and every woman was softly getting undressed. I followed suit and we all sat down.

We opened our eyes and looked at each other: without our uniform, our armour and our branding. We were resplendent, luminous, primal, beautiful. There was nothing crude about the moment; it seemed entirely pure and natural. That is truly inspiring – to know that when we are naked and seen, we are all deeply beautiful. Revelling in the integrity of the natural body.

Once we had settled, the workshop began to unfold. We split into threes. One woman sat with her legs crossed, the second lay down with her head in the first one's lap, the third sat cross-legged, between the legs of the woman in the middle. I can't remember if the woman lying down had something covering her hips, but I do remember feeling safe and not exposed at all.

First we were just held there. Still with our head on one woman's womb and the wings of our hips in the cups of another woman's palms. It was deeply soothing and grounding. Something about the energetic connection dropped you right down so you were held, contained and connected. Then we began stroking, first the hips and the tops of the shoulders, then around the breasts and the flanks of the thighs, then gently tracing our fingertips down the full length of the body.

I know, this is just what people think Tantra is – the seduction of the flesh and immersion in sensation. And of course, part of this is true, and these practices are nebulous and often haunted by desire and possession. But in this case, it was sacred and healing. The stroking was not charged with desire, as this touch normally is.

There was no goal, but the effect was brightening, as the body responded in the most natural way, creating a shimmer through the skin, sharpening the senses and awakening the intuition. When the event was over, I stepped out into the night air with my whole body humming in a state of receptivity. Every cell was vibrating. All my senses sharp and seeing. All of me was alive and interacting with the pulsating world around me.

If you feel safe and open enough, you could try this with some friends. If not, the practice below is a soft little opener.

### PLEASURE CATS

My friend Chloe Isidora taught this on our first Venus Day event a few years ago, which celebrated all the glorious things about being a woman. It was deeply indulgent, feminine and sensual event. We wanted everyone to leave feeling luscious and held.

We'd been hosting some curious events for a while, but I felt a little knot of anxiety tighten when our women burst into the room in a smack of clingy lycra, warming up their bodies in preparation for the type of class that was entirely the opposite to this offering...

Practise this with friends, and surrender into simple touch. If you are teaching, make sure that you are absolutely one hundred percent comfortable holding this practice. You need everyone in the room to trust you, so they can relax into receiving. They will follow your energetic invitation. Working in groups of three is ideal. Two is OK, if need be. Wear comfortable, cosy clothes and have blankets to hand.

Create a little nest of blankets on the floor. One woman lies down, coiled on one side. The other two sit one at her head and one by her hips. They are going to gently massage and stroke her. If you are one of those doing the stroking, ask her where she would like to be touched. Follow where she directs you. Harness your attention into the moment. Treat her like a treasure, a beloved. Like a queen. Be attentive, stroke her slowly, touch her hair, massage her head. Perhaps massage her feet. Be absolutely absorbed in the moment. Notice what comes up. See whether this feels natural or uncomfortable. Witness without judgment.

Take turns to receive. See how this feels. Do you find it easier to give than to receive? Are you impatient? Or do you find you drop right into the pleasure of being petted, like our beautiful feline friends?

If you are holding space, you must give people the option of being held energetically, as opposed to being touched. It's important that everyone feels safe: you never know what trauma there is in the room, so you must open the conversation for people to give their consent and create their own experience.

When the ritual has come to an end, thank each other for all of the sweet touch and attention.

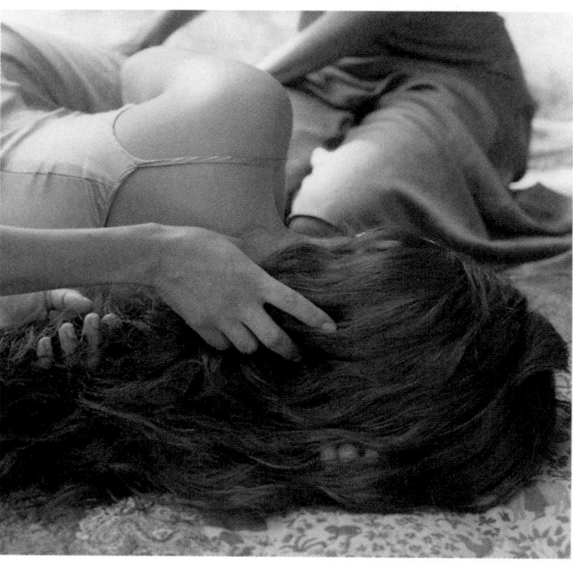

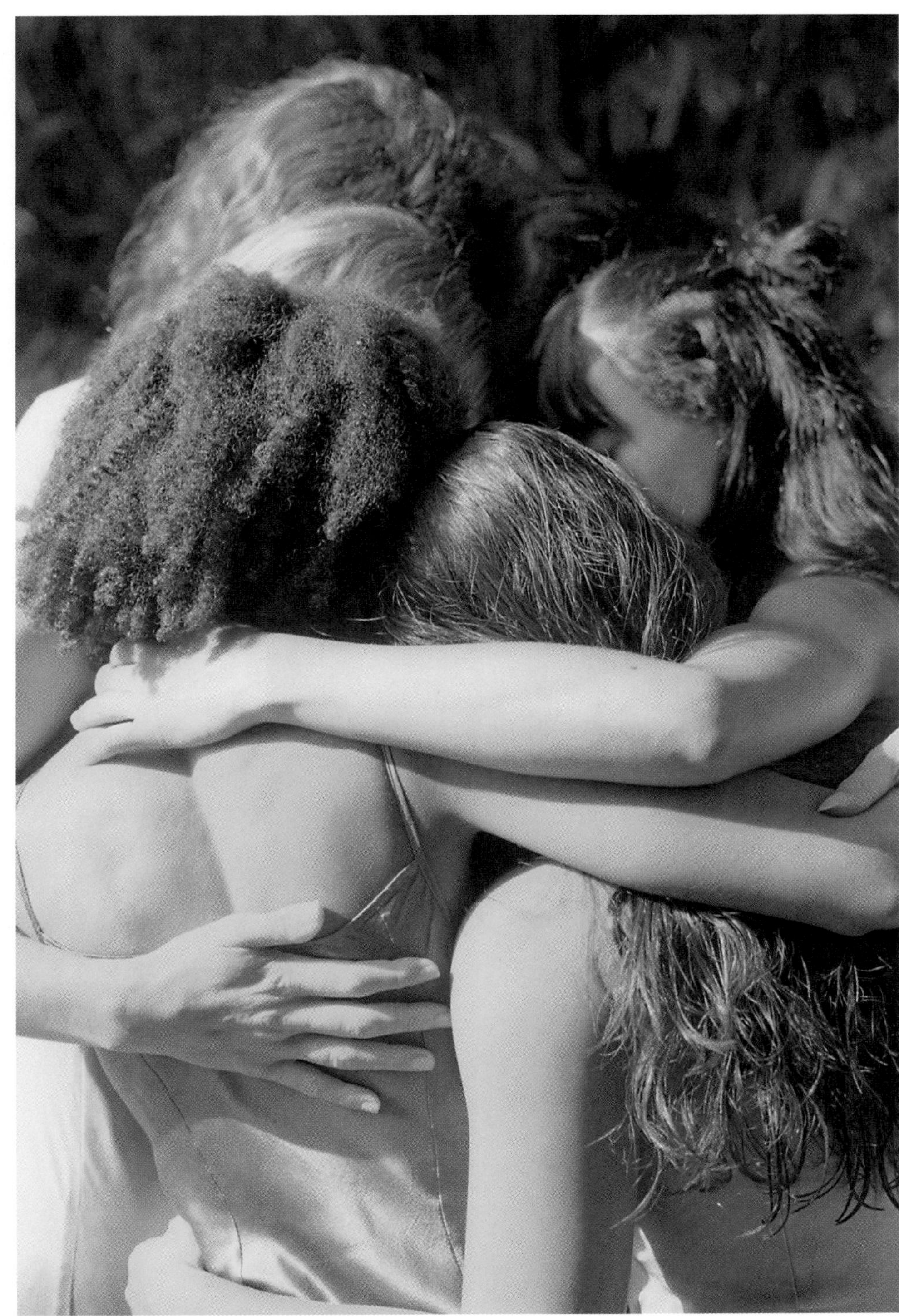

# PLEASURE MEDICINE

Absolutely everyone deserves raw pleasure. Good sex and transcendental orgasms are our birthright. Even if you don't feel it now, you're brimming with potential. My yoga practice guided me back to myself, so I could fully immerse myself in the poignancy of sensation. It resulted in me accepting and loving my body at all its stages and cycles. Whatever you've unlocked so far, there's more to discover. Your sexuality will continue to evolve, develop and deepen throughout your whole life – it's never too late to find your orgasm or have really cosmic sex. The more you uncover and weave your own map of pleasure, the more profound and life-enhancing your experiences will become.

If you look at the history of sex, you'll begin to see that women's sexuality was universally celebrated until biblical times. The vulva was honoured as being deeply sacred. Symbols of the yoni were carved into caves by the very earliest humans. According to Naomi Wolf, "From the beginning of recorded history, every culture that has been studied has a version of a sex goddess."

A long journey of changing attitudes at the hands of a patriarchal society has seen women demoted and the glorious potential of the vulva, the potency of female sexuality and the healing powers of the female orgasm extricated from our identity. The sexual script became masculine, medicalized and is still longing for wisdom and poetry.

I've always been fascinated by sex. As a child, I remember playing games with friends, exploring each other under the guise of doctors and nurses. Even at a young age, these games felt charged. When I look back to my childhood, there was also an awareness of my parents' sexuality. Nude swims, long weekends in bed and walking around without clothes when they thought we were out. Sex and skin were a part of life.

At some point, though, the narrative changed. Contradiction is my mother's privilege, and one that I've inherited. When I was a rebellious teenager, my mother was worried about me. Catholic shame and guilt regarding everything pleasurable became the dominant sentiment at home. My mum was always on guard, fearful of the worst thing that could ever befall a good Catholic mother: her daughter could become a "slut"...

My mother's attitude was not unusual. Many young women assimilate shame as a result of their dominant cultural, religious and political narrative. For me, the idea that female sexuality was somehow bad, or that female pleasure was unimportant, took a long time to shift. Although I enjoyed myself, it took ages for me to learn how to worship my own body, to cultivate and harness my sexual energy for myself.

So, despite having been aware of my sexuality from a young age, I had to do a lot of work before I could feel that sexual pleasure was intrinsically good – a secret power for me to explore, own and brandish. I also had an incredibly restless mind, which meant it was challenging to be completely present, either on my own or with a partner.

As I coaxed myself out of my head and into my flesh, without even realizing it, I was extricating myself from what didn't feel good or true. The key to a pleasurable life with good sex is enjoying your own body and being able to inhabit sensation fully, moment to moment, to follow the pleasure.

## THE PLEASURE RESPONSE

Have you noticed what our bodies do when they're turned on? There are the obvious responses: we feel our heart quicken, a thread of arousal spools from our belly and blossoms into an awareness of sensation in our pussy, this electric tingle of anticipation might lead us to become wet and... To be honest, I've never thought much about the other mysterious processes in our body that prepare us for sex. But of course, some kind of magic happens for our pussies to be ready for receiving.

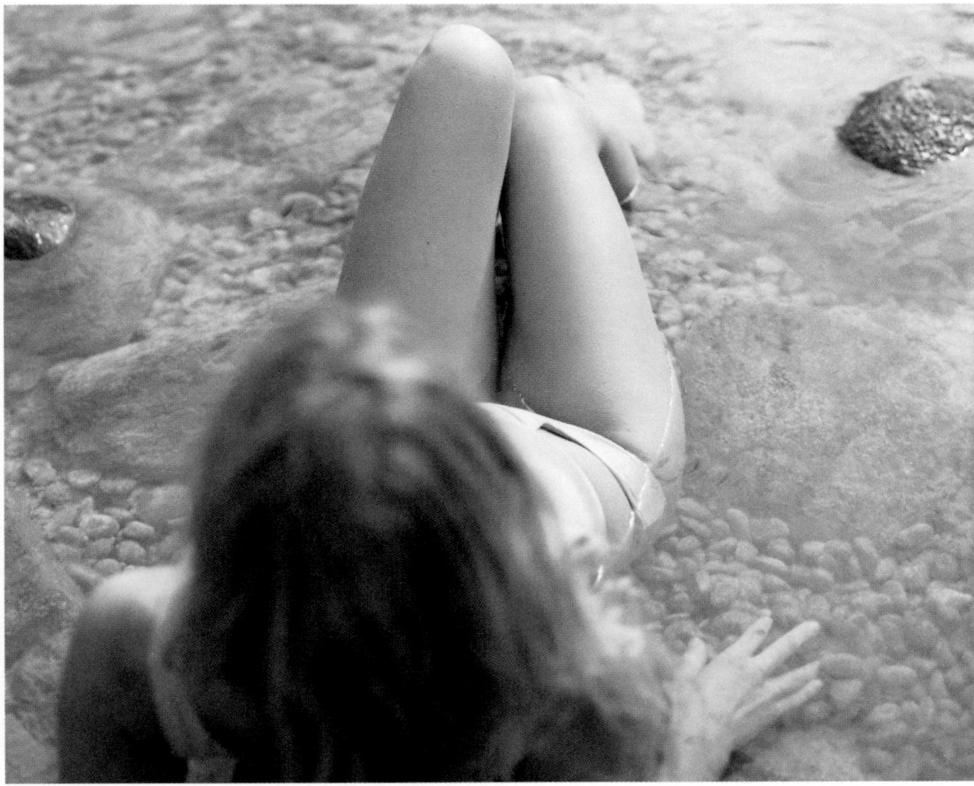

Once I began to research the biological wonders of our pleasure response, it renewed my sense of awe for the mystery of this visceral human portal. I hope that learning about what your body is doing will help draw your attention to it, to feel more profoundly and to be captivated by yourself.

### BECOMING AROUSED

We generally need to feel fully relaxed to become highly aroused and have glorious sex. In order for our body to undergo this mystical alchemical process, it needs to be uninterrupted by stress or anxiety, which will block the arousal process. Women need to feel safe enough with their partner to release their inhibitions, allowing the body to take over and carry them into an orgasmic trance.

The state of arousal is a profound psychosomatic cycle that signals to the body that it can relax, drop out of fight and flight, and allow a cocktail of sexy chemicals to work on the brain and permeate all the cells in the body.

This feedback loop between body and mind needs to be sensitively maintained in order for us to have incredible sex. Our mind must dissolve into our body, and our body must be continuously sensually engaged to harness the mind.

We've all had experiences when that magnetic incline of sexual hunger has suddenly evaporated, interrupted by an unwelcome intruder. If you struggle with surrendering into the realm of feelings, your sex response might also be arrested in elusive or abstract ways. A certain way of being touched might trigger this, or our thoughts could dance off on a critical tangent and kill our vibe.

It takes time, trust and practice to immerse in pleasure bathing. You need to begin teaching yourself the pleasure principle on your own. You are enough. You can find your own pleasure map without a human guide. You don't need a toy, a pornographic distraction or a vibrator. (These may initially help you to orgasm, but they're not a long-term solution and shouldn't become a habit.)

This is why it can take a long time for us to have fantastic sex. We need to be seduced. Eye gazing kick-starts a feeling of intimacy that will filter down through our body, initiating a neurological process that viscerally signals to us we are both safe and turned on. Deep kissing begins the steady release of delicious drugs like dopamine, oxytocin and serotonin, which help in the first flush of anticipation and affection. Caressing lights up the energetic body, vivifies the senses and preps the physical antennae for indulgence.

Physiologically, our heart rate and blood pressure rise. There's an increase in blood flow around the body, which causes our pupils to dilate. Our face might flush. Our body then releases nitric oxide, which relaxes our muscles and further increases blood flow. Our pussy grows wet and the external genitalia become engorged, a beautiful blossoming of exciting fullness that you will notice when you give your pussy your full gaze (see below). At this point, as your clitoris begins filling with blood, she wakes up and behaves in much the same way as a penis does when aroused. She's also made of the same tissue, becomes hard and increases in size – a clitoral erection.

### SEXUAL PLATEAU

As we brighten with electric arousal and experience a full body flush, our nipples harden and may feel tender. Our breasts may also increase in size. Once we become fully aroused, things that previously felt uncomfortable or painful can begin to feel pleasurable, so we may like to be touched or handled in a different way in order to be turned on. The changes in our bodies once we are fully aroused might translate into a hunger for more extreme experiences, which is why some people seek to amplify the sensation in other ways. There's a very interesting pleasure and pain connection with sex and the brain, which is the guiding principle for S&M.

In the build-up to orgasm, our muscles begin to tense, which is why we feel that incredible relief after we climax.

### PLEASURE TRANCE

At this stage, we're receiving a huge surge of dopamine and adrenaline to ensure we continue to enjoy ourselves and charge magnetically onward. Our clitoris is so highly sensitized that she retreats under her hood for protection, and our labia minora darken.

The Bartholin's glands on either side of the vagina (credited with playing a role in female ejaculation) release more vaginal lubrication to carry us through.

This is when the pulsations in our pussy deepen and expand through our body. Our muscles contract and we may start to shake involuntarily in anticipation.

By this point, our whole body is a pool of juicy hormones, we're totally electrified, the two main pleasure centres in the brain – the amygdala and the hippocampus – are engaged and the parts of the brain that deal with anxiety and fear have begun to deactivate. We have well and truly surrendered into a vibrating vortex of delicious sensation. We're in a trance, totally uninhibited, our mind engulfed by a euphoric drive.

### SURRENDER

As we now release all the sexual energy we have been kindling, we catch on to a wave and surrender into an eruption of euphoric tingles and bliss. We melt, maybe even ejaculate. Endorphins and oxytocin create a feeling of transcendence and then of deep love and affection. We might feel weightless, ripples of colourful warmth flowing through us as our uterus contracts to encourage sperm on the journey up the cervix.

Post-orgasm, we feel a deep sense of peace and relaxation: a heightened sensation of connection within and without. We can stay here and marinate, or go back for more.

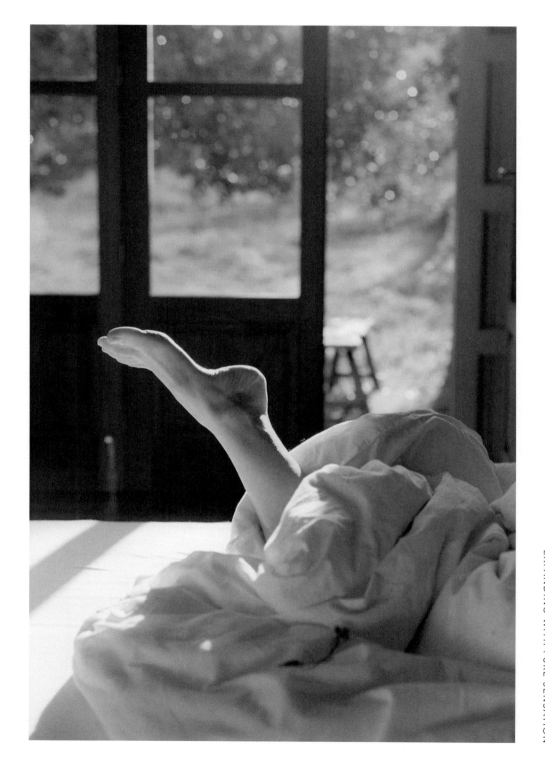

Unlike men, who require a refractory period and have to begin their journey towards arousal again, women are able to continue to receive pleasure. We can often have more intense second or third orgasms – we just keep firing them off! Our brain is conveniently wired to be always receptive to pleasure, so when we've orgasmed once, our pleasure antennae are already sensitized, ready for receiving, and our body-mind is tuned into an orgasmic frequency. Plus, orgasms heighten our sex drive. Our body knows what's good for it...

### OWN YOUR PLEASURE

Why don't we take sex more seriously? It's convenient to trivialize it, because when you actually ask people, almost everyone feels as if they aren't having enough, that it's too rushed or that they lack confidence in the bedroom. If you start talking about it at a deeper level, you have to acknowledge what's missing and then do the work.

This lack of discussion is either convenient for men in heteronormative relationships, or a curse. It relieves some of them of the duty to really get to know their woman, to put their ego aside, be humble and start from the beginning – spend more time, learn new tricks. For other men, absolutely nothing would make them happier than to pleasure their woman, but if you as a woman don't know how you like to be worshipped, how are you going to communicate what you enjoy to your lover? How are they supposed to bring you to orgasm?

It's important for you actively to take ownership of your pleasure. It's your power. It's your medicine. It can heal you.

If you're in a relationship, self-pleasure is still for you – it will enhance your sex with a partner. The more you know yourself, the more communicative you can be and the further you realize you can take it. Slowly stoke up your energy, tease yourself, bring yourself to the edge before tumbling into ripples, a weightless wash of kaleidoscopic bliss.

As lovers, it's important to dedicate enough time for pleasure. This may sound basic, but sometimes modern life is busy and exhausting, so we all need to remind ourselves. Especially if we're stressed and tired – that's when we most need the sense of euphoric transcendence, reconnection and relaxation. There's nothing more joyful than good sex.

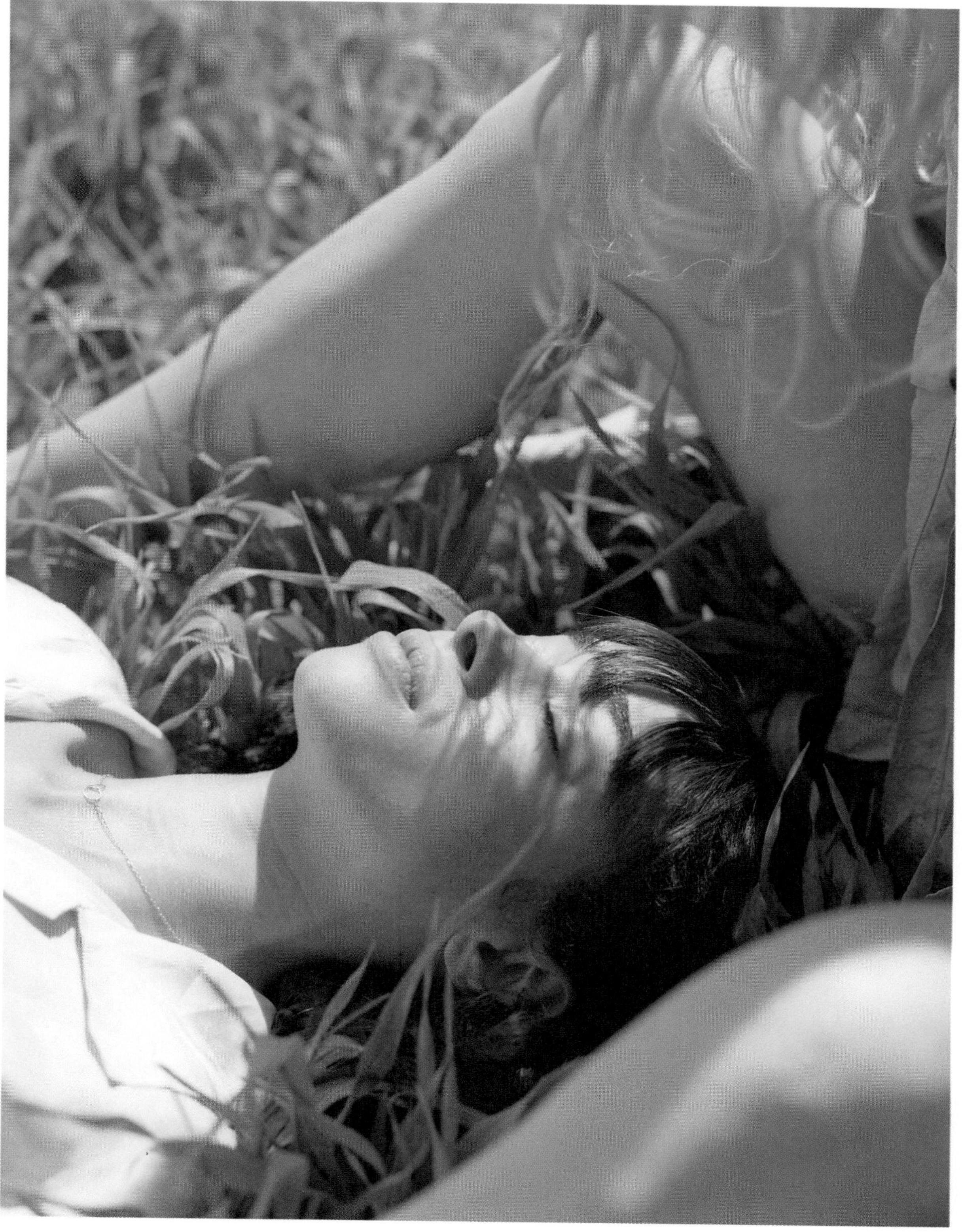

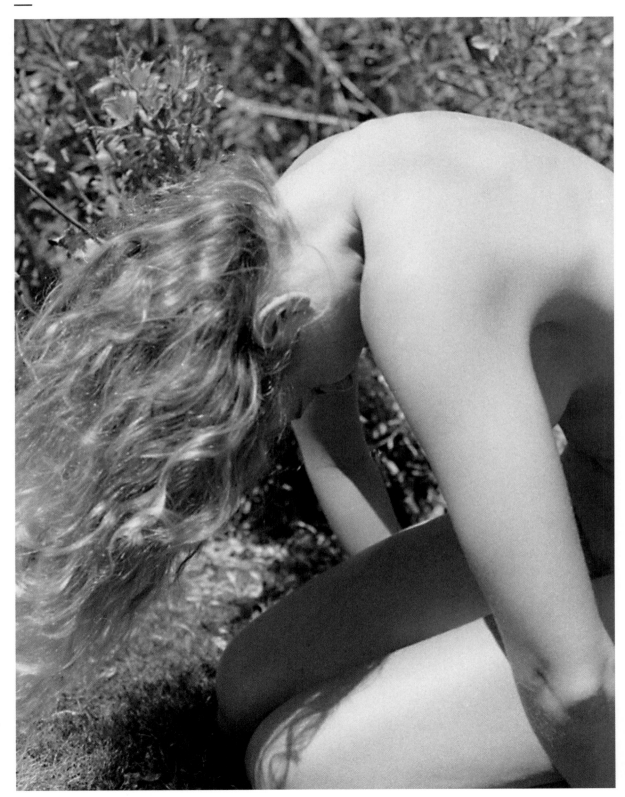

## SAY HER NAME

One of the first things you need to do to take ownership of your pleasure is to decide what to call her and become comfortable with the name you've chosen. It's important. Many of the words to describe her have devolved to take on negative connotations. I use the word pussy a lot in this chapter. You may find it triggering, as it has been co-opted for pornography. But if you use it, you are reclaiming it and instilling it with your own meaning. Cunt is generally considered to be the absolute worst name (wash your mouth out with soap and water immediately). But I love it. It was used by Chaucer, spelt queynte, and is defined as "a clever or curious device or ornament" in the Middle English Dictionary. It's strong, direct and satisfying to sound.

I'm not a huge fan of the words vulva or vagina: they're too clinical for me. I use yoni in a non-sexualized context. It's a beautiful Sanskrit word that's infused with the Eastern tradition of revering the divine, life-giving feminine energy. It feels appropriately sacred and beautiful.

Here are some names that came up in a workshop that SYC hosted with the brilliant Grace Hazel: pussy, yoni, vulva, flower, lady garden, Frida Kahlo... You get the picture.

## VENUS AND THE LOTUS

This practice is inspired by the wonderful Lacey Haynes, who holds "pussy gazing" events with the intention of reconnecting women to the beauty of their pussies in order to heal and empower.

You'll need a hand mirror and somewhere cosy and warm to sit. Wear a dress that you feel beautiful in, no need for underwear. Build a throne of cushions to support you, so you can feel comfortable and fully relaxed: a pleasure island for yourself. Light candles, burn some delicious smells, play some beautiful and peaceful music. These rituals will enhance your experience and give you time to land,

The beauty of this practice is the art of noticing, of settling into yourself, of giving yourself time and attention. As soon as you begin to really notice, something magical happens. Your pussy responds. She loves to be appreciated, she adores being seen and honoured. You might see her blossom and open, you could feel awed by her mysterious beauty and experience a natural shimmer of arousal as you deepen your vision and see the folds and caverns begin to bloom.

Seeing yourself in all your beauty is incredibly profound and moving, so don't be surprised if emotions surface. You might feel turned on, tearful, sad, hypnotized, peaceful. Know that everything is perfectly normal, honour all your emotions and allow them to rise.

○ Begin by sitting down in a comfortable, cross-legged position. Close your eyes and take some time to be with yourself and notice who you are today. Observe what lies beneath the surface, which emotions are colouring your body, whether you feel bright, light and alive, or dense and dull.

○ Witness your thoughts, notice them without judgment, then let them go. Allow time for your current stories to unfold – about five to ten minutes. It sometimes takes a while for the mind to sink into the felt sense, so keep bringing yourself back, anchoring the mind within the body by focusing on your breath.

○ Then let your awareness travel down and start to notice. Can you feel your pussy? As you breathe right now, do you notice sensation there? It's OK if there's a disconnect: just begin to tune in, refining your awareness and seeing if directing it into your pussy area can ignite an awakening.

○ As you inhale, draw energy down into your pussy. Focus on relaxing as you exhale, and see if you can imagine your pussy blooming open. Do this for about five minutes. Really try to drop into sensation, noticing how your feeling sense changes. Again, if there's a disconnect, that's OK. Just stay with the breath, witness what thoughts may arise, refrain from judgment and keep bringing yourself back.

○ Begin to introduce some sounds, a sigh or groan. A natural sound to honour how you're feeling right now. A sound not for anyone else, an audible release that is neither performative nor "attractive", just honest. Notice how it feels once you introduce that sound. It might help you to drop into sensation, as the sound vibrates through your body. Without any judgment, just notice if it's easy, or if you find some kind of resistance or challenge to using your voice. That's fine. This is for you to be with yourself, to explore. Do what feels good.

○ Come back to yourself with breath. Notice when the thoughts wander or disengage and bring them back. Do this for five minutes, hearing your own voice, being observant of sensations as they arise.

○ Place one hand on top of the other on your pussy. Hold her. Sit here and breathe, allowing the heat of awareness to gather. Do this for a few minutes. Then find a gentle movement from the pelvis, subtle, almost imperceptible, almost energetic, that translates into a rocking, gradually travelling up to inform gentle undulations of movement in the spine. Stay here for five minutes.

○ Maintaining the movement, slowly release your pussy and begin to reach your arms into the air to form a Y-shape – the sacred shape of the yoni. Return your hands into yourself. Place your palms over your face, touch your fingertips to your eyelids, trace your lips, run your palms down your neck and begin to caress your body, your breasts, your stomach and your hips.

○ Return your hands to your pussy. Notice how she is feeling. What is her energy, is she awake?

○ Take your mirror, hold it in front of you and look at your face. Look at you, see your face as a whole, drink her in. See your face as the perfectly imperfect vision that she is and smile. Look into your own eyes and hold your gaze. Be with yourself.

○ Witness and feel the intimacy of the moment. Allow the world fall away. Tell yourself that you are beautiful, out loud or without sound.

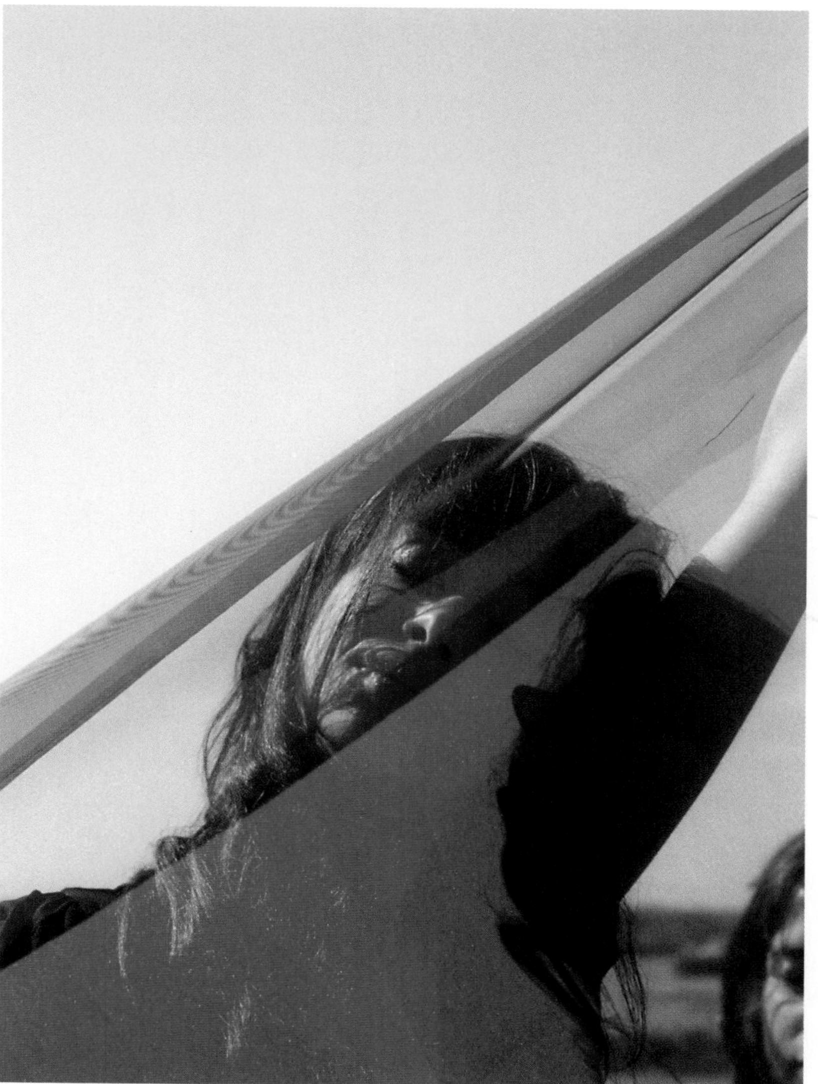

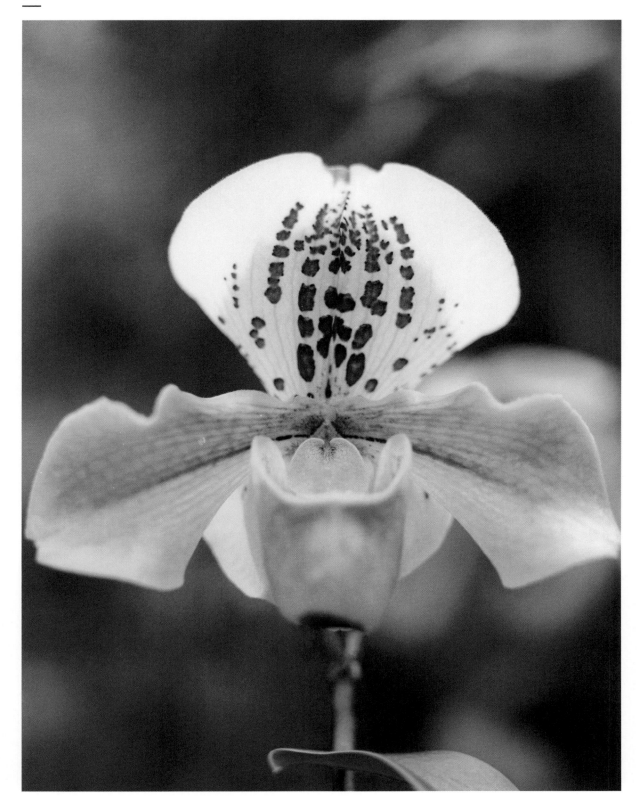

○ Take a deep five minutes looking, feel how different the experience is when you are there to witness and cherish, not critique. Say, "I love you. I am whole, I am perfect, I am the beloved." Repeat these mantras, mean them. Believe their truth.

○ Find a comfortable position, either lying down or sitting up. You're going to stay here for ten to fifteen minutes. Either stay free and open or cover yourself with a blanket to make your own little tent of discovery.

○ Travel your mirror down to your pussy and gaze at her. Let everything you've been led to believe is "normal" fall away. See her as she is, in her intricate beauty. Breathe into her. Observe a change in sensation, notice what effect your gaze has on her. See if her shape and colours change, notice if you become aroused or wet.

○ Tell her that she's beautiful, that you love her, that she's magical. Dwell in the moment, allow yourself to be awed. See if she opens, see what emotions surface in you, allow them to shift and change. Witness if you change the way you feel about her.

○ When you're ready, say goodbye and lie down. You can either continue into your own ritual of self-pleasure, or thank yourself and your yoni. Bathe in the afterglow for a few minutes, with one hand on your heart and one cupping your sacred yoni.

○ When you stir again, move slowly and try to keep the mind at bay so all the juicy presence and electricity sink into your cells, to carry you through the rest of your day.

## HONOUR YOUR BODY

Our life is an ongoing journey of self-discovery. We change with each day, each season, experience or lover, and so does our body. It's so important that we take time to witness ourselves, to cherish our flesh. To sense our own shifting landscape and be able to enjoy and communicate it. Our bodies move through the world inscribed with a catalogue of projections or expectations. Most of us inherited some sense of shame regarding our body or sexuality, so any journey of self-empowerment has to include worshipping our body and owning our pleasure. It's incredibly powerful and it's certainly political.

This does not mean that we need to be in a relationship, to constantly self-pleasure or have a high sex drive. There are many ways for our body to receive attention from ourselves or our partner, without even taking our clothes off. It's simply the commitment to honouring our body by being responsive to what it needs. By treating it tenderly, tuning into it enough to hear its longings, acknowledging the thrills, rushes and ripples as natural and deeply nourishing – all those juicy arousal hormones do wonders for rebalancing the levels of stress hormones in the body. For many women, this kind of respect and self care is new and very healing.

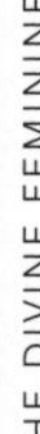
THE DIVINE FEMININE

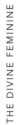

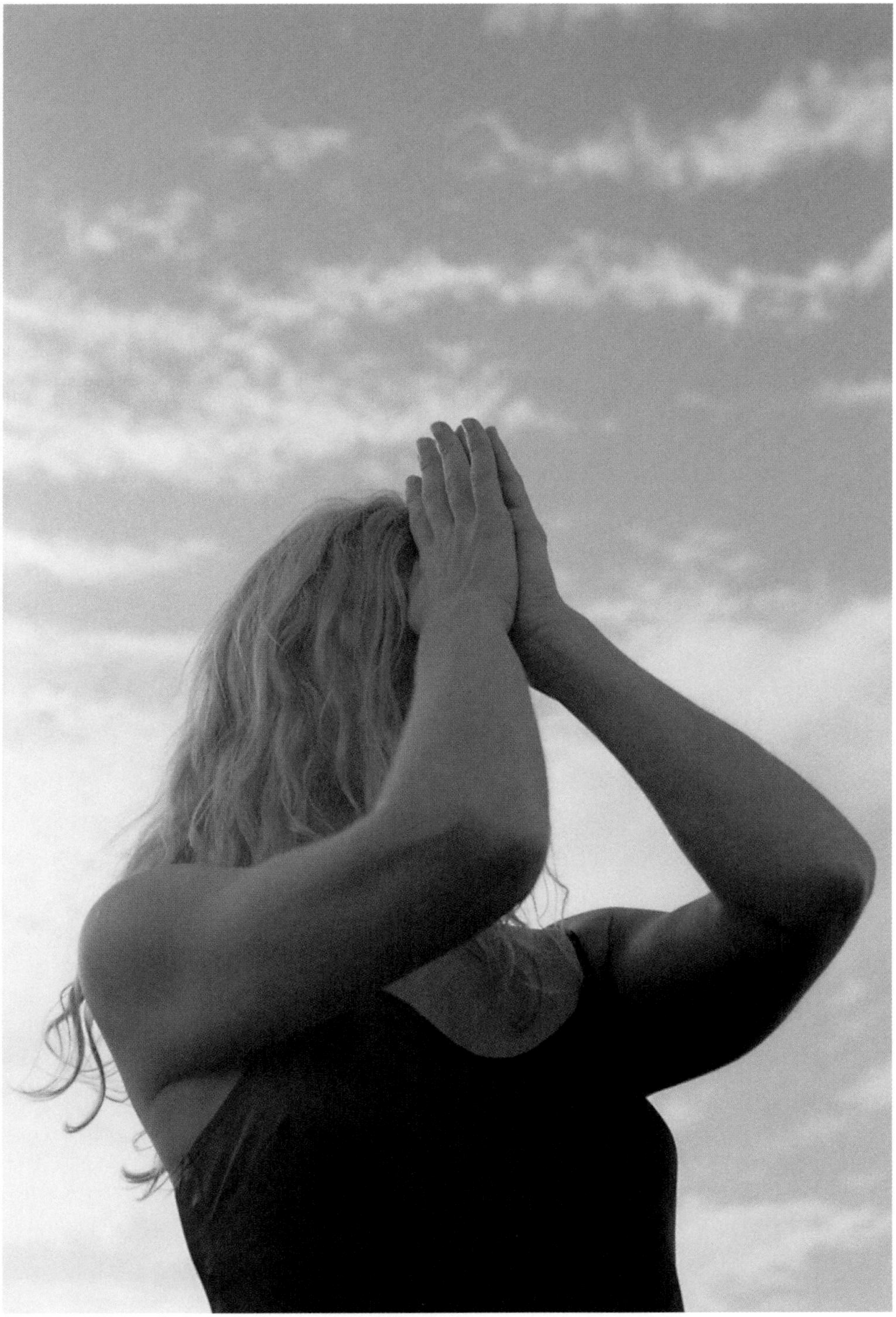

# THE DIVINE FEMININE

It's obvious to me from my personal practice that once you get in deep, yoga changes your relationship with yourself and the world around you.

I believe the practices found here are maps to awaken the multiple dimensions of our being human, and that we have the right to heal, vivify and enhance how we experience our body. I have found that through exploring all facets of our own unique bodies, we experience a profound sense of integration with the collective body. Through this felt sense of connection and community we can create more compassionate, joyful and sustainable behaviour.

From all the teachings I've had the privilege to access, all the conversations with friends who've steeped their lives in ancient yogic wisdom, I felt there was a yearning for a reclamation of the yoga lineage. A feminine interpretation for our times, one that creates an environment for everyone to flourish safely and have the freedom to explore their callings.

You can only offer what you know, and everything in this book is an ongoing process – what I needed to learn, what I am still and will always be learning. I taught myself to love my body, because I'd neglected it too long. I learned about my menstrual cycle, because I'd denied it too many years, I sought to empower myself because it was time I loved and trusted who I was becoming. I've included what carried me through the darkness, and now I appreciate the shadows that frame the light. I wanted to explore pleasure, because enjoying my sexuality and asking for what I want continues to inspire and embolden me.

Writing this book has opened my eyes again to wonder. I've experienced life-changing epiphanies and learned new ways to be with myself and my loved ones, especially my partner. The most precious gift is that learning about trauma healed my relationship with my mother. I will be forever grateful.

I hope you have found tools here to help you life a life of truth and pleasure.

If I can change, so can you.

Love,

Gabrielle x.

# BIBLIOGRAPHY/FURTHER READING

**It is hard to name all the many inspirations for this book, as I turned to many people, sources and platforms, but here is a list of some of the most informative books that guided me, which could serve as a starting point for your own adventure.**


Anodea, J., *Eastern Body, Western Mind: Psychology and the Chakra System as a Path to the Self*, Berkeley, CA: Celestial Arts, 2004

Broad, W.J., *The Science of Yoga: The Risks and the Rewards*, New York, NY: Simon & Schuster, 2013

Dinsmore-Tuli, U, *Yoni Shakti: A Woman's Guide to Power and Freedom Through Yoga and Tantra*, London: YogaWords, 2014

Feuerstein, G., *Tantra: The Path of Ecstasy*, Boulder, CO: Shambhala Publications, 1998

Feuerstein, G. and Wilber, K., *The Yoga Tradition: Its History, Literature, Philosophy and Practice*, Chino Valley, AZ: Hohm Press, 2001

Johari, H., *Chakras: Energy Centers of Transformation*, New York, NY: Destiny Books, 2000

Kempton, S., *Awakening Shakti*, Louisville, CO: Sounds True, 2013

Kuo-Deemer, M., *Qigong and the Tai Chi Axis: Nourishing Practices for Body, Mind and Spirit*, Mineola, NY: Ixia Press, 2019

Mallinson, J. and Singleton, M., *Roots of Yoga*, London: Penguin Classics, 2017

Myss, C., *Anatomy of Spirit: The Seven Stages of Power and Healing*, London: Bantam, 1997

Nagoksi, E., *Come As You Are*, London: Scribe UK, 2015

Odier, D., *Tantric Quest: An Encounter with Absolute Love*, Rochester, VT: Inner Traditions, 1997

Pope, A. and Hugo Wurlitzer, S., *Wild Power: Discover the Magic of your Menstrual Cycle and Awaken to the Feminine Path to Power*, Carlsbad, CA: Hay House, 2017

Scaravelli, V., *Awakening the Spine: Yoga for Health, Vitality and Energy*, London: Pinter & Martin, 2011

Singleton, M., *Yoga Body: The Origins of Modern Posture Practice*, New York, NY: Oxford University Press, 2010

Winston, S., *Women's Anatomy of Arousal: Secret Maps to Buried Pleasure*, Kingston, NY: Mango Garden Press, 2010

Wolf, N., *Vagina*, London: Virago, 2013

# INDEX


Poses and exercises are in *italics*

acupuncture 45
*adho mukha svanasana variation* 100
adrenaline 45, 50, 208
altars 143
*alternate nostril breath* 130
anger 54–5
  *simhasana: lion's breath* 129
anxiety 43
  *bhramari: bee breath to soothe anxiety* 130
  *Carolyn Cowan's Vagus nerve stretch* 132
arms: massage 199
arousal 207–10
asana 14, 19, 34, 36–7
astanga 34
authenticity 26–7
autonomic nervous system 50–3
avidya 22

back: massage 199
*back to the source* 108
bandhas 124–5
*bee breath to soothe anxiety* 130
Begley, Sharon *The plastic mind* 157, 161, 164
*bhramari: bee breath to soothe anxiety* 130
Blackaby, Peter 65
Blavatsky, Helena 32
the body 38–9, 60–1. *see also* movement
  the energy body 42–6
  natural rhythms 15
body-building and yoga 37
Bowman, Katy 64
brahma nadi 47
the brain
  brain-gut connection 158
  and breathing 123
  and the mind 158–64
  neuroplasticity 157

breath control 34, 47, 120–1, 142
  bandhas 124–5
  breathing patterns 122–3
  deep breathing 123
  frequency of breathing 47
  and movement 66
  oceanic yogic breathing 53
  and rest/relaxation 53
breathing exercises
  *bhramari: bee breath to soothe anxiety* 130
  *Carolyn Cowan's Vagus nerve stretch* 132
  *drop into peace* 126
  *exhalation: soothe into sleep* 135
  *global breathing for beginners* 129
  *kapalabhati: skull-shining breath* 128
  *kumbhaka: breath retention* 126
  *nadi sodhana: alternate nostril breath* 130
  *pauses as portals* 126
  *simhasana: lion's breath* 129
  *sitali: breath to cool and relax the body* 130
  *ujjayi* 127
  *viloma inhalation: alert* 134
  *viloma: interrupted breathing patterns* 126
*the bridge* 96

*camatkarasana: modified wild thing* 98
*Carolyn Cowan's Vagus nerve stretch* 132
cat/cow posture 54
cells 37, 45
chakras 48
change 147–51
chanting 53
chest: massage 199
clitoris 208
cognitive behavioural therapy 161–4
concentration (dharana) 34
consciousness 158
*corpse pose* 18, 118
cortisol 45, 50, 196
craniosacral therapy 56

depression 154–7
dharana (concentration) 34
dhyana:(deep meditation) 34
Dinsmore-Tuli, Uma 174
disassociation 50–2, 57
dopamine 123, 207, 208
dreams 142
*drop into peace* 126

*eagle pose* 100
*earthly constellations* 110
eightfold path 34
*electric body* 91
emotions 48, 56–7, 167
endorphins 123, 195, 208–10
the energy body 42–6
  and emotions 56–7
  and trauma 54–5
enlightenment 22, 34
enteric nervous system 158
*exhalation: soothe into sleep* 135

face & head: massage 200
feet: massage 197–8
*fertile ground* 96
fight or flight 45, 50–3
flow yoga 61, 66–7, 121
  poses & and practices 77, 98, 115
*free movement: electric body* 91
freeze response 50–2

*garudasana: eagle pose* 100
*global breathing for beginners* 129
glutes: massage 199
Goldheart, Jayne 15
gratitude 142
guilt and shame 166–8
gunas 32–3
gut and brain connection 158

*half surya namaskar* 78
hand gestures (mudras) 136–8
hands: massage 200
hatha yoga 35, 66
heart-opening exercises 53
Hinduism 14, 30, 32–3, 38, 43
holistic approach to wellbeing 42, 45–6
*human ocean* 106

ida nadi 47
Indian roots of yoga 36–7
inhalation 120
- *viloma inhalation: alert* 134

injuries 68
intuition 14, 15

jalandhara bandha 125
*janu sirsasana* 110
*Jessi sequence* 98
Johari, Harish 47
Judith, Anodea 46, 48

kaivalya 34
*kapalabhati: skull-shining breath* 128
*kinetic poetry* 77
Krasnow, Mark 123
kriya yoga 32
*kumbhaka: breath retention* 126
*kumbhaka with ujjayi* 127
kundalini 47, 48

legs: massage 198
Levine, Peter 54–5
lifestyle 63–4, 147–51
*lion's breath* 129
*lizard pose* 98

Mallinson, James 30
mantras 140–1, 163
massage 196
- *pleasure cats* 202–3
- self-massage 197–200

meditation (dhyana) 15, 18, 22, 34, 142, 158
menstrual cycle 15, 26, 174–83
- awareness of 182–3

mental health 154–65
- shadow work 166–8

microbiome 158
the mind 158–64
mindfulness 68, 161–3
mood changes. *see* depression; menstrual cycle
morning rituals 142–3
*mountain pose (tadasana)* 72–4
movement 57, 61
- and the body 68–9
- finding rhythm 66–7
- rewilding 64–5
- and sedentary lifestyles 63–4
- and trauma 55

mudras 136–8
mula bandha 124
Myss, Carolyn 46, 48
*mystic moon* 92–5

*nadi sodhana: alternate nostril breath* 130
nadis 47
neck: massage 200
negative thinking 163–4
the nervous system 50–5
neuroplasticity 157
niyama (observance) 34
non-duality 38
noticing 63–9

observance (niyama) 34
Om chanting 53, 140–1
orgasm 15, 27, 208
ovulation 179–80
oxytocin 195, 207, 208

parasympathetic nervous system 50–2, 53–4, 123
*pascimottanasana* 110
Patanjali's Yoga-sutras 14, 32–4, 161
pelvic floor 89, 124
Pert, Candice 56–7
pingala nadi 47
*plank pose* 86
*pleasant pose (sukhasana)* 74
Pope, Alexandra 174, 175, 182
poses & and practices 25
- *adho mukha svanasana variation* 100
- *back to the source* 108
- *bridge* 96
- *camatkarasana: modified wild thing* 98
- *earthly constellations* 110
- *fertile ground* 96
- *free movement: electric body* 91
- *half surya namaskar* 78
- *human ocean* 106
- *janu sirsasana* 110
- *Jessi sequence* 98
- *kinetic poetry* 77
- *mystic moon* 92–5
- *pascimottanasana* 110
- *plank pose* 86
- *remember the sky* 102–4
- *rock & roll* 113
- *savasana* 118
- *stoke your fire* 84–9
- *sukhasana: pleasant pose* 74
- *sun in my heart* 115–17
- *surya namaskar: sun salutation* 80–2
- *tadasana: breathe to move* 74
- *tadasana: root to rise* 72
- *tarasana* 110
- *upavista konasana* 110
- *utthan pristhasana: lizard pose* 98
- *your heart is ancient* 100

positive thinking 163–4
postural yoga 14, 19, 34, 36–7
prakrti 33
prana 43–6, 47
pranayama. *see* breath control; breathing exercises
pratyahara (sense-withdrawal) 34
present moment 68, 161–3
psychosomatic healing 56–7

rajas 33
relationships 168, 210
relaxation 60, 123
- *sitali: breath to cool and relax the body* 130

*remember the sky* 102–4
restraint (yama) 34

rewilding 64–5
rhythm, finding 66–7
rituals: morning rituals 142–3
*rock & roll* 113
rta 67

sacred spaces 143
Sakti 38
samadhi (ecstasy) 22, 28, 32, 34
Sandow, Eugen 37
satsang 15
sattva 33
*savasana: corpse pose* 18, 118
Secret Yoga Club 172–3, 184–8
  mission 6–9
  origins 16–17
sedentary lifestyles 63–4
self-massage 197–200
self-pleasure 27, 210–17
self-reflection. *see* svadhyaya
self-study. *see* svadhyaya
sense-withdrawal (pratyahara) 34
serotonin 157–8, 207
sex and sexuality 27, 205–6
  arousal 207–10
  owning your pleasure 210–17
shadow work 166–8
shame and guilt 166–8
shoulders: massage 199
siddhis 25
*simhasana: lion's breath* 129
Singleton, Mark 30, 36
*sitali: breath to cool and relax the body* 130
Siva 38
skin 194–6
skull-shining breath 128
sleep: exhalation: soothe into sleep 135
somatic experiencing 55
speaking your truth 151
*stoke your fire* 84–9
stress 43–5, 149, 158
  *Carolyn Cowan's Vagus nerve stretch* 132
  *nadi sodhana: alternate nostril breath* 130
*sukhasana: pleasant pose* 74
*sun in my heart* 115–17
sun salutation 80–2
*surya namaskar: sun salutation* 80–2
sushumna nadi 47, 124
svadhyaya 14–15, 26–7, 63, 147–51
sympathetic nervous system 45, 50–3

*tadasana: breathe to move* 74
*tadasana: root to rise* 72
tamas 33
tantra 37–9
  neo-tantric ritual of touch 201–2
*tarasana* 110
teachers, finding 65–6
technology 143
time out 178
touch 194–6. *see also* massage
  neo-tantric ritual of touch 201–2
transcendence 48
trauma
  and the body 54–5
  and disassociation 50–2
  and the emotions 56–7
truth, speaking 151

*uddiyana bandha* 125
*ujjayi* 53, 127
*upavista konasana* 110
Upledger, John 56
*utthan pristhasana: lizard pose* 98

vagus nerve 53–4, 158
  *Carolyn Cowan's Vagus nerve stretch* 132
the Vedas 14
*viloma inhalation: alert* 134
*viloma: interrupted breathing patterns* 126
visualization 54
*visualization with ujjayi* 127
Vivekananda 32
Vranich, Belisa 123

*wild thing (modified)* 98
women's circles 184–90
  creating 188–90
women's groups 172–3

yama (restraint) 34
yoga. *see also* poses & and practices
  ancient practice 22–5
  authenticity 26–7
  definitions of 28
  as a journey & destination 12–13
  philosophy 18–19
  questing 14–15
  and rest/relaxation 53–4
  roots of 30, 36–9
  teaching 16–17
yoga nidra 54, 178
yoga-sutras 14, 32–4, 161
yogasana 142
*your heart is ancient* 100

# WITH GRATITUDE

So many people have been part of the journey of SYC, and this book. It's hard to name all of the wonderful souls who have contributed to the story since 2013. Those of you who have joined our events and retreats – you are the reason we are here today, so thank you.

I am grateful to the kind team at Aster. I'm thankful to Kate Adams, my wonderful publisher, for her kindness, vision, inspiration and ongoing encouragement. With huge thanks to Alex Stetter, Yasia Williams, Miranda Harvey and Caroline Alberti.

Thanks to my agent Charlie Brotherstone for so much guidance, above and beyond.

With a huge amount of gratitude to Natasha Marshall, the wonderful photographer who has captured so much of the magic of SYC over the years. It is always a joy to see the world reinvisioned through her lens, capturing and crystallizing secret moments.

A huge thank you to Sarah Cleaver, for styling and art directing the shoots and helping bring the words and pictures to life.

The women in the photos are our friends. Some of the images were taken on retreats over the years and capture happy memories. We had a wonderful adventure in Jersey, thanks to the hospitality and generosity of Helen and India Hamilton. I also stayed in their studio for a month or so writing – it was the perfect little nest, and a privilege to spend time together. Thank you to all our wonderful models and friends that made each shoot a precious experience: Sarah June Wells, Jessica Brown, Sarah Benmerrah, Duha Sinada, Jonelle Lewis, Ava Riby-Williams, Sara Zaltash, Omotayo Akingbola, Charlotte Forsyth and Ziver Irkad.

I'm incredibly grateful to Jordan Maxwell for all her support on SYC, particularly over the writing period. Also to Jaz Teoh, for her valuable contribution a few years ago.

Thank you, thank you. Beautiful humans.

To my mamma, Marlyn Hales. For everything. For the reading, the cheer-leeding, the feeding and the inspiration. To the kindest brother, Henry Hales.

To my teachers: Janice Helens (my first yoga teacher), Sharon and David Life for the Jivamukti method. Although I have ventured from this path, I am grateful for the initiation and the early discipline. Carolyn Cowan (my guardian Kali) who has inspired so much of our work with women and helped me find my own voice. Zephyr Wildman, for her combination of mysticism and humour and anatomical precision. Finally, Jean Hall, for the creative sequencing, the detail, the delicacy and poetry. All fantastic women, with excellent minds and huge hearts. They have contributed so much to the yoga community and changed the lives of many of their students. I am awed and humbled by your teachings.

I'd also like to list some of the teachers who continue to inspire me from afar, online, in print and via podcasts: Elena Brower, Tara Judelle, Meghan Currie, Seane Corne for her activism and taking a chance with SYC in the early days. Max Strom, the gentle giant and breath wizard. Mollie McClelland Morris, Mimi Kuo Deemer, Fern Trelfa. Uma Dinsmore-Tuli and Sally Kempton for their incredible work introducing practices specifically for women's bodies and seasons. Alexandra Pope and Sjanie Hugo Wurlitzer for their brilliant work on the menstrual cycle. Krista Tippett's *On Being* podcast, Esther Perel, Juliet Allen, Michaela Boehm, Vanessa Scotto and Brooke Thomas for two of my favourite podcasts: *Bliss and Grit* and *Liberated Body*. Thank you to Rusty Taylor, Darryl Lim, Lucy Haygarth and Sabrina Kraus Lopez, for their kindness and vision.

Thank you to all the strong women who illuminate my life: Madeleine Botet de Lacaze, Charlotte Hall, Rachel Johnston, Romy Finbow, Chloe Isadora, Rikke Brodin, Ella Bowman, Nicola Atkins, Josie Flight, Sophie Gaten, Antonia Shaw, Maria Yat, Jess McMenemy, Jayne Goldheart, Jessi and Sarah. You are my family and inspiration.

Finally, to my partner, Ben. I adore you. Thank you for growing with me. My oak tree.